T0399510

Youth, Sexuality and Sexual Citizenship

Sexual citizenship is a powerful concept associated with debates about recognition and exclusion, agency, respect and accountability.

For young people in general and for gender and sexually diverse youth in particular, these debates are entangled with broader imaginings of social transitions: from 'child' to 'adult' and from 'unreasonable subject' to one 'who can consent'. This international and interdisciplinary collection identifies and locates struggles for recognition and inclusion in particular contexts and at particular moments in time, recognising that sexual and gender diverse young people are neither entirely vulnerable nor self-reliant.

Focussing on the numerous domains in which debates about youth, sexuality and citizenship are enacted and contested, *Youth, Sexuality and Sexual Citizenship* explores young people's experiences in diverse but linked settings: in the family, at school and in college, in employment, in social media and through engagement with health services. Bookended by reflections from Jeffrey Weeks and Susan Talburt, the book's empirically grounded chapters also engage with the key debates outlined in its scholarly introduction.

This innovative book is of interest to students and scholars of gender and sexuality, health and sex education, and youth studies, from a range of disciplinary and professional backgrounds, including sociology, education, nursing, social work and youth work.

Peter Aggleton is an emeritus professor at UNSW Sydney, Australia; an honorary distinguished professor at The Australian National University in Canberra, Australia; an adjunct professor in the Australian Research Centre in Sex, Health and Society at La Trobe University, Melbourne, Australia; and a visiting professor at University College London, UK.

Rob Cover is an associate professor in media and communication in the School of Social Sciences at The University of Western Australia.

Deana Leahy is a senior lecturer in health education in the Faculty of Education at Monash University in Melbourne, Australia.

Daniel Marshall is a senior lecturer in literature in the School of Communication and Creative Arts at Deakin University in Melbourne, Australia.

Mary Lou Rasmussen is a professor of sociology in the College of Arts and Social Sciences at The Australian National University in Canberra, Australia.

Sexuality, Culture and Health series

Edited by Peter Aggleton, UNSW Sydney, Australia
Richard Parker, Columbia University, New York, USA
Sonia Corrêa, ABIA, Rio de Janeiro, Brazil
Gary Dowsett, La Trobe University, Melbourne, Australia
Shirley Lindenbaum, City University of New York, USA

This series of books offers cutting-edge analysis, current theoretical perspectives and up-to-the-minute ideas concerning the interface between sexuality, public health, human rights, culture and social development. It adopts a global and interdisciplinary perspective in which the needs of poorer countries are given equal status to those of richer nations. Books are written with a broad range of readers in mind, and will be invaluable to students, academics and those working in policy and practice. The series also aims to serve as a spur to practical action in an increasingly globalised world.

Understanding Global Sexualities
New Frontiers
Edited by Peter Aggleton, Paul Boyce, Henrietta L. Moore and Richard Parker

Men who Sell Sex
Global Perspectives
Edited by Peter Aggleton and Richard Parker

Sex and Sexualities in Contemporary Indonesia
Sexual Politics, Health, Diversity and Representations
Edited by Linda Rae Bennett and Sharyn Graham Davies

Culture, Health and Sexuality
An Introduction
Edited by Peter Aggleton, Richard Parker and Felicity Thomas

Gay Science
Intimate experiments with the problem of HIV
Kane Race

Youth, Sexuality and Sexual Citizenship
Edited by Peter Aggleton, Rob Cover, Deana Leahy, Daniel Marshall and Mary Lou Rasmussen

https://www.routledge.com/Sexuality-Culture-and-Health/book-series/SCH

Youth, Sexuality and Sexual Citizenship

Edited by Peter Aggleton,
Rob Cover, Deana Leahy,
Daniel Marshall and
Mary Lou Rasmussen

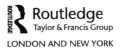

Routledge
Taylor & Francis Group

LONDON AND NEW YORK

First published 2019
by Routledge
2 Park Square, Milton Park, Abingdon, Oxon OX14 4RN

and by Routledge
711 Third Avenue, New York, NY 10017

Routledge is an imprint of the Taylor & Francis Group, an informa business

First issued in paperback 2021

British Library Cataloguing-in-Publication Data
A catalogue record for this book is available from the British Library

Library of Congress Cataloging-in-Publication Data
Names: Aggleton, Peter, editor. | Cover, Rob, editor. |
Leahy, Deana, editor.
Title: Young people and sexual citizenship / edited by Peter Aggleton, Rob Cover, Deana Leahy, Daniel Marshall and Mary Lou Rasmussen.
Description: First Edition. | New York: Routledge, 2019. |
Series: Sexuality, culture and health | Includes bibliographical references and index.
Identifiers: LCCN 2018023000 | ISBN 9780815379874 (hardback) |
ISBN 9781351214742 (ebook)
Subjects: LCSH: Youth—Sexual behavior. | Identity (Psychology)
Classification: LCC HQ27 .Y679 2019 | DDC 306.70835—dc23
LC record available at https://lccn.loc.gov/2018023000

ISBN: 978-0-815-37987-4 (hbk)
ISBN: 978-0-367-52226-1 (pbk)
ISBN: 978-1-351-21474-2 (ebk)

Typeset in Baskerville
by codeMantra

Contents

Acknowledgements

This book is one of several outputs from the *Belonging and Sexual Citizenship among Gender and Sexual Minority Youth* (Queer Generations) research project, which was supported by the Australian Government through the Australian Research Council's Discovery Projects funding scheme (project DP150101292).

The views expressed herein are those of the editors and authors, and not necessarily those of the Australian Government or the Australian Research Council.

Parts of Chapter 18 appeared in an earlier form in Talburt, S., ed., (2018). *Youth Sexualities: Public Feelings and Contemporary Cultural Politics*. Santa Barbara, CA: Praeger.

The editors would like to thank the UNSW Sydney Arts and Social Sciences Practical Justice Initiative for its support of the project, Tim Wong for his help in liaising with the contributors to this volume, and Sarah Hoile for her administrative assistance preparing the manuscript for publication.

Foreword

Jeffrey Weeks

Sexual citizenship (and its sister idea intimate citizenship) is a Janus-like concept. It offers a critical look backwards at earlier ideas of citizenship and their occlusions, particularly in relation to race, gender, sexuality, young people and other exclusions. And it looks forward to a wider ideal that is more inclusive, especially in relation to the rights, recognition and belonging of diverse subjectivities, identities and communities. This book provides a welcome range of contributions that takes sexual citizenship seriously and deploys the concept to explore the experiences, needs and agency of young people battling to make the concept meaningful to them.

Despite the nostalgic, sepia-tinted memories of cultural conservatives of all political persuasions, there has never been a golden age of adult/youth harmony. The boundaries between the generations that have full, at least theoretically, civil, economic, social and sexual citizenship and those younger people still aspiring to it may vary historically across time and place, but they are frequently fragile, fought over and policed. The social history of different peoples, periods and cultures is dotted with generational conflict, sometimes fought on the streets, more often fought in the families, communities and classrooms where young people learn their values, hopes and aspirations, and find that adults seem to exist to thwart them, while adults regularly see their offspring as threats to the ways of life they have so painfully sustained or constructed.

This bald description may seem too much a caricature, but like all caricatures it follows the outlines of reality. Young people are always the future, but the future is a foreign country that has to be searched and fought for. Since the Second World War in both the Global South and North, and the fluid areas in between, young people have presaged and propelled the changes that have remade the world, from the pushiness of the post-war baby boom generation that helped undermine the hidebound traditions of Europe, the Americas and Australasia over the past 50 years to the millions of young people involved in the independence, Arab Spring and similar movements in the postcolonial South. The results of their efforts may not always have been what young people desired or struggled for, but the drama of their interventions is undeniable, and the effects have often been transformative. And the contemporary 'youth-quake' observed by pollsters, advertisers and politicians is surely a harbinger of conflicts to come, especially in those parts of the world where a demographic revolution has produced vast populations of young people, often without jobs, good quality education or political voice but tuned into global conversations by the Internet and social media.

Sexuality is regularly a particular site of conflict, perhaps not surprisingly. It touches on recurrent contestations over norms, values, standards, patterns of life and identities. As the contributions to this book show in vivid detail and careful analysis, the mobile frontiers between young people's sexuality and full sexual citizenship and social belonging continue to be fraught and fiercely fought over. The eruptions of anxiety about the unruly behaviour of young people (or at least the perception of that behaviour) that have punctuated recent history in many countries inextricably link sexuality with other sources of fear and loathing, such as racial and class difference. The potent brew has regularly given rise to moral panics – a concept used by the sociologist Stanley Cohen (1972) in his analysis of battles between youthful 'mods' and 'rockers' but soon deployed to describe and explain more overtly sex-related crises. Implicit in the concept is the exploitation of inchoate anxieties by the media, moral entrepreneurs and the agents of social control.

Most sexualised panics since the 1960s play on the dialectic of dangerous agency (embodied in the behaviours and practices of young people) on the one hand and often frenetic attempts at social regulation on the other. Recurrent anxieties exist around teenage pregnancy, homosexuality, porn, video 'nasties', sexually transmitted infections, AIDS, the perils of sex education, the wild frontier of social media and the Internet, the 'sexualisation' of young people, trafficking and, most potent of all, paedophilia: these speak of a culture which remains deeply uncertain about where to draw the lines about what young people feel is desirable and what adults feel is acceptable behaviour. To a remarkable degree these tensions continue to focus, despite great advances in social liberalisation in many parts of the world, on lesbian, gay, bisexual and transgender (LGBT) young people, as various contributions to the book illustrate. Tropes around the corruption of youth into queer ways of life continue to circulate, from countries in Africa to Russia, but not excluding more ostensibly liberal jurisdictions, as in recent campaigns in Australia against anti-bullying education to make schools safe for LGBT young people. And as the Lawrence (Larry) King case in the USA vividly illustrates, the disruptive example of a queer/trans subject of colour can unsettle inclusive-based arguments of sexual citizenship – what Ricky Gutierrez-Maldonado in Chapter 4 of this book calls 'too-muchness'.

As I have suggested, there is little that is historically new in these tensions, but what makes them especially toxic in the contemporary world is the curious mixture of growing sexual awareness and experience of young people at ever younger ages on the one hand and their increased emotional, social and economic dependence on the adult world on the other. Surely no earlier generations can have become aware so early of such an enormous, highly eroticised environment in both the virtual and 'real' worlds, or had easier access to it, as a result of the digital revolution. It is not surprising that a number of the essays in this book are deeply preoccupied with the opportunities – and risks – for young people offered by the Internet and social media for everything from identity affirmation, dating, friendship and sociality to political mobilisation around sexualised issues: a site of subjectivity, resistance and autonomy as well as of pleasure and possible exploitation and pain. Yet at the same time, lengthening years of public education, poor job opportunities, the cost of housing, delayed marriage and parenting, the growing tendency for young people to continue to live with their parents in the family home into their 20s and even 30s has increased the emotional and financial dependence of many young people on their families. This is a powerful source of uncertainty for both adults and young people. It is one of the paradoxes of the new world of sexuality that as the old categorical distinctions that shaped sexual life in Western countries, between masculinity and femininity, and heterosexuality and homosexuality are challenged and undermined by more fluid understandings of sexuality and gender, new kinds of categorisations and distinctions are constructed between adults and young people.

In trying to understand these issues it is important that we recognise the significance of what Ken Plummer (2010) has called 'generational sexualities'. He has written about 'generational narratives', through which perspectives and standpoints derived from changing social worlds give rise to different stories about the past and present. This does not mean that age cohorts necessarily think alike. The most famous generation in recent history, those post-war baby boomers, was sharply divided, even as their stories came to dominate sexual and gender discourse. Many of the leading lights in the powerful waves of social conservatism that fought against family and sexual change in the name of traditional values were of the same age cohort as feminists and gay liberationists, shaped by the same experiences but ending up with radically different perspectives. Not only are there divisions amongst those of the same chronological generation, but different sexual generations coexist so that in the contemporary world conservative traditionalists and nostalgists of all ages, radicals now growing old (and less radical?), the AIDS generation marked by sexual fear and backlash, young erotic explorers, libertarians, dissidents, queer activists, liberals and fundamentalists jumble together in uneasy coexistence. Each generation, and each fragment or subgroup of a generation, brings different understandings to the complex and shifting world of sexuality. Crucially, we live our sexual lives in a particular place, and at a particular time, alongside others living in different temporalities (Weeks 2016, pp. 19–22). At any particular time there are a multiplicity of temporalities, delicately intertwined, which can have profound implications for thinking about different sexual histories. 'Queer-time' has different rhythms and imperatives from conventional time, as Judith/Jack Halberstam (2005) famously argued, marked and made by specific histories of exclusion, oppression and resistance.

Generational distinctiveness is a key element in Brian Heaphy's contribution to the book. His analysis of the narratives of two cohorts of young LGBT people, barely a decade apart, shows an element of continuity but also unprecedentedly

rapid change, shaped by the unexpectedly speedy embedding of civil partnerships and same-sex marriage in Britain in the first two decades of this century.
For the older cohort, there was still a sense of embattlement as the scars of
thwarted citizenship animated their sense of identity. There was a characteristic
uneasiness in relations between LGBT youth and families of origin, and a strong
narrative of social exclusion. For the younger cohort, hopes of equal citizenship
had become more or less 'ordinary', everyday and taken for granted. Young
LGBT people were now entering a changed world – where coming out as a personal and social process seemed less relevant because it was not so necessary. A
same-sex preference or gender fluidity were less goals that had to be struggled
for. They were aspects of 'just being'. Alongside this were new emphases on
emotional and social aspirations – less on 'friendship as family' and community
connectedness that were characteristic of the earlier days of LGBT struggles for
citizenship and increasingly on more conventional family relationships, marriage and parenting. The couple had reasserted itself as a relational ideal, and a
sense of the future was embodied in child-rearing.

But if this ideal was becoming hegemonic in newly liberal and tolerant Britain,
it was not the whole story, Heaphy argues. Weaker narratives of continuing social
exclusion are in danger of being marginalised within a liberal consensus. There
continue to be sharp limitations to full recognition and autonomy in different
communities, marked by classic divisions of class, geography, race and ethnicity,
and increasingly religion. There are very definite limits to choice about identities
and relationships. This is sharply illustrated in the chapter by Louise Boon-Kuo,
Erica R. Meiners and Paul Simpson, focussing on Australia and the USA. They
explore how young people's sexual citizenship is shaped by interactions with the
criminal legal system, especially amongst queer youth of colour, where, it is argued, 'all facets of belonging' are shaped by the carceral state. A disproportionate
percentage of queer youth are in detention in the USA, and the figure is heavily
racialised: African American youth are five times as likely as white youth to be
imprisoned, while in Australia 55% of all young people in detention centres are
of indigenous origin. Racial exclusion and criminalisation are compounded by
heterosexism and cissexism in families and schools, and all these factors impact
adult possibilities so that for many young people citizenship is 'an emergent and
contingent condition' rather than a right or a destiny. Inevitably, there is a danger
of the emergence of new divides, between the good queers, moving towards forms
of social integration, and the bad queers, in danger of being excluded again from
full sexual citizenship.

But if the carceral state illustrates the continuing fracture and ultimate failure
of full sexual and intimate citizenship, it cannot be seen as the defining characteristic of the contemporary liberal state in relation to queer youth. More
common, indeed pretty universal, are the myriad interactions between individuals, communities and state authorities in the education, health and care systems
which work to marginalise 'vulnerable' queer youth. In their chapter Adrian Kin
Cheung Yan and Denise Tse-Shang Tang highlight how, in Hong Kong, a 'trinity

of governance' – consisting of sexual morality, cultural tradition and religious conservatism – organises a sex education system which continues to stigmatise LGBT young people. Anna Bredström and Eva Bolander explore the limits of a Swedish 'norm-critical' sexual education programme. Crystal Abidin and Rob Cover warn of the dangers of 'homonationalism', which does not challenge heterosexuality. For Jessica Fields and colleagues neo-liberal pressures produce markets that expect lesbian, gay, bisexual, transgender and queer (LGBTQ) youth to be self-regulating actors and prioritise some youth over racialised others. Deeply rooted religious traditions that cannot be reduced to neo-liberal imperatives are often as potent, however – see Yvette Taylor's article. To my mind it is clear that the state's role is characterised by ambivalence, ambiguity, *ad hoc* pragmatism and opportunism as much as intentionality and clear strategy. It is often difficult to argue for a coherent state response, even within its own organs, let alone across many different jurisdictions. But incoherence tells its own story.

The end result of confused messages from the state is the accentuation of a sense of the vulnerabilities and uncertainties of individual and social life for many queer youth ('precarity'), which undermines the hope for full sexual citizenship and belonging. Set against this are many examples of resilience, resistance and alternative forms of conviviality. Faced by homophobic teachers, some queer people go beyond the subjectivity of resistance to take up 'expert' subjectivities on sexuality and gender issues (see the chapter by Katie Fitzpatrick and Hayley McGlashan). Pre-existing scripts can be interrupted in new alliances across different sexual and gender experiences, whilst distinctive subjectivities and needs can at the same time be affirmed. Tiffany Jones argues for divergent pathways to inclusion for trans and intersex youth. Samia Goudie emphasises also the fluidity of Aboriginal forms of kinship, disrupted by invasion, colonisation, displacements and schisms, but argues for the reclaiming of lost or abandoned stories through poetry and language. Building on a vitalist perspective that emphasises affect, Pam Alldred and Nick J. Fox argue for a process of 'citizen-ing': the processual character of becoming a citizen.

A, perhaps the, key element in reimagining and reclaiming alternative paths to conviviality and citizenship for queer youth is the cyber world and the new forms of connectivity it offers. And here there have been truly remarkable changes, paralleling the changes Heaphy explored. Twenty years ago, as Brady Robards and colleagues argue, there was a sharp distinction between the virtual world and the real world. You went there as a visitor, exploring an alternative space. Today this particular binary divide has all but disappeared. The digital world is fully embedded in the lifeworld. But digital social spaces can still be important because they carry with them 'different heteronormative/homophobic burdens' and offer vital opportunities: for the affirmation of self, links with like-minded others, access to knowledge, a place to challenge stereotypical assumptions, sites to explore identities, health information, the transfer of subcultural capital and a performative space. And the chance of sexual contact, pleasure and love.

Robards et al. identify clear age-cohort differences in the use of cyberspace and how young people see their genders and sexuality. There is increasing use of non-binary and gender-fluid definitions, more identification with bisexual rather than lesbian or gay identities, less use of queer as a self-description and a proliferation of more personalised descriptions. For many, involvement in the cyberworld is itself an act of citizenship and a form of 'everyday activism'. It points, as Kath Albury and Paul Byron suggest, to a more participatory culture, with young people actively producing forms of knowledge, solidarity, identification and mutual support that are important in health education. Involvement in the digital world also brings new risks and vulnerabilities, as Christopher Pullen reminds us in relation to the youth refugee crises, but with a much wider resonance.

The crucial point, however, is that the digital revolution has made possible new links across the chasm of difference and distance that are transforming the possibilities of LGBT youth in their various paths to sexual citizenship and in the process querying/queering the meanings of citizenship itself. This book overall offers important new insights into these and other developments that are remaking the life chances of young people.

References

Cohen, S., 1972. *Folk Devils and Moral Panics*. London: MacGibbon and Kee.

Halberstam, J., 2005. *In a Queer Time and Place: Transgender Bodies, Subcultural Lives*. New York: New York University Press.

Plummer, K., 2010. Generational Sexualities: Subterranean Traditions and the Hauntings of the Sexual World: Some Preliminary Research, *Social Interaction*, 33 (2), 163–191.

Weeks, J., 2016. *What Is Sexual History?* Cambridge: Polity.

Editors and contributors

Crystal Abidin is a sociocultural anthropologist with an interest in vernacular Internet cultures, particularly young people's relationships with Internet celebrity, self-curation and vulnerability. She is a postdoctoral fellow with the Media Management and Transformation Centre (MMTC) at Jönköping University in Sweden, a lecturer in the School of Communication and Creative Arts at Deakin University in Australia and an adjunct researcher with the Centre for Culture and Technology (CCAT) at Curtin University in Australia.

Peter Aggleton is a sociologist and educationalist who has worked on gender, sexuality and health for over 30 years. He is an emeritus professor at UNSW Sydney, Australia, and a distinguished honorary professor in the College of Arts and Social Sciences at The Australian National University in Canberra, Australia. He is the editor of several book series and of the peer-reviewed journals *Culture, Health & Sexuality* (Routledge), *Sex Education* (Routledge) and *Health Education Journal*.

Kath Albury is a professor of media and communication at Swinburne University of Technology, Australia. Her research focusses on young people's practices of digital self-representation, and the role of user-generated media (including social networking platforms) in formal and informal sexual learning. She leads an Australian Research Council Linkage Project on *Safety, Risk and Wellbeing on Digital Dating Apps* with industry partners ACON Health (formerly the AIDS Council of New South Wales [NSW]) and Family Planning NSW.

Pam Alldred is a reader in education and youth studies at Brunel University in London, UK. Her interests include sexualities and sexual health, gender diversity, education for equality and research methods. She has recently published *Sociology and the New Materialism* (N. J. Fox, 2017) and is lead editor of the *Handbook of Youth Work Practices* (F. Cullen, K. Edwards and D. Fusco, 2018). She has led European projects on gender-related violence, homophobia and responding to sexual violence in universities.

Eva Bolander is a senior lecturer in pedagogic practice in the Department of Social and Welfare Studies at Linköping University in Sweden. She has extensive experience researching sexuality education in Sweden using multiple methods, including ethnographic field research and visual and text analysis. Related research interests include intersectional perspectives on schooling and teaching materials, values in education and critical pedagogies.

Louise Boon-Kuo is a lecturer in the University of Sydney Law School, Australia, where she conducts research in the areas of border control, criminalisation, race, gender, sexuality and citizenship. She is author of *Policing Undocumented Migrants: Law, Violence and Responsibility* (Routledge, 2017) and the book review editor for *Current Issues in Criminal Justice*. She collaborates on community projects focussed on diverse forms of incarceration.

Anna Bredström is a senior lecturer in the Institute for Research on Migration, Ethnicity and Society (REMESO) at Linköping University, Sweden. Her research, informed by feminist intersectionality theory, critical race theory and science and technology studies, focusses on bodies, health and medicine, and youth and sexuality. Her publications include work on HIV policy and sex and alcohol. She is particularly interested in developing methods for a critical multicultural sexuality education.

Paul Byron is a research associate in media and communication at Swinburne University of Technology, Australia. He researches digital media cultures of care, particularly LGBTIQ+ young people's practices of peer-based support and information sharing. He has an interest in the everyday use of digital media for practices of health, intimacy and friendship.

Brendan Churchill is a research fellow in sociology in the School of Social and Political Sciences at the University of Melbourne, Australia. His research focusses on the intersections of work and family life, and is driven by the desire to understand the ongoing impact of changes in the nature and structure of work as well as the transformation of family life, especially for women. He has also researched how young people negotiate life course transitions, relationships and intimate life.

Kyra Clarke is a lecturer in media studies at Massey University in New Zealand. Her research intersects the areas of feminism, affect, pedagogy and queer theory, exploring a range of popular textual forms, particularly film and television. Her publications include *Affective Sexual Pedagogies in Film and Television* (Routledge, 2017).

Rob Cover is an associate professor at The University of Western Australia. He has received Australian Research Council funding for projects on youth sexuality (2015–2018) and gender diversity in Australian film (2018–2020). He has published widely on topics in digital media, youth sociology, health communication and resilience. Recent books include *Queer Youth Suicide, Culture and*

Identity: Unliveable Lives? (Routledge, 2012), *Digital Identities: Creating and Communicating the Online Self* (2016) and *Emergent Identities: New Sexualities, Genders and Relationships in a Digital Era* (Routledge, in press).

Tania Ferfolja is an associate professor in the School of Education at Western Sydney University, Australia. She is an experienced pre-service teacher educator and researcher. Her work focusses on gender and sexuality diverse subjectivities in education, policy and curriculum. She is currently co-authoring (with Jacqueline Ullman) a book entitled *Sexuality and Gender Diversity in a Culture of Limitation: Student and Teacher Experiences in Schools* (Routledge).

Jessica Fields is a professor of sociology and sexuality studies at San Francisco State University, California, USA, and the author of *Risky Lessons: Sex Education and Social Inequality* (2008). With Laura Mamo, Nancy Lesko and Jen Gilbert, she leads *The Beyond Bullying Project* (funded by the Ford Foundation), which aims to understand and interrupt ordinary hostility in high schools to LGBTQ sexualities. Jessica is currently writing her second book, *Problems We Pose: Feeling Differently about Qualitative Research*.

Katie Fitzpatrick is an associate professor in health education and physical education in the Faculty of Education and Social Work at the University of Auckland, New Zealand. Her research focusses on health education in schools and is supported by a Royal Society of New Zealand (RSNZ) Rutherford Discovery Fellowship. Katie has published numerous articles and book chapters, and two books on health education and physical education: *Critical Pedagogy, Physical Education and Urban Schooling* (Peter Lang, 2013) and *Health Education: Critical Perspectives* (Routledge, 2014).

Nick J. Fox holds an honorary chair in sociology at the University of Sheffield, UK. He has researched and written widely on materialist and post-human social theory as applied to health, environment, embodiment, sexuality, creativity and emotions, and is co-editor of the journal *Health*. His most recent book (with Pam Alldred) is *Sociology and the New Materialism* (2017).

Jen Gilbert is an associate professor of education at York University in Toronto, Canada. Her research focusses on the challenges that LGBTQ sexuality and gender pose for schooling. She is a co-investigator on *The Beyond Bullying Project*, a digital media storytelling project that collects narratives of LGBTQ sexuality and gender in high schools, and is currently working on a study of discourses of consent in sexuality education. Her most recent book is *Sexuality in School: The Limits of Education* (2014).

Samia Goudie uses the term Blak Rainbow to describe her identity as a proud Bundjalung woman. She recently left a position as a senior lecturer in Aboriginal and Torres Strait Islander health at The Australian National University in Canberra, Australia, to develop a consulting business. In 2006–2007, she received a Fulbright award, which enabled her to visit a number of US universities and share research with First Nations communities and Tribal colleges. Prior to this, she worked as a community development leader and as an Aboriginal Health Worker. She is an author, a filmmaker and a mother.

Ricky Gutierrez-Maldonado is a doctoral candidate in the Department of Education Culture & Society at the University of Utah, USA. His dissertation is on the relationship between queerness, childhood and education, with a focus on queer and transgender youth of colour. He is also currently serving as a student program specialist with the Pride Center at San Joaquin Delta College in Stockton, California, USA. He works with queer and transgender students to advance social justice and LGBTQ+ advocacy.

Benjamin Hanckel is a researcher at King's College, London, UK, and holds a university associate role at the University of Tasmania, Australia. He has experience working in the Asia-Pacific and England on community development projects, health promotion and youth-related research. His work focusses on the design of new technologies for well-being and the role they play in young people's lives, particularly those marginalised by mainstream society.

Brian Heaphy is a professor of sociology in the School of Social Sciences at the University of Manchester, UK. He has undertaken research on social change with respect to lesbian, gay and bisexual family and couple relationships, ageing sexualities, living with HIV, friendships and personal life. His most recent publications draw on his research with Carol Smart and Anna Eisensdottir on the everyday experiences of same-sex partnership and family recognition.

Tiffany Jones is an Australian Research Council-supported early career research fellow in the Department of Educational Studies at Macquarie University, Australia, and an adjunct associate professor at the Australian Research Centre in Sex, Health and Society at La Trobe University, Australia. She is the author of *Intersex: Stories and Statistics from Australia* (2016) and other books. She has consulted on LGBTI issues for the United Nations and government and non-governmental organisations.

Deana Leahy is a senior lecturer in health education in the Faculty of Education at Monash University in Melbourne, Australia. She has undertaken research that critically examines the politics and practices of school health education, with a particular focus on sexuality education, drug education and food education.

Nancy Lesko is Maxine Greene Professor of Education at Teachers College, Columbia University, New York, USA, where she works in the areas of curriculum, social theory, gender studies and youth studies. She is co-editing *Feeling Education: Affect, Encounters, Pedagogy,* and her current research project, *Public feelings toward teachers,* maps the changing perceptions of teachers across the decades of the testing and accountability movement.

Laura Mamo is a professor of health education and associate director of the Health Equity Institute at San Francisco State University, USA, where she studies the intersections of gender and sexuality with science, medicine and health. She is the author of *Queering Reproduction: Achieving Pregnancy in the Age of Technoscience* (2007), co-editor of *Biomedicalization: Technoscience, Health, and Illness in the U.S.* (2010) and co-author of *Living Green: Communities That Sustain* (2009).

Daniel Marshall is a senior lecturer in literature in the School of Communication and Creative Arts at Deakin University in Melbourne, Australia, and the convenor of Deakin University's Gender and Sexuality Studies Major. He previously held positions as a research fellow in the Australian Research Centre in Sex, Health and Society at La Trobe University, Australia, and as an invited visiting scholar at the Center for LGBTQ Studies (City University of New York, USA) and at the Weeks Centre for Social and Policy Research (London South Bank University, UK).

Hayley McGlashan is a professional teaching fellow in the Faculty of Education and Social Work at the University of Auckland, New Zealand, where she teaches and researches in health education, sexuality and physical education. Hayley has a background in teaching health and physical education in secondary schools and is currently completing doctoral research into how schools support LGBTQ+ youth.

Erica R. Meiners is the Bernard J. Brommel Distinguished Research Professor at Northeastern Illinois University, USA, where she teaches justice studies, education, and gender and sexuality studies. She also works in multiple other sites, including a high school she co-started, prisons and community workshops. She is the author of several books, including *For the Children? Protecting Innocence in a Carceral State* (2016), and articles in a wide range of academic journals, magazines, blogs and anthologies.

Sujith Kumar Prankumar is a doctoral student in the Centre for Social Research in Health at UNSW Sydney, Australia, with special interests in race and ethnicity, gender and sexuality, young people and sexual health. His research concerns sexual citizenship and belonging among queer and minority ethnic young people in Sydney. He has worked in higher education, diversity training and health advocacy in Singapore and the USA.

Christopher Pullen is a principal academic in media theory at Bournemouth University in the UK. He is published widely on sexuality and the media, with a particular focus on LGBT identity. His recent work includes a focus on HIV-related narratives and the significance of personal autobiography, and forthcoming work on the therapeutic potential of television drama focusses on the representation of addiction narratives.

Mary Lou Rasmussen is a professor of sociology in the College of Arts and Social Sciences at The Australian National University in Canberra,

Australia. She is co-editor, with Louisa Allen, of the *Palgrave Handbook of Sexuality Education* (2016). Her well-cited monograph entitled *Progressive Sexuality Education: The conceits of secularism* (Routledge, 2016) has recently been published in paperback.

Brady Robards is a senior lecturer in sociology in the School of Social Sciences at Monash University, Melbourne, Australia. He studies digital culture, with a focus on how people use and produce social media and how social media platforms operate as memory archives. He has studied social media use among particular groups, such as LGBTIQ+ people, young people and tourists, and in the context of alcohol consumption.

Paul Simpson is a research fellow in the Kirby Institute for Infection and Immunity in Society at UNSW Sydney, Australia. His research focusses on health, marginalisation, ethics and identity in state institutional and civil society contexts, with a focus on Indigenous and sexual- and gender-minority people. He is currently working on projects including the *Health Research in Prisons Project* and the *Second Sexual Health and Attitudes of Australian Prisoners Survey*.

Susan Talburt is professor of Women's, Gender, and Sexuality Studies and interim director of the *Institute for Women's, Gender, and Sexuality Studies* at Georgia State University in Atlanta, USA. She recently edited *Youth Sexualities: Public Feelings and Contemporary Cultural Politics* (2018).

Denise Tse-Shang Tang is an assistant professor in the Department of Cultural Studies at Lingnan University, Hong Kong. Her research focusses on gender and sexualities, visual culture, urban spaces, migration, youth programmes and service delivery. Apart from academic work, she has an extensive background in programme management and advocacy in the areas of violence against women, juvenile justice, queer youth, Aboriginal issues, mental health, substance use and HIV in Canada and the USA.

Yvette Taylor is a professor of education at the University of Strathclyde, Glasgow, Scotland. She is interested in intersectional inequalities, and her projects include the Norface-funded Comparing Intersectional Life Course Inequalities amongst LGBTQ Citizens in Four European Counties study and the Economic and Social Research Council (ESRC)-funded Making Space for Queer Identifying Religious Youth project. Yvette edits the Palgrave Gender and Education Series of books and she co-edits the Routledge series on Advances in Critical Diversities.

Son Vivienne is a lecturer and researcher in digital media at RMIT in Melbourne, Australia, and works as an activist and media-maker with expertise in digital self-representation, online activism, queer identity and rhetorical strategies/feminist practices for speaking and listening across difference. The author of *Digital Identity and Everyday Activism: Sharing Private Stories with Networked Publics* (2016), Son curates several collective storytelling websites for queer and gender-diverse communities.

Jeffrey Weeks is an emeritus professor of sociology at London South Bank University, London, UK, and author of numerous articles and 25 books, many focussing on the history and social organisation of sexuality in general and LGBT identities and intimate life in particular. He has been closely involved in the debates over sexual citizenship since the 1990s. His most recent monograph is *What is Sexual History?* (2016). He was awarded a WAS (World Association for Sexual Health) gold medal for his outstanding contribution to the study of sexuality in 2017.

Adrian Kin Cheung Yan is a graduate research student in the Department of Sociology at the University of Hong Kong. His research interests include the sociology of education, the sociology of emotions, citizenship education and gender studies.

Youth, sexuality and sexual citizenship

An introduction

*Peter Aggleton, Sujith Kumar Prankumar,
Rob Cover, Deana Leahy, Daniel Marshall
and Mary Lou Rasmussen*

In popular scientific and policy discourse ideas about childhood and youth tend to elicit two rather contradictory responses. On the one hand, children and young people may be seen as the nation and a family's future, full of promise and good things to come. Their creativity, vibrancy and youthfulness are to be valued, holding the potential both to rejuvenate the present and to lead to a better future. In political discourses as diverse as fascism (Kater 2004), social reformism (France 2007) and communism (Gorsuch 2000, Yang 2016), children and young people are afforded special status as adults-in-waiting and future citizens. On the other hand, there is a darker side to childhood and youth. Children in general, and 'adolescents' in particular, are often construed as willful, irresponsible and feckless – in need of adult tutelage, discipline and control. In the absence of guidance and restraint, things can go wrong – children may cease to apply themselves to study, young people can go off the rails and adolescents in particular may turn delinquent. It is the tension between these competing ideologies – the good and the bad, the hopeful and the more pessimistic – that makes it so difficult to take a balanced view of young people and their future.

Youth, rights and citizenship

Despite the widespread ratification of the United Nations Convention on the Rights of the Child in 1989, and the broad range of political, economic, civil, social and cultural rights which it affords to children, rarely if ever are these rights realised and protected in the manner intended. All too often, children and young people are denied a meaningful say in the education they are offered, in future employment, in the kinds of health provision they access, in whether or not or who to marry, and in countless other spheres of life, even in some of the richest countries of the world.

For youth, the process toward full participation, citizenship and adulthood is not just ritual but also liturgy: young people are expected to establish a respectful – and respectable – relationship not only with their parents and elders but with the state, imbibing its customs, beliefs and traditions, preparing for participation in the workforce and practising self-responsibility and control. A principal objective of this liturgical process is for young people to gain the favour of the all-knowing, paternalistic, omnipresent state and its full citizen-members in order to complete their transition to full membership. If they fail to do so, they remain liminal citizens, only able to participate to the extent deemed convenient by others. But the existence of the liminal (or quasi) citizen presents a thorn in the state's project of projecting power and benevolence, so efforts to mould its subjects into citizens acquiescent to national interests become especially pronounced. Through activities as diverse as compulsory schooling and community service, state and community powers pull young people's lives into their disciplinary orbit in the hope of moulding these adults-in-waiting into responsible, self-correcting citizens of benefit to future society and country.

As the future of the world is so firmly organised around the figure of the child, considerable energy is expended in ensuring their charges' discipline, well-being and 'protection', with no shortage of assumptions made about what might lead to the best possible outcome. Children are the *tabulae rasae* onto whom are projected the anxieties and insecurities of the body politic. As Hatch (1995) observed,

> The notion was that if we can somehow intervene in the lives of children, then poverty, racism, crime, drug abuse, and any number of social ills can be erased. Children [thereby become] instruments of society's need to improve itself.
>
> (p. 119)

A counterpoint to this (i.e., children's ignorance) lies in the assumption of their inherent wisdom by some media and cultural studies research, which 'seeks to celebrate the sophistication of the "media-wise" child' (Buckingham 2009, p. 355).

The preservation of youth and childhood 'innocence' is central to the project of mitigating a volatile, uncertain and shameful world. Paraphrasing the literary theorist Jacqueline Rose, who reflects on children in philosophy and literature – in this case *Peter Pan* – 'the child has access to a lost world or primitive state denied to the social-contaminated adult, a state which the child then restores to the adult' (Rose cited in McGillivray 2015, p. 104). In this way, our contemporary obsession with children is but one consequence of panic over the perceived breakdown of the economic, social, cultural and political order.

The literary critic Lee Edelman has described this reproductive futurism as 'the fascism of the baby's face' (Edelman 2004) – which pervades much of the political activism underpinned by this vision of a heteronormative future. He explains the mechanics of the image of a child in the following way:

> the image of the Child, not to be confused with the lived experiences of any historical children, serves to regulate political discourse – to prescribe what will count as political discourse – by compelling such discourse to accede in advance to the reality of a collective future whose figurative status we are never permitted to acknowledge or address... That figural Child alone

embodies the citizen as an ideal, entitled to claim full rights to its future share in the nation's good, though always at the cost of limiting the rights 'real' citizens are allowed.

(Edelman 2004, p. 11)

Edelman suggests that in this fixation with securing the moral borders so that emerging generations can spring forward to create a future utopia, the rights and desires of current citizens are curtailed. This can be seen most graphically in earlier concern over the growth of juvenile delinquency (Cohen 2002) and current sexualisation panics concerned with enforcing antediluvian images of childhood innocence, despite clear historical and sociological evidence of young people being sexually aware, interested and even engaged (Waites 2005, Bhana 2007, Egan and Hawkes 2010, Elliott 2012).

In many societies, the periods of life we know as childhood and youth are increasingly extended, denying children and young people the opportunity to enter into citizenship for longer periods of time while simultaneously promoting the idea that their 'innocence' must be protected. Where once (in Western societies) adulthood began when a child left school (aged 12, 13 or 14, perhaps), entered the workforce and/or left home, now it begins at the end of secondary education or only after the completion of a university degree. Yet at the same time, somewhat contradictorily, there are pressures on young people to become full consumers in their own right (of ideas, things and selves) that the modern-day economy requires. As the Slovenian sociologists Mirjana Ule and Tanja Rener (2001) put it,

Given the tendency towards a prolonged youth moratorium, what we have here is both the acceleration and the slowing down of childhood and adolescence. In general, the entrance into the areas of principal social positions and continual and permanent employment now occurs later in life. At the same time some activities typical of adulthood, for example, becoming a competitive consumer, forming their own lifestyle autonomously, and so on, are being assumed at an earlier age.

(Ule and Rener 2001, p. 273)

Crucially, young people are trained for the exigencies of the state not just at school but also through activities such as youth skills and youth empowerment programmes run by educational and non-governmental organisations that, while ostensibly supporting young people's agency and interests, conscript them to serve state interests by training them to be better 'democratic subjects' (Kwon 2013, p. 127). Under the guise of empowerment and social justice, the state's duties are increasingly outsourced to young people and their communities, who are but minimally compensated for their labour and time, other than by being patted on the back for being 'good citizens'. As Wyn and White (1997) observe, what we are seeing in most advanced capitalist countries is the forfeiture of basic citizen rights for an increasing proportion of the youth population. Citizenship is increasingly contingent upon labour market position, and what 'rights' and 'claims' one can make is dependent in practice upon whether or not they are connected in some way to educational or labour market institutions.

(p. 138)

The figure of youth, then, straddles a number of complex cultural formations and social changes that underpin the assumed need for discipline and the expectations of their creative potential. In this book we are particularly concerned with exploring the combination of two elements of this complex constellation, sexuality and citizenship, with the hope that refracting young people's experiences through the lens of sexual citizenship may help us better understand the affective, political and moral aspects of their lives.

Sexual citizenship

Sexual citizenship, broadly defined, refers to sexual claims of belonging; it considers both the intimate and sexual aspect of a person, together with aspects of their identity, in their participation – or lack thereof – in the rights and responsibilities of being a citizen. The concept was perhaps first coined in the early 1990s by David Evans (1993), who argued that sexual citizenship is materially constructed within capitalist societies by the relationship between the state, sexual morality and the market. More recently, Rasmussen and colleagues (2016) have considered how sexual citizenship rests on shifting bodies and shifting embodiments, a perspective which highlights the many exclusions inevitably associated with the notion of sexual citizenship.

The historian and sociologist Jeffrey Weeks (1998) has written that sexual citizenship shares features with other claims to citizenship, including enfranchisement, inclusion, belonging, equity and justice, tempered by new responsibilities. It lies as 'the fateful juncture of private claims to space, self-determination and pleasure, and public claims to rights, justice and recognition'. Weeks highlights a major tension though between the sexual as a private and often personal domain, and citizenship, with its connotations of the public, implying involvement and participation in rights and recognition struggles within the wider community and society.

Sexual citizenship's focus on rights claims has, however, had a patchy history, and the concept of citizenship has been questioned as being an imposition from the West that is inflexible and othering. Legal scholars Kessler and Robson (2008) argue that the concept places 'citizenship over personhood, thus excluding members of our own communities and allies' (p. 571), a line of argument Richardson (2018) summarises as a focus on 'the violence of (sexual) citizenship' (p. 94). In a more radical move, Plummer (2001) argues for the use of the term intimate citizenship, which he sees as implying not 'one model, one pattern, one way or one voice' (p. 243) but rather '*a plurality of public discourse and stories about how to live the personal life in a late modern world where we are confronted by an escalating series of choices and difficulties around intimacies*' (p. 238, emphasis in original). This more in-dividual and person-centred approach aligns with geographer Michael Brown's (2006) plea for a concept of sexual citizenship 'grounded in a caring, relational, and grounded notion of obligation – and one sensitive to the political ecologies of disease' (p. 894).

According to Ara Wilson (2002), opponents of sexual, reproductive and wom-en's rights strategically charge sexual rights advocates with 'ethnocentrism and cultural imperialism', 'promoting the breakdown of the family (hence the erosion of community, peoples, and nations)' and 'exacerbating materialistic individu-alism' (p. 257). Further, as Angelia Wilson (2009) points out, 'if articulated out-side a liberal democratic frame, the claim to human rights has little purchasing power. Deployment of political signifiers makes the most strategic sense when this happens within the frames that give them meaning' (p. 82). Acknowledging such critique, political scientist Carol Johnson and sociologist Tara Atluri have argued for a wider, more fluid and inclusive interpretation of sexual citizenship so as to be adaptable to 'non-Western social and political constructions' (Johnson 2017, p. 160), and which moves outside the 'market-driven cultures of sex as prop-erty and legal entitlement' (Tagore cited in Atluri 2012, p. 734).

Nevertheless, sexual citizenship is useful in that it recognises and situates individuals and society as intrinsically sexual, thereby contesting more tradi-tional notions of citizenship that have relegated the sexual to the private and the domestic in favour of new possibilities. 'The division between socio-economic and sexual issues is false', notes anthropologist Carole Vance (1982, p. 40). Their inter-dependency is reaffirmed 'in domesticity, reproductive politics, and the split between public and private, fantasy and action, male and female' (Vance 1982, p. 40). In a related vein, David Bell and Jon Binnie write, 'We consider all citizenship to be sexual citizenship, as citizenship is inseparable from identity, and sexuality is central to identity' (Bell and Binnie 2000, p. 67). And while sex-ual citizenship's basis in rights language may be a source of contention, it is also filled with the potential that has seen it successfully adapted in studying various non-Western contexts – from Africa (Bhana 2007, Oduro 2012, Pieterse 2015) to Asia (Farrer 2006, Kong 2011, *Sexualities* 2017). The anthropologist Sally Engle Merry has called the process of appropriating global ideas of human rights and translating them into local terms vernacularisation (Merry 2006), and successful efforts to vernacularise concern for sexual, reproductive and women's rights can be found across a variety of contexts (Levitt and Merry 2009).

An especially convincing account of the relationship between sexual citizen-ship and sexual rights can be found in the work of Diane Richardson (2000), who highlights three main ways in which sexual rights are understood within sexual rights discourse: as conduct-based ('rights to various forms of sexual practice in personal relationships'), as identity-based ('rights through self-definition and the development of individual identities') and as relationship-based ('rights within social institutions: public validation of various forms of sexual relations') (pp. 107–108). All are interconnected: 'the right to sexual pleasure', Richardson says,

> is complex and inextricably linked to other rights of citizenship. For example, it is difficult to envision what it would mean to speak of women's rights to sexual pleasure, without at the same time recognising rights that enable women's control over their sexuality and reproduction.
>
> (p. 114)

In her more recent writing, Richardson (2018) encourages thinking more broadly about sexual citizenship: the historic focus on lesbian, gay, bisexual and trans (LGBT) communities in sexual citizenship literature and advocacy, she argues,

> narrows the lens of (sexual) citizenship in ways that direct attention away from thinking about groups of people whose rights of (sexual) citizenship may also be contested, for example people with HIV and AIDS, post-trafficked women, refugees, migrant workers and so on.
>
> (p. 95)

It may therefore be useful to think about citizenship more broadly as belonging 'where, rather than civic inclusion, social relations and [the] practices of daily life inscribe citizenship status' (p. 97). Taking such a perspective as a starting point, we turn now to examine the thorny issue of youth sexual citizenship.

Sexual citizenship and youth

If controversy exists with respect to 'youth, rights and citizenship' as well as in relation to the concept of 'sexual citizenship' itself, matters become more complex when it comes to the relationship between sexual citizenship and youth. Kerry Robinson (2012) has drawn attention to especially 'difficult citizenship' that exists within this domain, with notions of childhood innocence trumping efforts to provide young people with an education about gender, sex and relationships that is equitable, honest, evidence informed and fair. More generally, Nikolas Rose (1999) has written that childhood is one of the most intensely governed aspects of human existence. Ultimately, the realisation of children's citizenship rights (be they linked to sexual citizenship or otherwise) exists in tension with the adult exercise of power to determine who does what, when, where and why.

There is a small but growing body of conceptual and theoretical research describing young people's navigations of sexuality using citizenship frameworks. Robinson (2013, 2016), for example, argues for the importance and relevance of sexual citizenship in children's and young people's lives as a matter of social justice, while Waites (2005) offers ways of thinking about the rights and obligations young people should have in relation to sexuality, specifically as it relates to age of consent legislation. Tsaliki (2016) examines childhood sexualisation in politics, academia and the media, while Farrer (2006) has looked at the politics of sexual storytelling in reform-era China. While these early signs of activity around youth sexual citizenship are encouraging, much existing writing remains limited in its scope, focussing on particular topics, such as young people's lack of access to comprehensive, inclusive sexuality education (Illes 2012, Carmody and Ovenden 2013, Honkasalo 2017, Shah 2017), or more general issues, such as the challenges young people face in growing to become informed and responsible citizens capable of making independent decisions around sexual identity and well-being (Fonseca et al. 2012, Oduro 2012, Moore 2013).

There remain major gaps in understanding how young people articulate their own views of citizenship and belonging (especially in relation to gender and sexuality as identities, selfhoods and life projects), their opinions concerning rights-based discourses and what is most important to them. This is significant given shifting sociopolitical dynamics globally and the impact of these developments on youth life prospects. Important questions to be answered include how are the meaning(s) and value(s) of citizenship changing, and how do young people position themselves (or not) sexually (or otherwise) within the global citizenship matrix? Who do young people regard as the best translators, mediators and arbiters of what counts as youth and sexual citizenship? In what ways might changing experiences of youth life alter the constituent elements of what we gather together to call 'citizenship'? And in the increasingly post-nation state experience of life fostered by transnational knowledge flows and global ecological crisis, even if young people might still (yet?) find some resonance in a claim to citizenship, what are they imagining they are becoming a citizen of?

The situation with respect to belonging, recognition and right to participation claims is especially problematic for lesbian, gay, bisexual, trans* and queer (LGBTQ) youth whose opportunities and whose sexual and/or gender identities and practices often differ from hegemonic ideals and whose lives are often made difficult (unbearable even) by misunderstanding, prejudice, discrimination and fear.

The latter part of the twentieth century saw an increasing acceptance of sexual and gender diversity, moving away from earlier historical understandings which understood such diversity in a host of problematic ways – including as sinful, abnormal, socially deviant, sick or a 'passing phase' to be got through en route to heterosexual marriage – and then only in uneven ways around the world. In much of the majority world today, there remains deep hostility towards those who are gender and sexually 'different' or diverse, be they adults or young people. Four countries still retain the death penalty for homosexual acts between men, and many more (through their legal and administrative systems or otherwise) fail to recognise the existence of lesbians, trans* and intersex people, among others (Carroll and Mendos 2017, p. 8). And Indonesia and Bermuda have recently taken steps to rollback the rights of LGBTQ citizens, a salient reminder that citizenship is not a fixed state.

Yet at the same time there has been an ongoing and profound diversification of gender and sexual identities and practices among youth, with various websites, social media and Tumblr pages presenting lists of between 37 and 300 gender labels, and between 35 and 84 sexual orientations as of March 2018 (genderfluidsupport.tumblr.com, safespacenetwork.tumblr.com and the critical/satirical site ageofshitlords.com). A new language of gender and sexual identification has emerged in these online sites, built on the interactive and co-creative contributions of young people in dialogue with each other, prompting calls for greater freedom for identifying gender, sexuality and romantic/sexual possibilities from some and substantial criticism from others. Although older models of identity labelling as well as newer frameworks of citizenship are the basis for this new range of sexual and gender categories, they present unprecedented challenges to masculine/feminine and hetero/homo binaries, and the exclusions these have sometimes produced.

In this kind of context, how best can we recognise and respond to children and young people's different circumstances, interests and needs? Can the concept of sexual citizenship carry the weight of so much diversification, or might this diversity occasion a wholesale renovation of the term? What kinds of alliances need to be built, and what kinds of knowledge can help move matters forward? All too frequently moralism and misleading forms of 'common-sense' substitute for research and evidence-informed debate.

Two prevailing views of gender and sexual minority youth continue to dominate recent writing and scholarship. First, there is the view that these young people are vulnerable (Fenaughty and Harré 2003) and best understood as victims (see Talburt et al. 2004, Marshall 2010, Payne and Smith 2016 for critiques of this view). On the other hand, LGBTQ youth may be seen as unusually resilient, the avid users of tools of social participation, such as social media and the Internet (Driver 2008). When these differences are exaggerated, as is often the case in popular discussions of the topic, their limitations become obvious: not all gender and sexual minority young people are vulnerable, nor are they all self-reliant. Instead, their agency, both individual and collective, is influenced by the material and discursive resources available. What is required, as signalled earlier, are studies and accounts that investigate young people's struggles for recognition and inclusion – in particular contexts and at particular moments in time – from the perspective of competing claims in relation to sexual citizenship.

The aim of this book therefore is to explore young people's understandings and experiences of sex, sexuality and citizenship – on their own terms and in diverse but linked settings – in the family and through kinship, at school and in tertiary education, in work and employment, and through engagement with health services, among other topics. Our interest here is largely but not exclusively on the experience of gender and sexually diverse youth. This choice of focus is deliberate because we believe it holds the potential to reveal not only the uniqueness of LGBTQ youth identities, subjectivities and practices but also the normative backcloth against which these experiences must be set. For above all else, gender and sexuality are relational, intersecting with hegemonic structures of ethnicity, ability, class, religion and age – among other influences – and it is in the hegemony of heterosexism and its 'wicked brothers' (sexism, genderism, racism, disablism and ageism) and the counter-hegemony of diverse young people's responses that our interest lies. In the remainder of this book, young people's experiences in these domains will be examined through chapters prepared by leading authors in the field.

This book

Our book begins with a foreword by Jeffrey Weeks, whose historical analysis of the origins and development of LGBTQ politics laid the foundations for concepts of sexual citizenship today. In reflecting on the relationship between citizenship and youth, it draws attention to the continuing tension between adult and youth perspectives on how the world should be. In an age of lengthening public education, poor or non-existent job opportunities, spiralling costs of housing and delayed marriage and parenting, young people struggle for the future, not necessarily on the terms 'given to them' by past generations but informed by perspectives of their own. Simultaneously, however, there has been a growing awareness of the diversity of ways of feeling/doing gender, sex and sexuality, attributable at least in part to the increased visibility and circulation of information related to these topics. In such a context, new generational subjectivities are being formed, especially among LGBTQ and other gender and sexual minority youth. What the consequences of this interaction between constraint and possibility will be for future claims to sexual citizenship remains to be seen. But it is a project worth contemplating, both conceptually and empirically, as the chapters in this book set out to do.

The first section of this book focusses on questions of kinship as it might be understood across a number of domains. We begin with a chapter by Brian Heaphy, who examines personal narratives of family and kinship as told by LGBQ people in their 20s and 30s in two studies, the first undertaken in the mid-1990s and the other undertaken more recently in 2009–2010. Set against the backcloth of sociocultural and legal change in LGBQ rights in Britain, the chapter highlights how strengthened notions of family and intimate citizenship in the 2000s co-exist with accounts of compromised citizenship more distinctive of the earlier period. There follows a chapter by Louise Boon-Kuo, Erica R. Meiners and Paul Simpson, which has a focus on carceral politics. The concern here is on how queer young people's sexual citizenship and affective belonging is impacted by the criminal justice systems of the USA and Australia. The chapter highlights both the damage caused to young lives and the creativity, refusal and resilience of queer youth as they resist the imposition of power and policing by the carceral state. This first section ends with a more personal account of what it might be to reimagine, reclaim and rename sexual citizenship and selfhood in Australia today. The power of Samia Goudie's poetry and reflections reveals what kinship and self-making imply for a proud Bundjalung woman living in Australia today. Her writing points to the need for intersectional analyses in which history, ethnicity and race are given place.

Section 2 of this book turns its attention to schooling and education – settings in which LGBTQ young people often encounter non-recognition, social exclusion, genderism, homophobia, transphobia, violence and abuse. It begins with an chapter by Ricky Gutierrez-Maldonado which revisits the murder of Lawrence 'Larry' King in Oxnard, California. Focussing on the ways in which this was reported in advocacy and media discourses, the chapter highlights how efforts to advance sexual rights in and through schooling must move beyond a concern for rights alone to engage with the bodily practices and the embodied subjectivity of queer and trans students of colour. Writing in a European context, and from a different theoretical perspective, Anna Bredström and Eva Bolander's chapter looks at the form and content of current sexual education in Sweden. Their writing highlights how the 'Swedishness' inherent in such an approach sets limits on what can be engaged with and talked about, and by whom. It signals the need to adopt an anti-racist perspective, which can accommodate conflicting values, while treating culture in a non-essentialist way. Finally, Adrian Kin Cheung Yan and Denise Tse-Shang Tang, in their chapter, examine the forms of social control to which lesbian, gay and bisexual (LGB) youth in Hong Kong are subjected in schools. Sexual morality, cultural 'tradition' and religious conservatism constitute the 'trinity of governance' that stigmatises and sets limits on the inclusion of gender and sexual minority youth in modern-day Hong Kong. Their chapter signals the value of a home-grown sexual citizenship framework for advancing LGB young people's recognition, participation and rights.

In Section 3 of the book, we focus in on issues of well-being and health. Tiffany Jones begins the section with a chapter highlighting the importance of commonality and difference as part of sexual citizenship claims. Drawing on recent research into the experiences, inclusion and well-being of trans* and intersex youth, her chapter stresses the importance of distinguishing between each of these groups in efforts to advance sexual citizenship and rights. In the next chapter, Pam Alldred and Nick J. Fox advance a new materialist approach to understanding sexualities education and sexual citizenship. Focussing on efforts to promote sexual health and well-being in school, they identify two competing discourses concerning young people and gender/sexuality education: the first, which identifies children and youth as 'innocent' presexual beings at risk of corruption by sexual knowledge, and the second, which sees them as active sexual citizens with legitimate sexual health concerns and needs to be empowered through social intervention. Alldred and Fox's analysis extends this perspective to examine the sexuality-education assemblages emerging in relationships between young people and professionals, and the capacities (both sexual and otherwise) that these produce in bodies. The third contribution to this section, from Jessica Fields, Jen Gilbert, Laura Mamo and Nancy Lesko, shifts the focus to mental health and well-being. Drawing on the work of *The Beyond Bullying Project*, a storytelling and research initiative in the USA, it turns once again to questions of intersectionality, showing how racialised expectations of assimilation and responsibility shape efforts to promote inclusion, diversity and respect in US schools. This chapter identifies possibilities for new alliances that can interrupt damaging neo-liberal perspectives on youth, sexuality and citizenship.

Past decades have witnessed recurrent moral panics concerning young people, sexuality and the media. Section 4 engages with some of these concerns through its focus on communication technologies, including 'new' social media and young people's creative uses of communication technologies. In their chapter Brady Robarts, Brendan Churchill, Son Vivienne, Benjamin Hanckel and Paul Byron examine how the digitally mediated spaces inhabited and used by lesbian, gay, bisexual, trans, intersex and queer (LGBTIQ) people have evolved over the last 20 years, drawing on data from four age cohorts. Kath Albury and Paul Byron highlight how young people's social and mobile media use is often construed by adults as controversial and/or problematic. Rejecting risk-based narratives, and drawing on their recent work with teachers and health professionals (among others), they advance an understanding of media practice which recognises young people's rights to access technologies as forms of digital and sexual citizenship. The last chapter in this section, by Christopher Pullen, adopts a slightly different stance by looking at the representation of refugee and proto refugee queer youth in recent television documentaries. Through a study of three recent films – *Exodus: Our Journey through Europe*, *Exiled: Europe's Gay Refugees* and *Hunted: The War Against Gays in Russia* – this contribution analyses how documentary depictions of queer youth are shown to be inspirational and often resilient figures who, through their actions, help bring into focus new social justice and civil rights contexts for renegotiating an understanding of youth sexual citizenship.

Section 5 changes the focus to inclusion and sexual citizenship in the world of work. Tanya Ferfolja, in her chapter, looks at the experiences of a group of LGBTQ queer-identifying young people as they navigate entry to a teaching career. Stressing that schools are largely heteronormative environments in which silence relating to diverse gender and sexuality prevails, the chapter examines how trainee teachers navigate these workplace challenges so as to develop forms of school citizenry aligned to LGBTQ subjectivity. The task is not easy but can be successfully accomplished through processes of affirmation, accommodation and adjustment. Crystal Abidin and Rob Cover, in the next chapter, engage with a different set of work-related concerns: namely, those pertaining to the micro-celebrities working in the new earning environment of social media. Analysing the work of the gay-identified YouTube influencer Troye Sivan, in particular, the authors show how the development of content fostering gay support succeeded in promoting both rights-based sexual citizenship activism and Sivan's own career. Yvette Taylor's contribution to this section shifts the focus yet again to look at an under-researched group and set of issues: namely LGBTQ religious youth. Her concern here is with anticipated future forms of employment and the role that religiosity, gender and sexuality may play in current-day imaginings of these.

Taylor also illustrates how religion and sexuality still collide in legislative and popular imaginations, and realisations of citizenship status in the UK context, where the supposed decline of religion may be conflated with an increased entitlement to sexual citizenship for LGBTQ groups. Such a conflation sidelines the citizenship possibilities and realities negotiated and imagined by queer religious youth in imagining future forms of employment and family formations.

The final section in this book looks at sex as a set of media narrations and identifications, as providing the foundation for new subjectivities, categories and labels, and as the basis for contestations around whose knowledge counts most in schools. In the first of these chapters, Kyra Clarke analyses representations of youth and sexualities in the millennial television series *Skins*. Tracing the coming of age of three groups of young people in their final year of college/school, the series was controversial for its explicit portrayals of drug use and sex. Queer characters, pleasures and desires figure in all six seasons, and Kyra's chapter looks at key moments of transgression and what these might imply for notions of sexual citizenship and broader relational possibilities. Katie Fitzpatrick and Hayley McGlashan look to future possibilities, drawing on findings from two studies of LGBTQI youth (re)imagining teacher-student relationships and the positioning of young people in schools. Their work raises important questions about where 'expertise' on issues of gender and sexuality really lies: in the expert knowledge that teachers and the curriculum promulgate or in the lived experience of diverse groups of young people (including queer youth) themselves? At the end of this section, Rob Cover's chapter on youth micro-minorities homes in on the proliferation of labels, identities and categories (of gender and sexuality) that can currently be found in young people's use of social media. It considers how this new taxonomy or lexicon of identities and identifications – which moves well beyond traditional masculine/feminine and hetero/homo dichotomies – has emerged and what it might signal for the future. Does the inclusion of terms such as heteroflexible, asexual, homoflexible, sapiosexual, nonbinary, aromantic, pansexual and others signal a new openness in young people's self-identifications and socio-sexual relations or a yet more insistent surveillance of the self and others?

Our book concludes with an afterword by Susan Talburt. Here, she reflects not only on the contributions this book contains but also on the wider terrain in which citizenship in general and sexual citizenship, in particular, may be understood. Like Jeffrey Weeks, she identifies both transgressive and citizenship moments in recent sexual politics, but she points to the multiple ways in which sexual citizenship is lived out through conscious-raising, protest and rights claims as well as in more everyday spaces provided by the park, the bar, the bedroom and, increasingly, in social media. Her analysis is salutary in its signalling of how sexual citizenship and neo-liberalism interrelate: through claims to normality and inclusion; through entry into the mainstream; and through the reification of the liberal, sovereign queer subject who (at last) is capable of self-governance. Her essay concludes with some reflections on who (and what) remains excluded from the 'relentless normalisation and entrepreneurialism of neoliberalism' – children and youth, the poor and the dispossessed, the unmarried and those who do not wish to be married, and people of colour, among many others.

It has been an enormous pleasure to work closely with a wide range of contributors over the past 12 months to develop this book. Their insights into questions of sexual citizenship and youth have raised important questions for our own work on the ongoing Australian Research Council-funded 'Queer Generations' (Belonging and Sexual Citizenship among Gender and Sexual Minority Youth) project. Here, we have been examining the experiences of two different generations of gender and sexual minority youth in Australia. Our interest has been in the sources of support found most useful by young people and the ways in which formations of participatory sexual citizenship are useful to young people in making sense of sexual and gender differences, lived realities of subjectivity and identity, and perspectives on growing up. The project has involved archival, policy and media research as well as focus groups and interviews with LGBTQ respondents in three Australian states (Western Australia, New South Wales and Victoria), in both state capitals and regional areas, with two generations: those born in the 1970s and those born in the 1990s.

Among the key questions raised by this work and by the chapters that make up this book are the following:

- How might the concept of sexual citizenship be informed – and altered – by the different experiences and perspectives of different generations of queer people?
- Recalling the discussion earlier in this introduction regarding the critiques of rights-based approaches, and the difficulties of applying these approaches in diverse geopolitical locations, how might the expanded diversification of sexuality and gender witnessed at the contemporary moment play out? Will it help sponsor more tailored, context-specific understandings of sexual citizenship, or will it sponsor a new iteration of colonialist endeavour?
- What kinds of demands do these new forms of sexual citizenship place on the nation and the community?
- What forms or mechanisms of governance or justice will be required to bestow (or remove) citizenship rights and adjudicate competing citizenship claims – or will the sexual citizenship of the future disarticulate itself from acts of external bestowal, removal and adjudication?

While it is too early to suggest answers to these questions, and while one should always be suspicious of an immediate response or 'quick fix', we can see in both past and contemporary youth responses to gender and sexual politics creativity, contestation, resistance and agency (both individual and collective). These, therefore, are far from tangential issues in many young people's lives, nor are they issues on which younger people and adults necessarily agree. For it is in the everyday responses of young people as they navigate the complex web of desires, 'freedoms', rights and citizenship claims that we can catch glimpses of both the past and the future: the past in the sense that the struggles of today are not without their own history, indeed they are in many ways the legacy of tasks left undone in former times, and the future in the sense that the ground is changing under our feet so quickly. What does citizenship mean in the context of an exploding world population, increased transnational movement and growing statelessness? How might citizenship endure as a primary concern as people's affinities with global communication platforms grow to outstrip national identifications? How can we identify a citizen at all when identity itself is being constantly refashioned? Little is certain, beyond the forcefulness of this transitional moment, and youth sexual citizenship is being forged in the heat of all this change, taking shape before us.

References

Atluri, T., 2012. The Prerogative of the Brave: Hijras and Sexual Citizenship After Orientalism. *Citizenship Studies*, 16 (5–6), 721–736.

Bell, D. and Binnie, J., 2000. *The Sexual Citizen: Queer Politics and Beyond*. Cambridge, MA and Malden, MA: Polity.

Bhana, D., 2007. The Price of Innocence: Teachers, Gender, Childhood Sexuality, HIV and AIDS in Early Schooling. *International Journal of Inclusive Education*, 11 (4), 431–444.

Brown, M., 2006. Sexual Citizenship, Political Obligation and Disease Ecology in Gay Seattle. *Political Geography*, 25 (8), 874–898.

Buckingham, D., 2009. Children and Television. In: J. Qvortrup and W. A. Corsaro, eds. *Palgrave Handbook of Childhood Studies*. Basingstoke: Palgrave Macmillan, 347–359.

Carmody, M. and Ovenden, G., 2013. Putting Ethical Sex into Practice: Sexual Negotiation, Gender and Citizenship in the Lives of Young Women and Men. *Journal of Youth Studies*, 16 (6), 792–807.

Carroll, A. and Mendos, L. R., 2017. *State Sponsored Homophobia 2017: A World Survey of Sexual Orientation Laws*. Geneva: International Lesbian, Gay, Bisexual, Trans and Intersex Association. Available from: http://ilga.org/downloads/2017/ILGA_State_Sponsored_Homophobia_2017_WEB.pdf

Cohen, S., 2002. *Folk Devils and Moral Panics* (3rd ed.). London and New York, NY: Routledge.

Driver, S., 2008. Introducing Queer Youth Cultures. In: S. Driver, ed. *Queer Youth Cultures*. Albany, NY: SUNY Press, 1–18.

Edelman, L., 2004. *No Future: Queer Theory and the Death Drive*. Durham, NC and London: Duke University Press.

Egan, D. R. and Hawkes, G., 2010. *Theorizing the Sexual Child in Modernity*. New York, NY: Palgrave Macmillan.

Elliott, S., 2012. *Not My Kid: What Parents Believe About the Sex Lives of their Teenagers*. New York, NY: New York University Press.

Evans, D., 1993. *Sexual Citizenship: The Material Construction of Sexualities*. London and New York, NY: Routledge.

Farrer, J., 2006. Sexual Citizenship and the Politics of Sexual Story-Telling among Chinese Youth. In: E. Jeffreys, ed. *Sex and Sexuality in China*. London and New York, NY: Routledge, 102–103.

Fenaughty, J. and Harré, N., 2003. Life on the Seesaw: A Qualitative Study of Suicide Resiliency Factors for Young Gay Men. *Journal of Homosexuality*, 45 (1), 1–22.

Fonseca, L., Araújo, H. C., and Santos, S. A., 2012. Sexualities, Teenage Pregnancy and Educational Life Histories in Portugal: Experiencing Sexual Citizenship? *Gender and Education*, 24 (6), 647–664.

France, A., 2007. *Understanding Youth in Late Modernity*. Maidenhead and New York, NY: Open University Press.

Gorsuch, A. E., 2000. *Youth in Revolutionary Russia: Enthusiasts, Bohemians, Delinquents*. Bloomington and Indianapolis: Indiana University Press.

Hatch, J. A., 1995. Studying Childhood as a Cultural Invention: A Rationale and Framework. In: J. A. Hatch, ed. *Qualitative Research in Early Childhood Settings*. Westport, CT and London: Praeger, 117–133.

Honkasalo, V., 2017. Prevention, Prevention, Prevention. It's All About Prevention and Diseases. In: B. Formark, H. Mulari, and M. Voipio, eds. *Nordic Girlhoods: New Perspectives and Outlooks*. Cham, Switzerland: Palgrave Macmillan, 103–105.

Illes, J., 2012. Young Sexual Citizens: Reimagining Sex Education as an Essential Form of Civic Engagement. *Sex Education*, 12 (5), 613–625.

Johnson, C., 2017. Sexual Citizenship in Comparative Perspective: Dilemmas and Insights. *Sexualities*, 20 (1–2), 159–175.

Kater, M. H., 2004. *Hitler Youth*. Cambridge, MA: Harvard University Press.

Kessler, T. and Robson, R., 2008. Unsettling Sexual Citizenship. *McGill Law Journal*, 53, 535–571.

Kong, T. S. K., 2011. *Chinese Male Homosexualities: Memba, Tongzhi and Golden Boy*. London and New York, NY: Routledge.

Kwon, S. A., 2013. *Uncivil Youth: Race, Activism, and Affirmative Governmentality*. Durham, NC and London: Duke University Press.

Levitt, P. and Merry, S., 2009. Vernacularisation on the Ground: Local Uses of Global Women's Rights in Peru, China, India and the United States. *Global Networks*, 9 (4), 441–461.

Marshall, D., 2010. Popular Culture, the 'Victim' Trope and Queer Youth Analytics. *International Journal of Qualitative Studies in Education*, 23 (1), 65–85.

McGillivray, A., 2015. A Child's Mind as a Blank Book: Myth, Childhood, and the Corporation. In: A. Diduck, N. Peleg, and H. Reece, eds. *Law in Society: Reflections on Children, Family, Culture and Philosophy: Essays in Honour of Michael Freeman*. Leiden and Boston, MA: Brill Nijhoff, 101–124.

Merry, S. E., 2006. *Human Rights and Gender Violence: Translating International Law into Local Justice*. Chicago, IL: University of Chicago Press.

Moore, A., 2013. For Adults Only? Young People and (Non)participation in Sexual Decision Making. *Global Studies of Childhood*, 3 (2), 163–172.

Oduro, G. Y., 2012. Children of the Street: Sexual Citizenship and the Unprotected Lives of Ghanaian Street Youth. *Comparative Education*, 48 (1), 41–56.

Pieterse, M., 2015. Law, Rights, Space and Sexual Citizenship in South Africa. *Social Dynamics*, 41 (3), 482–501.

Payne, E. and Smith, M. J., 2016. Gender Policing. In: N. M. Rodriguez, W. J. Martino, J. C. Ingrey, and E. Brockenbrough, eds. *Critical Concepts in Queer Studies and Education: An International Guide for the Twenty-First Century*. New York, NY: Palgrave Macmillan, 127–136.

Plummer, K., 2001. The Square of Intimate Citizenship: Some Preliminary Proposals. *Citizenship Studies*, 5 (3), 237–253.

Rasmussen, M., Cover, R., Aggleton, P., and Marshall, D., 2016. Sexuality, Gender, Citizenship and Social Justice: Education's Queer Relations. In: A. Peterson, R. Hattam, M. Zembylas, and J. Arthur, eds. *The Palgrave International Handbook of Education for Citizenship and Social Justice.* Basingstoke: Palgrave Macmillan, 73–96.

Richardson, D., 2000. Constructing Sexual Citizenship: Theorizing Sexual Rights. *Critical Social Policy,* 20 (1), 105–135.

Richardson, D., 2018. *Sexuality and Citizenship.* Cambridge, MA and Medford, MA: Polity Press.

Robinson, K. H., 2012. Difficult Citizenship: The Precarious Relationships Between Childhood, Sexuality and Access to Knowledge. *Sexualities,* 15 (3/4), 257–276.

Robinson, K. H., 2013. *Innocence, Knowledge and the Construction of Childhood: The Contradictory Nature of Sexuality and Censorship in Children's Contemporary Lives.* Oxford and New York, NY: Routledge.

Robinson, K. H., 2016. Children's Sexual Citizenship. In: S. Seidman and N. L. Fischer, eds. *Introducing the New Sexuality Studies* (3rd ed.). London and New York, NY: Routledge, 485–493.

Rose, N., 1999. *Governing the Soul: The Shaping of the Private Self* (2nd ed.). London: Free Association Books.

Sexualities, 2017. Special Issue: Rethinking Sexual Citizenship: Asia-Pacific Perspectives. *Sexualities,* 20 (1–2), 143–257.

Shah, S., 2017. Disabled People Are Sexual Citizens Too: Supporting Sexual Identity, Well-being, and Safety for Disabled Young People. *Frontiers in Education,* 2. Available from: www.frontiersin.org/articles/10.3389/feduc.2017.00046/full

Talburt, S., Rofes, E., and Rasmussen, M. L., 2004. Introduction: Transforming Discourses of Queer Youth and Educational Practices Surrounding Gender, Sexuality, and Youth. In: M. L. Rasmussen and S. Talburt, eds. *Youth and Sexualities: Pleasure, Subversion and Insubordination.* New York, NY: Palgrave Macmillan, 1–13.

Tsaliki, L., 2016. *Children and the Politics of Sexuality: The Sexualization of Children Debate Revisited.* London: Palgrave Macmillan.

Ule, M. and Rener, T., 2001. The Deconstruction of Youth. In: A. Furlong and I. Guidikova, eds. *Transitions of Youth Citizenship in Europe: Culture, Subculture and Identity.* Strasbourg, France: Council of Europe Publishing, 271–288.

Vance, C. S., 1982. *Diary of a Conference on Sexuality.* New York, NY: Barnard Women's Center.

Waites, M., 2005. *The Age of Consent: Young People, Sexuality and Citizenship.* Hampshire and New York, NY: Palgrave Macmillan.

Weeks, J., 1988. The Sexual Citizen. *Theory, Culture & Society,* 15 (3), 35–52.

Wilson, A., 2002. The Transnational Geography of Sexual Rights. In: M. P. Bradley and P. Petro, eds. *Truth Claims: Representation and Human Rights.* New Brunswick and London: Rutgers University Press, 251–265.

Wilson, A. R., 2009. The Neat Concept of Sexual Citizenship: A Cautionary Tale for Human Rights Discourse. *Contemporary Politics,* 15 (1), 73–85.

Wyn, J. and White. R., 1997. *Rethinking Youth.* Sydney, NSW: Allen & Unwin.

Yang, G., 2016. *The Red Guard Generation and Political Activism in China.* New York, NY: Columbia University Press.

Section 1

Kinship

Chapter 1

Family, kinship and citizenship

Change and continuity in LGBQ lives

Brian Heaphy

Introduction

Historically, lesbian, gay bisexual and queer (LGBQ)[1] relationships have been constructed as the antithesis of 'good', 'healthy' and 'legitimate' family and kin. Indeed, family and kin have played a key role in regulating LGBQ lives (Altman 1979, Bozett and Sussman 1989, Calhoun 2003). Often in the interests of protection from stigma, LGBQ people have been ostracised by or have distanced themselves from their family of origin (Davies 1992, Patterson 2000, Saewyc et al. 2006). From the 1970s onwards studies have explored LGBQ 'alternative' families that were made up of friends, partners, other associates and children (where they existed) (Macklin 1980, Allen and Demo 1995, Buell 2001). These were often conceived as 'replacement', 'surrogate' or 'fictive' kin that provided material, emotional and social resources in the absence of support from biological and legal kin.

By the 1990s, the language of 'chosen' families had entered the lexicon of research on LGBQ life (Weston 1991, Weeks et al. 2001). Chosen families were viewed less as necessary replacements for families of origin, but more as self-defined elective kin that could include friends, partners, ex-partners, accepting families of origin and children that were conceived both within and outside of heterosexual relations. These families, together with demands for the protection of same-sex partners' next-of-kin, parenting and caring 'rights', became the basis of what some viewed as a (radical or conservative) turn to intimacy in LGBQ politics (Seidman 2001, Weeks 2007). This, in turn, contributed to what some deemed to be the moment of LGBQ 'equality' (Blasius 1994) or 'sexual citizenship' (Weeks 1995).

Against this backdrop, this chapter considers the difference that more recent sociocultural and legal developments have made for LGBQ experiences of family, kinship and citizenship in Britain. British developments are thought to be amongst the most globally advanced in terms of LGBQ 'rights' and experiences in this context provide a point of reference for the possible implications of similar developments elsewhere. Specifically, the chapter examines the personal narratives of family and kinship as told by LGBQ people who were in their 20s and 30s in the mid-1990s and in 2009/2010. These narratives, as explored by two different studies of LGBQ relational life that I will discuss,[2] formed part of the cultural context in which two separate cohorts of LGBQ youth entered their mid-teens and early 20s in Britain. They can be conceived as generationally specific narratives of experience that have provided young people with a sense of the possibilities of living and relating as LGBQ.

The first study focussed on the personal narratives of family and intimacy told by self-identified LGBQ people in the mid-1990s. The analysis here focusses on the narratives of those who were in their 20s and 30s at the time of the interview. The second study focussed on the personal narratives of couples and individuals who entered into a civil partnership[3] between 2005 and 2010. The focus here is also on the narratives of those who were in their 20s and 30s at the time of interview. The chapter explores 'strong' and 'weaker' personal narratives of family and kinship that contributed to cultural understandings of LGBQ life at the time that they were told, and how generation and formal partnership status structured them. To do this, it focusses on interviewees' personal definitions of family and kin, their accounts of family distance and belonging, friendship and chosen families and the perceived possibilities for parenting. This enables consideration of the ways in which the family expectations of some LGBQ youth can radically change across generations, while such expectations remain unchanged for others.

Family, kinship and LGBQ lives

Family, stigma and social relocation

At the end of the 1970s Dennis Altman (1979, p. 47) claimed 'straight is to gay as family is to no family'. Prior to that the Gay Liberation Front Manifesto (1971/1978) stated 'The very form of the family works against homosexuality'. Underpinning these statements was the political belief that family and LGBQ lives were incompatible. This was in large part due to the role the family had played in enforcing compulsory heterosexuality (Rich 1983) through socialisation, regulation and even violence. Indeed, Bruce Voeller (1980, cited in Muller 1987, p. 140) noted: 'Nowhere has the hostility to homosexuality been more frightening to large numbers of gay men and lesbians than their own families'.

In the UK in the 1970s and 1980s, as in most parts of Europe and North America, 'compulsory' heterosexuality implied growing up in families in which heterosexuality was still assumed or 'enforced' from birth. The majority of those aged between the mid-teens and mid-20s in the mid-1990s would have grown up in a family context where heterosexuality was viewed as an inevitable outcome. Unsurprisingly, identifying as lesbian, gay or bisexual could lead to a sense of personal crisis with respect to self-identity, family and kinship relations. Family responses ranged across a continuum from wholehearted acceptance to confused tolerance to overt hostility and violence (Bozett and Sussman 1989).

Sexual difference could lead to ostracism or self-imposed social, emotional and geographical distance between young LGBQ and their 'given' kin in a quest to create a non-heterosexual life of their own (Davies 1992).

As Mark Blasius (1994) has argued, one of the defining characteristics of compulsory or institutionalised heterosexuality is that the spaces, places and representations of everyday life are purged of LGBQ visibility. One explicit legal example of this in Britain is what was commonly termed Section 28 of the Local Government Act 1988, which prohibited local authorities from 'promoting' homosexuality or gay 'pretended family relationships'. It also prevented more progressive local government councils from financing educational materials and projects perceived to promote a gay lifestyle. LGBQ sexual identities, lifestyles and practices were deemed to be risky (for example through their association with HIV) and morally dangerous. They carried a high degree of stigma and fear.

It is against the backdrop of stigma, the risks of hostility and of sociocultural (including legal) representations that denigrated LGBQ relationships that we can understand the uneasy relationships between LGBQ youth and their families of origin in the 1980s to the mid-1990s. Coming out at that time often implied coming into new identities and the social relations and communities that supported them as well as geographical relocation to urban areas that were perceived to be more anonymous and accepting of sexual/gendered difference (Cruickshank 1992, Blasius 1994, Weston 1995). These identities, communities and places provided the basis for new support networks, new families and new definitions of kin.

Chosen families, parenting and intimate citizenship

In the 1990s the language of chosen and friendship families had become established in the lexicon of academic and community discourse about LGBQ life (Weston 1991, Nardi 1992, Weeks et al. 1999). In North America, for example, Nardi (1992) was discussing gay friendship families and Weston (1991) was discussing families we choose. Weeks et al. (1999) were also discussing 'families of choice' in the UK. Weston's research and analysis were especially insightful into how LGBQ families were constructed less by need and more by choice: where friends, partners, ex-partners, close associates and accepting families of origin were included in family definitions and practices. At the same time, partly as an aspect of AIDS activism, and partly as a response to so-called lesbian 'baby-boom', LGBQ politics had begun to focus more intensely on intimate 'rights' (Weeks 1995). This was often focussed on rights to family status through partnership and next-of-kin recognition, parenting and co-parenting rights, pensions, inheritance and so on. Developments in same-sex partnership recognition in a small number of Nordic and European jurisdictions also provided an impetus for focussing on civil unions and same-sex marriage 'rights'.

Additionally, LGBQ identities, lifestyles, relationships and families began to be increasingly and more widely represented in the culture, and the so-called pink pound had been 'discovered' by marketing companies and the media.

Combined, these dynamics gave rise to a sense of future possibilities for living openly as LGBQ people and claiming citizenship in law and in everyday life. Citizenship in this sense could be understood as concerning what Plummer (1995) termed 'intimate citizenship': 'the *control (or not)* over one's body, feelings, relationships: *access (or not)* to representations, relationships, public spaces etc.; and *socially grounded choices (or not)* about identities, gender experiences' (Plummer 1995, p. 151; emphasis in the original). Thus, LGBQ intimate citizenship is not merely a question of legislative 'rights' but goes well beyond those.

Legal equality, family and citizenship

By the end of the first decade of the 2000s the LGBQ politics of relational rights, together with greater cultural visibility of same-sex relationships and changes in social attitudes, as well as a more liberal government in the UK, led to a range of legal and policy initiatives that reflected a notable shift in how LGBQ identities and relations were perceived, including those linked to same-sex partnership and LGBQ parenting (Heaphy et al. 2013, Nordqvist and Smart 2014).

LGBQ youth in the late 2000s were privy to how same-sex marriages were being claimed and recognised in parts of Europe, North America and elsewhere. In the UK, much of the discriminatory legal initiatives of the previous decades had been repealed. In the 2000s alone, the ban on lesbians and gay men in the military was lifted; Section 28 was repealed; discrimination against LGB people in the workplace was made illegal; discrimination in the provision of goods, facilities, services, education and public functions was legally forbidden; transgender recognition was legally enacted; and homophobic abuse was included in the definition of hate crime. In addition, social attitudes to homosexuality continued to change in the direction of greater acceptance (Harding 2017).

Linked to this latter point, it could be reasonably assumed that families of origin were more likely to be accepting and supportive of their children in coming out as LGBQ, and young women and men were less likely to believe that LGBQ lives implied childlessness and stigma (Gabb 2005, Ryan-Flood 2009, Taylor 2009). Thus, the need for geographical and social distance from family of origin, and need to escape the 'heterosexual world', was not as likely to be experienced as essential as was previously the case. To come out in the 2000s, was to come into a world where it was a reasonable expectation of many young LGBQ people to continue to participate and have an unaltered sense of connectedness to family of origin. This is the distinctive context in which the latter of the two studies I discuss should be understood.

Generationally situated personal narratives

The personal narratives considered in this chapter were generated by two studies. The first, undertaken by Weeks, Heaphy and Donovan (see Weeks et al. 2001), and funded by the UK Economic and Social Research Council (ESRC), was based on a non-age specific sample. It explored the structure and meaning of 'non-heterosexual' intimate relationships, including family, friendships, sexual and community relationships. Interviews were undertaken in 1995 and 1996 (see Heaphy et al. 1998 for an account of the methodology). The analysis in this chapter focusses on the narratives of 63 individuals aged under 40 at the time of the interview, the youngest being aged 22. The second study was based on joint *and* individual interviews with 50 couples (100 partners) in 2009 and 2010. Partners were aged up to 35 when they entered a civil partnership and were aged under 40 at the time of the interview, the youngest being aged 21. The study, also funded by the ESRC, was undertaken with Heaphy, Smart and Einarsdottir (see Heaphy et al. 2013 and Heaphy and Einarsdottir 2012 for accounts of the methodology). Both studies included equal numbers of women and men.

Drawing from this data the chapter focusses on personal discourses of LGBQ families and kin that were likely to have shaped the relational expectations of two cohorts of LGBQ youth: the first, which was aged between their mid-teens and mid-20s in the mid-1990s, and the second, which was aged within the same range in 2009/2010. The different foci and samples of the two studies mean that direct comparisons cannot be made. However, discussing them together provides a way of thinking about how the possibilities open to different cohorts of LGBQ in terms of family, kinship and intimate citizenship have radically changed for some but remain unchanged for others. This can be usefully conceived in social generational terms.

Social generations are linked to cohort experiences, and the constraints and opportunities that shape life chances and world views. Generations do not necessarily share one world view, as they contain internally differentiated 'generation units' (what I term generational sub-sectors) (Mannheim 1952, quoted in Edmunds and Turner 2002, p. 9). As far as sexualities and relationships are concerned, there is no 'one' generational experience in any given national or legislative context, and within any generation there may be diverse experiences. The experience that most successfully articulates itself as *the* generational one is the one that is best supported and resourced to do so (*cf.* Edmunds and Turner 2002). Put another way, in Plummer's (1995) sociological vocabulary of personal stories, the story that establishes itself as *the* strongest (or dominant) story of a generation is that which is listened to and reproduced by a range of expert, political, policy, media, everyday listeners and validated by accounts of personal experience.

LGBQ narratives of family in the 1990s

There is a wealth of work on the extent to which self-recognition as LGBQ can be a personally challenging but also an enriching experience. As Davies put it in the 1990s,

> the man [sic] in the brink of coming out…inhabits a social matrix, a social structure which assumes, expects and enforces heterosexuality …the individual is faced with a psychic dilemma: the contradictions between the experiences of society and its creation: himself.
>
> (Davies 1992, p. 76)

In our 1990s study, the troubling implications of recognising oneself as lesbian, gay or bisexual were a common theme in personal narratives. As Juliet[4] (aged 39) remarked: 'I was about 16, 17, 18 by which time I realised clearly … that I was a lesbian – although I struggled with that for a long time – I didn't discuss it with anybody'. Sam (aged 31) also recounted 'My family had very fixed ideas… you meet someone [of the 'opposite' sex], you get married and have kids… subconsciously, I was working towards that'.

While some individuals braved the risk of family disappointment or hostility by being open about their sexuality at a relatively young age, for many being closeted from family was a more favourable option. Peter recounted that coming out 'was very easy and it was a good experience for me…I can't think of anybody who reacted in a way that upset me'. But, as he acknowledged, he 'was one of the lucky ones'. Luke (aged 30), for example, told a very different story:

> I got engaged and it came to the point where I was either having to deny what I was and continue to feel as bad as I felt, and run the risk of ruining [my fiancée's] life. So I chose to leave [Name of Town]…because if I had stayed in my hometown, it was only a matter of time before [my parents] would know.

As Cant (1997) suggests, moving away from the family home is most acutely experienced as freedom when the relationships and values that reside there are experienced as a prison. In our 1990s study we found plentiful examples of the need 'to escape the shame which you believe your homosexuality will bring you and your family' (Cant 1997, p. 6).

Moving out of the family home or moving away could be a key step in providing the opportunity to shape a new life. For individuals like Luke, quoted earlier, this could entail developing new ways of being in the world, and engaging with others who were seen as a new 'family'. As put it, his friends 'call each other family… they're family…I have a blood family, but I have an extended family… my friends'. Juliet (aged 39) also stated, 'I think that the way I think about [my friends] is the way that …generally people would regard as family'. For some, friends were 'more important than family' (Paul, aged 36).

As these personal narratives attest to social, emotional and geographical distance from family of origin were a culturally strong narrative amongst LGBQ people in the 1990s study, as were the possibilities that existed for creating friendship and chosen families – so much so that the latter became a strong feature of academic, therapeutic and broader cultural discourse. The latter families could be based on 'a feeling of belonging to a group of people who like me' (Simon, aged 32), and a sense of connectedness to 'people who you can rely on if you're in trouble, or just if you need help [or] the people you love, I suppose' (Rachel, aged 36).

One facilitator of connectivity to family of origin could be the existence of children, although this could increase social distance where family of origin disagreed with the 'lifestyle choice' of an LGBQ relative on the basis of social and moral risks to the child. In the 1990s study participants' narratives of parenting included accounts of impossibilities, opportunities and choice (Weeks et al. 2001). In talking about a sense of parenting impossibilities, Pat (aged 34) recalled her brother telling her 'once you become gay, you give up the right to have children'. David (aged 24) also recounted thinking 'Oh God, I'm never going to have children…I can have everything, I can live with somebody, but I'm never going to have children'. Inevitably, men tended to see parenting as a greater impossibility than women. As John (aged 37) put it, 'I could not conceive of having children now. But…I don't think it's an option anyway, in this country. I think it's a option for women, for lesbians'. Many gay men recounted giving parenting little thought.

Those LGBQ interviewees who did have children in the 1990s tended to have conceived through previous heterosexual relationships. However, in the 1990s new narratives of choosing to be a sole legal parent through adoption or donor insemination were beginning to emerge (legal recognition of parenting as a same-sex couple was unavailable). Some women had entered into parenting arrangements with gay male donors, a choice that could work well or prove troublesome for both parents over time. While surrogacy was sometimes acknowledged as providing the possibility for gay male parenting, a sense that the legalities in the UK were unclear and that the financial costs of overseas surrogacy were prohibitive, meant that most gay men saw this as an unrealistic option.

Personal narratives of the risks entailed in coming out, estrangement or social and geographical distance from family of origin, and the possibilities that LGBQ communities offered for friendships, chosen family and a sense of belonging (as well as emerging narratives of lesbian and gay parenting) were strong narratives circulating within LGBQ cultures and beyond in the 1990s. As such, they formed a part of the cultural background in which LGBQ youth in the 1990s sought to make sense of their sexualities and the implications for their relationships with others. These narratives were likely to be especially influential as they came from and circulated within LGBQ communities and were grounded in experiences of everyday life. They were well positioned to gather audiences to them, and powerful in representing the generationally grounded constraints and possibilities encountered by LGBQ in negotiating their family lives.

LGBQ narratives of family in 2009/2010

If culturally strong stories of LGBQ family relations in the 1990s focussed on the personal consequences of coming out for a sense of exclusion from mainstream families, an alternative story was on the cusp of emerging which became a powerful one by 2009/2010: that of family inclusion, connectedness, uncompromised belonging and the incorporation of same-sex couples (and their children) into mainstream family life. Partners in our 2009/2010 study often noted the long distance that had been travelled in LGBQ representation in a short time. As Cori (aged 31) put it, 'I was fifteen …sixteen years ago it was like there weren't really open gay people on TV, no one ever talked about it, [it] was completely different...just a million miles away from where things were when I was a kid'.

LGBQ stories of increasing sociocultural recognition and increasing family acceptance could go hand in hand. For some, there had been a shift from 'assumed heterosexuality' to an 'assumed acceptance' of sexual difference, to the extent that same-sex attraction was often not perceived as a critical personal issue to be grappled with. As Theresa (aged 31) recounted, 'I never really had...this kind of realisation that I'm gay, or discussions with people...I don't see it as an issue'. In narrating their relational biographies, roughly one-third of the women and half of the men made little or no reference to their coming out as a critically significant moment in their lives. Theirs were fairly straightforward stories of 'just' being LGBQ and relating to others on that basis.

About one-third of women and a quarter of men talked about coming out to their families in ways that suggested that they had assumed and experienced it to be unproblematic. The final third of women and quarter of men had experienced coming out as personally difficult or problematic. Even amongst the latter, many personal stories were of family acceptance, as Nancy (aged 29) recounted: 'I've never been confident about coming out...even though my mum was really fine and my dad ... he hasn't appeared fazed at all and my mum's really supportive of everything I do'. While Jeremy (aged 29) had assumed that living a fulfilling gay life would entail distancing himself from his family and community of origin, his experience proved otherwise:

> I got a job...next to where my parents live. That's where I met Stewart and things sort of went from there really... beforehand it wasn't something that I ever thought was possible... I didn't think I could ever, in my wildest dreams, come out in [that community] I don't think I actually existed until I came out to my parents.

The most common narrative that emerged in the 2009/2010 study was of straightforward family acceptance of non-heterosexual identity and relationships. Such acceptance could lead to a sense that the differences between heterosexual and same-sex relationships and lifestyles were relatively insignificant and that LGBQ and their heterosexual families of origin ultimately shared the same relational values. As Hanna (aged 26) put it, 'I think I share the same [relationship] values as [my] parents: you try and work things out...and I think sometimes that's all you need if you've got the love of your family'.

Friendships were a regular feature of our partners' previous single lives. Some partners in the 2009/2010 study deemed their current friendships to be as important as family, and many couples and partners valued socialising friendships. However, unlike interviewees in the mid-1990s study, those in the 2009/2010 study tended to prioritise couple and family relationships over friendships when it came to intimate connectedness, caring commitments and the preferred source of emotional, social and material supports. The general tendency was to see 'mature' couple commitments (such as those thought to be involved in civil partnerships) and a sense of belonging to a family of origin as enduring ties and friendships and friendship networks as more transitional bonds.

In a minority of cases, friendships continued to be deemed family after the participant entered a partnership. These included friendships that were seen *as* family or as 'better than' family. In discussing their relational lives, 10 out of 100 partners in the 2009/2010 study referred to friendship in this way. Veronica (aged 34) stated: 'I think it, friends are probably more important to me I think than my, than my family'. Friends were clearly significant to these partners, but only in the minority of cases did they seem to be as centrally significant as suggested by studies of previous generations of lesbians, gay men and bisexuals. This, I suggest, is in large part due to the dominance of the couple as a relational ideal and the extent to which, because participants had formalised their relationships within the last five years, they were likely to be especially invested in the couple when we interviewed them. Nevertheless, in the earlier mid-1990s study about two-thirds of participants aged in their 20s and 30s, who were also in committed couple relationships, told very different stories of family. In this respect, the possibilities for family relationships seem to have changed between the earlier and later generation, with the latter moving towards the incorporation of LGBQ into mainstream family life. Such changing possibilities were also evident when it came to parenting and children.

Couples in the later study tended to see their formalised relationships as part of settling down into a committed 'life-long' relationship, as did their parents and broader families or origin. Inevitably this raised questions about plans for parenting and almost all the partners had had some conversation about their desires and the possibilities in this respect. As Louise (aged 35) who had one child with her partner Kathryn recounted, on first meeting Kathryn (aged 40), she was struck by the fact that they 'just happened to be similar, because of the similar type of... middle class upbringing...very similar values'. She further recounted, 'I think that linked, very much to ...family life and whether we wanted children or not. I know that was a very early conversation we had... I certainly knew I wanted children'. Following an informal commitment ceremony, both partners 'went to the doctors and said, "We're gay...where do we need go to about having a baby"'. They then recounted that they went 'complete NHS [National Health Service] just the same as anyone else having [assisted insemination] treatment' and had what they described as very positive experiences.

The existence of children could strengthen the bonds between LGBQ people and their families of origin (especially, but not only, with those of the biological parent) who were often keen to be involved as grandparents, aunts, uncles and so on. One-third of the female participants in the 2009/2010 study co-parented (compared to about one-sixth in the earlier study), the majority of whom had conceived within the same-sex relationship. Of the remaining female couples, half had clear plans to parent through donor insemination or adoption at a point in the future. Only four female couples had decided not to parent. None of the male couples in the 2009/2010 study had children. While some had vague plans for parenting, the majority did not include parenthood in their concrete plans for the future. Some men did very much want to have children but felt that the process of becoming parents was beyond their capacities and/or resources. As Oliver (aged 30) put it, '[It] seem[s] fraught with difficulties'. Despite the legal, practical and social difficulties that men (and some women) assumed they would encounter in attempting to have a child within a same-sex relationship, the majority ultimately viewed this as a choice that *could* be made if both partners were invested enough in it and had the financial resources to afford it.

Taken together, the personal narratives considered so far may seem to attest to the ways in which LGBQ family relationships in Britain have changed dramatically between the mid-1990s and 2009/2010. Combined with surveys that indicate changing social attitudes and the host of legal and policy developments that came to fruition in that period it could seem LGBQ people had all but achieved the equality with heterosexuals and citizenship. For those entering into their mid-teens to mid-twenties at the end of the first decade of the 2000s then, one of the strong cultural narratives they would have been exposed to, that emerged in tandem with personal narratives of the new experiences of LGBQ, was of more or less wholly transformed possibilities for LGBQ living and relating. However, this is only part of the story.

Intimate citizenship: strong and weaker stories

As discussed earlier in this chapter, when considering LGBQ family and kin relations we need to move beyond legal rights and equalities legislation and consider what Plummer terms intimate citizenship. It is worth highlighting the issues Plummer deems to be important to this, namely (i) the control over one's body, feelings, relationships; (ii) access to representations, relationships, public spaces; (iii) and socially grounded choices about identities and relationships. Culturally strong narratives from the earlier and later studies that I have considered suggest that there has been a dramatic and relatively recent generational shift in these regards. However, a more situated perspective that takes into account diverse LGBQ experiences of family is important to acknowledge that while new opportunities exist for some, they are not available to all. In this respect, culturally weaker stories also exist that risk being sidelined by what might be seen as more mainstream developments.

In terms of control over one's body, feelings and relationships, some participants' narratives from the 2009/2010 study pointed to how their specific religious and cultural backgrounds shaped their family experiences and expectations in less than positive ways (see Taylor 2007, 2009, Yip and Page 2016). In terms of her experience of recognising herself as a lesbian Veronica recounted, 'It took me a long time to get over feelings of guilt about my sexuality because of all this baggage associated with Christianity'. With respect to her relations with her partner and her family of origin, and her expectations for future, Josha (aged 22) said,

My parents will expect me to marry [a Muslim man]. At some point I will get married. And that will be my life… if my parents knew of this relationship and were accepting of it, then this would be my proper life…because of these restrictions, I know it's not realistic to continue this.

Veronica and Josha were not alone in recounting how specific cultural and familial expectations impacted the control they had over their feelings and how they could express them. While their stories resonate strongly with the personal narratives of family and community stigma, regulation and hostility that were told in the 1990s study, they were relatively uncommon amongst participants in the 2009/2010 study. In this sense, they could be seen as 'weaker' stories of the continuing ways in which living and relating as LGBQ could be felt to be problematic, experienced as difficult and perceived to be outside of one's own control.

In terms of access to representations and public spaces, personal narratives of increasing family acceptance, as told in the 2009/2010 study, often went hand in hand with accounts of broader social acceptance as was thought to be evidenced by increasing representations of LGBQ lives, new opportunities for relationships and greater visibility in public spaces. While many interviewees pointed to the ways in which LGBQ were almost 'fully' represented in law, others pointed to the greater visibility of LGBQ in traditional and 'new' media as well as the opportunities that social media presented for networking and forming new relationships. Participants also noted the opportunities that were now open to them in terms of increased access to commercial LGBQ spaces, as well as mainstream spaces that were previously deemed to be heterosexual. In terms of mainstream space, for example, Peter (aged 38) said, 'you look around and you see things now, like you go into shops and there are civil partnership cards and all that kind of stuff'. Nathan (aged 39) also recounted that because a civil partnership is now an official category most people accept it: 'like I said most everybody does, most people do'. However, strong stories of increased social acceptance coexisted with weaker stories of the fairly constrained terms on which LGBQ had access to representations of their relationships, opportunities for relationships and visibility in public spaces.

Some participants commented on (or had internalised) what they perceived as 'negative' representations of LGBQ relationships. For example in discussing LGBQ family commitments, Maria (aged 33) recounted the well-known myth that 'In the gay community, if a relationship doesn't work then you just leave and that's that'. Also, some suggested that LGBQ relational cultures had developed in ways that left them feeling alienated. They perceived that such cultures had been reduced to commercial scenes, and as Louise put it, such scenes 'were very different from what was right for me… [I was] thinking well "I know I'm gay and I like women but I'm not like that so what am I?"'

Where participants in the 2009/2010 study believed LGBQ communities to be synonymous with LGBQ 'scenes', they suggested that participation was dependent on how you looked and that such communities could be exclusionary. Similarly, how LGBQ families looked could be important in determining their comfort in, and access to, mainstream public spaces *as* families. As Maria, a Black woman, recounted in discussing the schooling of the child she co-parented with her white female partner, the fact that they were same-sex parents meant the 'system wasn't set up' to deal with them. Like some other co-parents Maria and her partner felt pressure to perform or display their family in a way that made them recognisable to others *as* a family. This could entail a greater demand than existed for heterosexual parents to conform to culturally determined 'ideal' (white, middle class, heterosexual) standards of family respectability.

In terms of socially grounded choices about identities and relationships, it is clear from the 2009/2010 study that many LGBQ interviewees believed they were well-supported by their families of origin and personal networks in making socially grounded choices about their identities and relationships. Nevertheless, Josha's narrative that was considered earlier points how such choices could be constrained. Also, it is important to remember that, while three-quarters of the men and two-thirds of the women in our sample appeared to suggest that their sexualities and relationships were unproblematic for their family of origin, kin and friends, culturally weaker accounts of anxiety, caution and trepidation about coming out were narrated by a significant portion of the sample. These feelings did not come from 'nowhere', and signify continuing hostility towards LGBQ people (from kin, heterosexual friends and in the broader culture). Overall, weaker narratives from the study, such as these, highlight the need for interventions at the everyday level where LGBQ lives are lived that are aimed at enhancing informal 'rights' so as to enable diverse LGBQ to fully access intimate citizenship.

Conclusion

This chapter has examined personal stories of LGBQ experience in Britain to consider strong (and weaker) narratives that influence young people's generationally situated sense of the possibilities that exist for their family and kin relations. By considering strong, if not wholly dominant, narratives told by two cohorts it has sought to illuminate generational change with respect to the enhanced possibilities and expectations that exist for LGBQ relational life. Strong personal stories chime with political, expert and broader cultural discourses about increasing equality and citizenship, and because they are grounded in experience, they appear to evidence how the possibilities for LGBQ relational lives have changed dramatically in a relatively short time. They suggest that in countries such as Britain, LGBQ have reached the moment of 'equality'.

However, as has been argued in the chapter, legal equality does not equate with 'full' citizenship. Intimate citizenship in everyday life is a crucial aspect of the latter. Weaker stories about continuing hostility from family of origin, social distance and constrained family choices (such as those linked to men's same-sex parenting) continue to be told alongside strong stories of generational change. These narratives of compromised intimate citizenship, or the everyday limits to citizenship, can be more difficult to hear in LGBQ and mainstream cultural contexts where more positive stories dominate. They trouble our sense of the 'inevitable progress' towards full equality and legalistic conceptions of citizenship. And from the perspective of intimate citizenship they highlight that LGBQ rights is not a 'job done', as well as the continuing need for political, policy and personal interventions at the everyday level in which LGBQ family lives are lived, so as to enhance informal 'rights'. Such rights concern the extent to which *diverse* LGBQ can live socially connected lives in ways that respect their bodies, feelings and relationships; enable them to influence the diverse ways in which they would choose to be represented; and enable them to present and 'do' their identities and relationships in the diverse ways of their choosing.

Notes

1   This chapter uses the acronym LGBQ because the studies it discusses did not include trans people.
2   Both of these studies were generously funded by the UK Economic and Social Research Council. The first study was entitled Families of Choice: The Structure and Meaning of Non-heterosexual Relationships (Ref L315253030), and the second was entitled 'Just Like Marriage?' Young Couples' Civil Partnerships (Ref RES-062-23-1308).
3   Civil partnership is a legal arrangement that came into force in 2005 to recognise same-sex couple relationships. It affords much of the same rights as marriage. Despite the legal availability of same-sex marriage since 2014, civil partnerships are still available to same-sex couples today.
4   Pseudonyms are used for interviewees.

References

Allen, K. R. and Demo, D. H., 1995. The Families of Lesbians and Gay Men: A New Frontier in Family Research. *Journal of Marriage and Family*, 57 (1), 111–127.

Altman, D., 1979. *Coming Out in the Seventies*. Sydney, NSW and Eugene, OR: Wild and Woolley.

Blasius, M., 1994. *Gay and Lesbian Politics: Sexuality and the Emergence of a New Ethic*. Philadelphia, PA: Philadelphia University Press.

Bozett, F. W. and Sussman, M. B., 1989. Homosexuality and Family Relations. *Marriage & Family Review*, 14 (3–4), 1–8.

Buell, C., 2001. Legal Issues Affecting Alternative Families. *Journal of Gay and Lesbian Psychotherapy*, 4, 75–90.

Calhoun, C., 2003. *Feminism, the Family, and the Politics of the Closet*. Oxford: Oxford University Press.

Cant, B., ed., 1997. *Invented Identities? Lesbians and Gays Talk about Migration*. London: Cassell.

Cruickshank, M., 1992. *The Lesbian and Gay Liberation Movement*. New York, NY: Routledge.

Davies, P., 1992. The Role of Disclosure in Coming Out Amongst Gay Men. In: K. Plummer, ed. *Modern Homosexualities*. London: Routledge, 75–84.

Edmunds, J. and Turner, B. S., 2002. *Generations, Culture and Society*. Buckingham: Open University Press.

Gabb, J., 2005. Lesbian M/Otherhood: Strategies of Familial-Linguistic Management in Lesbian Parent Families. *Sociology*, 39 (4), 585–603.

Gay Liberation Front, 1971/78. *Gay Liberation Front: Manifesto*. Available from: https://sourcebooks.fordham.edu/pwh/glf-london.asp [Accessed 22 October 2017].

Harding, R., 2017. Personal Freedom: The Continued Rise of Social Liberalism. In: *NatCen Social Research, British Social Attitudes 34* [online]. Available from: www.bsa.natcen.ac.uk/latest-report/british-social-attitudes-34/key-findings/personal-freedom-the-continued-rise-of-social-liberalism.aspx [Accessed 1 September 2017].

Heaphy, B., Donovan, C., and Weeks, J., 1998. "That's Like My Life": Researching Stories of Non-heterosexual Relationships. *Sexualities*, 1 (4), 453–470.

Heaphy, B. and Einarsdottir, A., 2012. Scripting Civil Partnerships: Interviewing Couples Together and Apart. *Qualitative Research*, 13 (1), 53–70.

Heaphy, B., Smart C., and Einarsdottir, A., 2013. *Same Sex Marriages: New Generations, New Experiences*. Basingstoke: Palgrave Macmillan.

Macklin, E. D., 1980. Nontraditional Family Forms: A Decade of Research. *Journal of Marriage and the Family*, Nov 1, 42 (4), 905–922.

Muller, A., 1987. *Parents Matter: Parents' Relationships with Lesbian Daughters and Gay Sons*. Tallahassee, FL: Naiad Press.

Nardi, P., 1992. That's What Friends Are For: Friends as Family in the Gay and Lesbian Community. In: K. Plummer, ed. *Modern Homosexualities*. London: Routledge, 108–120.

Nordqvist, P. and Smart, C., 2014. *Relative Strangers: Family Life, Genes and Donor Conception*. Basingstoke: Palgrave Macmillan.

Patterson, C. J., 2000. Family Relationships of Lesbians and Gay Men. *Journal of Marriage and Family*, 62 (4), 1052–1069.

Plummer, K., 1995. *Telling Sexual Stories*. London: Routledge.

Rich, A., 1983. Compulsory Heterosexuality and Lesbian Existence. In: A. Snitow, C. Stansell, and S. Thompson, eds. *Desire: Politics of Sexuality*. London: Virago, 212–241.

Ryan-Flood. R., 2009. *Lesbian Motherhood: Gender, Families and Sexual Citizenship*. Buckingham: Palgrave MacMillan.

Saewyc, E. M., et al., 2006. Hazards of Stigma: The Sexual and Physical Abuse of Gay, Lesbian, and Bisexual Adolescents in the United States and Canada. *Child Welfare*, Mar/Apr, 85 (2), 195–213.

Seidman, S., 2001. From Identity to Queer Politics: Shifts in Normative Heterosexuality and the Meaning of Citizenship. *Citizenship Studies*, 5 (3), 321–328.

Taylor, Y., 2007. *Working Class Lesbian Life: Classed Outsiders*. Basingstoke: Palgrave Macmillan.

Taylor, Y., 2009. *Lesbian and Gay Parenting: Securing Social and Educational Capital*. Basingstoke: Palgrave Macmillan.

Weeks, J., 1995. *Invented Moralities: Sexual Values in an Age of Uncertainty*. Cambridge: Polity Press.

Weeks, J., 2007. *The World We Have Won*. London: Routledge.

Weeks, J., Heaphy, B., and Donovan, C., 1999. Families of Choice: Autonomy and Mutuality in Non-heterosexual Relationships. In: S. McRae, ed. *Changing Britain*. Oxford: Oxford University Press, 297–315.

Weeks, J., Heaphy, B., and Donovan, C., 2001. *Same Sex Intimacies: Families of Choice and Other Life Experiments*. London: Routledge.

Weston, K., 1991. *Families We Choose: Lesbians, Gays and Kinship*. New York, NY: Columbia University Press.

Weston, K., 1995. Get Thee to a Big City: Sexual Imaginary and the Great Gay Migration. *GLQ: A Journal of Lesbian and Gay Studies*, 2 (3), 253–277.

Yip, A. K. T. and Page, S. J., 2016. *Religious and Sexual Identities: A Multi-Faith Exploration of Young Adults*. London: Routledge.

Chapter 2

Queer interruptions

Policing belonging in the carceral state

Louise Boon-Kuo, Erica R. Meiners and
Paul Simpson

Consider the following two snapshots from high-profile engagements between queer young people and police in Chicago, USA, and Sydney, Australia.

Chicago, USA

On July 6th, 2011, over 800 people crammed into a Chicago Alternative Policing Strategy meeting in the Boystown neighbourhood of Chicago. The predominantly white local homeowners and businesses, outraged by a summer of non-white queer youth roaming 'their' neighbourhood, formed a group: Take Back Boystown. A cell phone video of a fight that involved a knife between two young people, which had gone viral, prompted calls for increased policing with proclamations such as: 'Boystown is a danger zone' (Sosin 2011).

By the 1980s, 'Boystown', also known as Lakeview, a Chicago neighbourhood that was once home to working class Puerto Rican and Mexican migrant families, had morphed into Chicago's gay mecca. With dance clubs, bathhouses, coffee shops and a gay bookstore, Boystown drew queers, and queer dollars, from across the Midwest USA. Rents started to rise, and by the 2000s, while the sex clubs had been replaced with expensive wine bars, the neighbourhood was officially the 'gaybourhood'. Home to the city's LGBTQ Community Center, Boystown attracts many LGBTQ young people of colour – particularly those who are homeless. Even if old enough to frequent the many bars and clubs (admittance is restricted to those over 21 years old) these young people cannot pay for $US15 cocktails or a cover charge. Infuriating most local business owners and some of their clientele, clusters of young queers use parking lots, alleys and sidewalks as their free queer club space: dancing, eating, socialising and working (providing all manner of goods and services including sex services). The response from businesses and groups like Take Back Boystown to this influx of queer youth was to hire a uniformed private security force 'to create a safe and welcoming environment for all to enjoy' (GoPride.com News Staff 2012). Notably, this private security was for 'local residents and patrons'. Excluded of course, were the non-paying, largely non-white young queers that continued to use the neighbourhood (GoPride.com News Staff 2012). Through creative forms of direct action, including packing and interrupting community meetings, increased private policing was resoundingly rejected by queer youth, and their allies. According to queer youth of colour organisation Gender JUST, more police would simply augment existing practices of racial profiling, further marginalising young people in the neighbourhood, and not creating safety (Sosin 2011).

Sydney, Australia

At the 2013 Sydney LGBTQI Mardi Gras parade, a police officer slammed the slight-statured and handcuffed Jamie Jackson Reed, a white youth then aged 18 years, to the ground. The officer then held him down with his foot, later explaining this was because Reed was bleeding. Reed was charged with resisting arrest, assaulting police and offensive language in public, charges colloquially known as the 'trifecta'. Paradigmatic of the criminalisation of minority populations in public spaces, police have often used the trifecta to charge when the police themselves have behaved inappropriately in their interactions with Aboriginal people (Aboriginal and Torres Strait Islander Social Justice Commissioner 1996). In dramatic footage posted to YouTube, the sound of Reed hitting the footpath was audible. A year later the Local Court dismissed all charges against Reed and he was awarded $AUD 39,000 to cover legal costs (AAP 2014b).

'This is 2013 not 1978' – proclaimed a placard at the 2,000 person protest march to the Sydney Police Centre one week later – invoking the police violence associated with the inaugural 24 June 1978 Sydney Mardi Gras Parade which ended with 53 people being arrested (Sydney's Pride History Group 2015). This protest drew a diverse crowd including students, people from rural areas involved in campaigns such as the Beat Project, and Wiradjuri man and long-time Aboriginal deaths in custody campaigner, Ray Jackson, who spoke at the rally (Rose 2013). Police sought to position the violence as exceptional to their 'first-class' relationship with the local gay and lesbian community. The offending officers came from the western suburbs, it was said, where policing is a 'different kettle of fish' (Rubinsztein-Dunlop 2013). By invoking the term 'western suburbs', an Australian code for an area significantly populated by racialised minorities and people of lower socio-economic status, police also appealed to a white homonormative vision of Parade queers.

While many gays and lesbians in the USA and Australia have achieved some measure of formal equality, incidents such as Boystown and Mardi Gras remind us that queer youth continue to be policed and regulated by the criminal justice system, often in the name of protecting others and their property, including wealthier and whiter queers. New deviancy theorists have long proclaimed that neither our criminal codes, nor the institution of policing, are neutral or benign (Becker 1963, Taylor et al. 1973). Across Australia and the USA, policing is informed by a spectrum of cultural stereotypes and subjectivities of class, race, gender, sexuality and ability resulting in an uneven field of surveillance, punishment and criminalisation (Mogul et al. 2011, Rodgers et al. 2017). Policing not only functions as the gateway for young people's entry into the contemporary carceral, or punitive, state, but shapes both affective and legal registries of citizenship and belonging. By tracing facets of how young queers[1] are impacted by policing, and suggesting how these practices shape their *material* and *affective* modes of belonging, we can begin to explore the collateral consequences of a carceral state on young queers in the USA and Australia.

Drawing from an interdisciplinary body of work, our analysis is informed by critical scholarship in queer and carceral studies, and related organising, that highlights how narratives of citizenship in 'western liberal democracies', refracted through mainstream lesbian and gay organising, invest in legalisation, criminalisation and punishment systems to promote equality. Sustained by various criminal legal system myths (e.g. the system can 'fairly' deliver justice for all; prisons increase safety; marginalised people are not disproportionately targeted and punished; Lamble 2013) these investments ultimately afford acceptance and rights to 'good' queers at the expense of (sexualised and racialised) others (Puar 2013), including queer youth.

Queer criminal careers

While emerging research clearly illustrates an over-representation of queer youth, particularly queer youth of colour, in the criminal legal system and therefore the importance of an intersectional analysis,[2] current over-representation is invisibilised through a lack of available data, research and advocacy. In some jurisdictions, adult prisons collect data on transgender women and to a lesser extent gay and bisexual men, yet we have no reliable data on how many queer people are subject to policing, appear before the courts, or are under community supervision (Robinson 2011). Criminal legal systems in countries such as Australia and the USA currently 'fail to recognise, record, and therefore understand the multifarious factors contributing to the criminalisation' of queer people (Rodgers et al. 2017, p. 9), or in other words, fail to recognise what others have referred to as a 'queer criminal career' (Asquith et al. 2017).

Limited US data reveals an over-representation of young queers in juvenile detention facilities. The US Bureau of Justice Statistics recently surveyed 18,100 youths placed in juvenile facilities across the USA and reported 12% self-identified as 'non-heterosexual' (Beck et al. 2013). Belknap et al. (2013) reported 13% of young people sampled in juvenile detention facilities in one US state identified as lesbian, gay or bisexual (27% of girls; 5% of boys). In a study of seven different juvenile prisons across the USA, an anonymous survey reported particularly high rates of incarceration for gender non-conforming, lesbian, bisexual and queer girls: '39.9% – a remarkably high percentage of girls in the juvenile justice system – are LBQ/GNC' (Irvine and Canfield 2016, p. 249).

No Australian data exists on queer youth in juvenile detention settings. The only study to have collected reliable population data on queer people in custody in Australia is the Sexual Health and Attitudes of Australian Prisoners (SHAAP) study, which found that 37% of adult women prisoners identified as lesbian or bisexual (*vs* 3.8% in the community), 5% of male prisoners identified as gay or bisexual (*vs* 3.2% in the community) and 0.3% identified as transgender or sister-girl[3] (Butler et al. 2013, Table 2, Butler et al. 2010, Richters et al. 2014, Table 5).

Juxtaposed against this lack of data is stark evidence, in both the USA and Australia, that young people of colour are the most heavily impacted by policing and incarceration practices. Although Indigenous people account for only 2% of the Australian population, Indigenous people comprise 55% of all youth in juvenile detention across the country, and as of June 2018, 100% of young people in juvenile detention in the Northern Territory (AIHW 2016, p. 2, Vita 2015, p. 8, Northern Territory 2018, p. 64). Overall Indigenous children are 26 times more likely to be in juvenile detention than non-Indigenous children (AIHW 2016, p. 2). Although the recent introduction of diversionary measures for young people has contributed to the steady reduction in the number of non-Indigenous youth in detention, this has not translated for Indigenous youth (Cunneen et al. 2016).

In the USA, while the total number of non-adults locked up has continued to decline over the past 35 years, African American youth are still five times more likely than white youth to be behind bars (Annie E. Casey Foundation 2013, p. 2). At every level of the US criminal legal system, young people of colour are significantly more likely than white youth to be removed from the home, transferred to adult court and sent to adult prison (Annie E. Casey Foundation 2013). Colonialism continues to shape the life pathways of Native Americans: According to a 2015 report, state courts are twice as likely to lock up first Native American youth for crimes such as alcohol use and truancy than any other racial and ethnic group (Coalition for Juvenile Justice 2015).

Recognising similarities between struggles for full citizenship and belonging for queer young people and racial justice is not enough: in the 1970s a 'sexual underclass' of queers and sex workers were viewed in Australia as 'close in status' to Aboriginal and Torres Strait Islander people and the homeless, in relation to shared experiences of police violence and criminalisation (Dwyer and Tomsen 2016, p. 28). An adequate analysis requires understanding the over-policing and over-incarceration of queer youth in the USA and Australia as fundamentally *the same problem* as the over-policing and incarceration of non-white, specifically Aboriginal and Black, communities: for example, in Australia nearly one in three lesbian or bisexual women prisoners and one in five gay or bisexual male prisoners are Aboriginal or Torres Strait Islander.[4]

This over-representation is a direct result of the structural inequalities and social and institutional practices that (re)produce criminalisation. Heterosexism and cissexism in families and schools augment young people's precarity and homelessness and increase participation in the criminalised street economy. An Australian Bureau of Statistics General Social Survey reports that lesbian and gay people (34%) and people with 'other' sexual orientations (21%) were more likely to report at least one past experience of homelessness compared with their heterosexual counterparts (13%) (ABS 2014).

Specifically, policing in public spaces, including streets, parks, malls/shopping centres, parties, music festivals and schools, plays a critical role in and conveys important information about citizenship. In public spaces, queer youth of colour are often 'read' by authorities as bodies that disrupt normative ways of performing white and sexual subjectivity. In the USA, research suggests that authorities often construe their self-defence or even self-expression as defiance, aggression, or predation (Grant et al. 2011, Smith and Stanley 2011, Daniel-McCarter et al. 2017). Interviews with 35 queer young people in Queensland, Australia, revealed how young people's performance of queerness can inform their encounters with police, making them 'differently visible' and rendering, for example, public intimacy or verbal interactions as transgressive, and thus shaping police use of discretionary public order powers (Dwyer 2011).

In Australia, practices of reading and identifying certain forms of 'non-heteronormative embodiment constitute part of contemporary policing work' (Dwyer 2008, p. 423). Besides sexuality and sexual practices such as 'beat' sex[5] being directly policed and regulated, Dwyer's (2012, p. 16) research highlights the more nuanced ways in which young people's sexuality and gender is regulated, noting forms of constraint attached to how young people's 'bodies made their gender or sexuality visible in ways that transgressed heteronormative expectations'. 'If I'm not looking really gay they'll be a lot nicer' and 'under their breath' was how one 19-year-old trans person 'described the subtleties of constraint and punishment used by police and security' (Dwyer 2012, p. 23).

Young people are particularly impacted by policing because in both Australia and the USA, the juvenile justice system continues to produce categories of crime, illegality and power – truant, delinquent, runaway, detention for 'care and protection' – that are applied only to juveniles (these kinds of crimes are referred to as 'status violations' in the USA). Behaviour and mobility – generally in public – are constrained by laws which police young people's ability to drink alcohol, to smoke cigarettes, to assemble (loitering and curfew), to engage in sexual activities, to work, to travel, to sign a legal contract, to wear particular clothing, to vote and more. In both Australia and the USA, studies document that the powers of the police to stop, search, move-on, and in major US cities such as Chicago to 'card', are used against young people particularly poor non-white and Indigenous youth who are *not* breaking any laws (NSW Ombudsman 1999, pp. 228–232, Gorner 2015). These police interventions subsequently become part of police records. This matrix of laws, coupled with young people's lack of access to private space, means that public spaces become the terrain where claims to being and belonging are asserted, and policed.

The conditions for young people once locked up are dismal. In the Northern Territory (NT) of Australia, the treatment of young people in state custody has included the use of spit hoods, shackles and tear gas. Snapchat videos of guards using homophobic language, recording boys urinating and 'jokingly' requesting oral sex have surfaced (AAP 2017). In the USA, far from acting as a 'kind and just parent', as was the original aim of the juvenile justice system over a century ago, the conditions inside juvenile prisons continue to be gruesome – crumbling facilities, sexual violence perpetrated by guards, lack of services, excessive use of solitary confinement and restraint – and the number one predictor of adult incarceration is juvenile incarceration (Mendel 2011, Bernstein 2014).

Beyond incarceration in facilities that ensure what scholar Ruth Wilson Gilmore (2007) has named 'premature death', queer young people's involvement with the criminal legal system shapes attachments to at least two registers of 'citizenship' – formal 'legal' citizenship and affective belonging. For policed and incarcerated juveniles, the pathway to full legal and participatory citizenship can seem remote, contested and uncertain, placing particular importance on affective belonging.

Carceral productions of citizenship and belonging

Young people may be 'citizens' in terms of legal status but are better described as 'citizens-in-waiting' (Kennelly 2011) or 'citizens-in-development' (Bynner 1997 cited in Kennelly 2011, p. 340). Age functions as the border to formally exclude, sometimes temporarily, people from many of the legal rights – voting – and responsibilities – paying taxes – associated with citizenship. Young people's involvement with the criminal legal system clearly shapes their ability to access many of these future rights.

In the USA, the term 'civil death' is used to refer to the consequences of conviction and incarceration that extend beyond life in prison, and young people are not exempt. After being released from prison, those with drug-related convictions are routinely denied access to public housing and social assistance benefits (Mauer and Chesney-Lind 2003). Access to federal educational financial aid for higher education (including a grant, loan or work-study position) is blocked or significantly delayed for those with drug-related convictions (Page 2004). In some states, incarceration for any crime may also translate into losing the right to parent. Incoherent and cumbersome state laws surrounding voting rights, disenfranchisement and restoration create confusion and misidentify and disqualify many formerly incarcerated potential voters (Uggen et al. 2012). For youth in the USA, police contact often forms the first step in a pathway toward civil death. In Australia, the consequences of incarceration are not so formalised, but in practice the social stigma of a criminal record, and the well-documented poor health and social outcomes of those released from detention, indirectly produce many of the same effects (see for example Cutcher et al. 2014). The consequences of policing and incarceration suggest that the citizenship of young people should not be understood as an inevitable linear progression towards full adult citizenship. Rather, as Hepworth (2015, p. 37) explains in relation to migrants of varied status in Italy, citizenship is better understood as a contingent and 'emergent condition'.

Beyond the structured and indirect ways in which the criminal legal system constrains access to full citizenship, the sexual citizenship of queer young people may also be understood as being 'in waiting'. Building on T. H. Marshall's influential definition of citizenship as 'full membership of the community, with all its rights and responsibilities' (1950, cited in Yuval-Davis 2006, p. 206), the notion of 'sexual citizenship' aims to distinguish how sexuality and gender shape access to the rights associated with citizenship. Specifically, in many countries queers possess differential legal (and social) rights to access some of the key institutions and practices associated with citizenship: marriage, age of consent and gender recognition (see for example Richardson 2000, Lister 2002). Queer young people may not yet seek to make such rights-based claims. Yet as the snapshots at the start of the chapter illuminate, contestations over the use of public space can (and do) act as entry points for queer young people's involvement with the criminal legal system and in so doing highlight how, for young people, sexual citizenship is not only about legal rights conferred or withheld by the nation but also is constituted through the 'politics of belonging' (Yuval-Davis 2006).

'Belonging', as Yuval-Davis (2016, p. 369) explains, is 'about emotional attachment, about feeling "at home"', and is shaped by the political systems and practices which construct identities and categorical boundaries. The criminal legal system produces both the collective identity of the 'law-abiding, insider citizen' (Valverde 2010, p. 220) and those marked as outside. The use of policing to regulate young people in the opening snapshots highlighted who was marked as an 'insider' and 'outsider', and directly shaped affective belonging through queer youth's social and political organising and protest to policing. This mediation and the production of citizenship registers (formal and insider *vs* affective and outsider) can be more fully understood through the idea of homonationalism and its connection to carcerality.

The concept of homonationalism, first introduced by Jasbir Puar in *Terrorist Assemblages: Homonationalism in Queer Times* (2007), responded to a historical shift since the 1990s in nation-states from their 'insistence on heteronormativity to the increasing inclusion of homonormativity' (Puar 2013, p. 26). Here, the 'acceptance' and 'tolerance' of certain gays and lesbians come to act as a 'barometer by which the legitimacy of, and capacity for national sovereignty is evaluated' (Puar 2013, p. 35). No longer outsiders, certain groups of gays and lesbians are now state recognised and accepted. Formal recognition of civil partnerships or marriage were even deployed to ('pink') wash a blemished state to distract, and secure support from its citizens and local and transnational stakeholders (Morgensen 2012).

As a framework for critique, homonationalism interrogates the citizenship and rights-based narratives of mainstream queer and other organisations and institutions that provide legal and consumer recognition of some queers. Yet the cost is an accompanying restriction of the welfare state and immigrant rights; the continued naturalisation of colonial conquest of Indigenous peoples and the land theft; and the growing use of state-led surveillance, policing and detention of the poor and other marginalised groups (Morgensen 2012, Puar 2013). As LGBTQ organising became more professionalised, grass-roots mobilisations against poverty, police brutality and prisoner rights were decentred (Kunzel 2008).

Although having a long history of being punished for transgressing social norms, by the 1990s LGBTQ groups in the US invested the carceral state – policing and punishment – to address violence within their communities and to advance the goal of achieving equality. 'Hate crime' laws, anti-discrimination legislation, and added policing of gentrified and homonormative spaces, including gaybourhoods, illustrates how the carceral state has moved from a 'key target of queer protest to [a] celebrated guardian of sexual citizenship' (Lamble 2013, p. 229). While Aharonson (2010) casts these new expressions of sexual citizenship as 'pro-minority criminalisation', Lamble (2013) refers to the shift as a chilling new death logic behind citizenship claims.

The Boystown and Mardi Gras examples, in their own ways, illustrate responses that rely on and invest in a logic of citizenship reliant on the policing and punishment of others/outsiders to protect the imagined 'safety' and capital of respected insiders. While the Take Back Boystown response to hire a uniformed private security force to augment local policing efforts provides an explicit example of such investments, the eventual outcome of the Mardi Gras response demonstrates a more indirect investment: in the form of acquiescence to a policing agenda that normalises queerness as a site to be policed (Russell 2017) and a political commitment to affluent homonormativity as opposed to intersectionality. Distancing themselves from the community rally against police brutality, Mardi Gras organisers led the development of The Mardi Gras Festival Accord (AAP 2014a). The Accord, in reminding authorities of the pink economics at stake for the city, did not build on earlier calls by Mardi Gras and other community-based organisations such as *Community Action Against Homophobia* (CAAH) to end the use of drug detection dogs and institute independent investigation into police misconduct (see for example Mardi Gras et al. 2013, pp. 8–11). Instead, the Accord saw a renewed focus on police sensitivity training, the 'fair' and 'equitable' police enforcement of queer spaces, and community organisations assistance in promoting awareness that police will enforce laws regarding alcohol and other drug use. Thus, the myths behind carceral investments were retained.

Russell (2017) has written that mainstream queer organisers are: 'left with limited options for negotiating or resisting the close regulation of queer spaces by the state if they are to avoid further exclusion, rejection or violence' and thus 'must be grateful to those who extend it, even as the overarching conditions of unequal power remain fundamentally unchanged' (p. 288). This places importance on developing new social and political projects within this space in which intersectional thinking and new citizenship expressions may take form.

An intersectional approach is crucial as carceral investments and associated institutional arrangements ultimately afford acceptance and rights to some queers, those estimated 'good' and 'respectful' (namely white lesbians and gays from non-poor backgrounds). Those who are shut out are the (sexualised and racialised) other: the 'bad' 'sick' and 'angry' queers – people of colour, trans and genderqueer, Muslim, Indigenous, the poor – and other forgotten or invisible queers (Puar 2013), including young people. Paradoxically, investments in legislation, policing and punishment to advance liberal rights and recognition of sexual and racial 'diversity' result in the exploitation, obfuscation and invisibilising of the very subjects of this diversity discourse.

Homonationalism, as an assemblage linked to carcerality, makes the over-representation and invisibility of young queers within the criminal legal system intelligible. Importantly, it also contributes to understanding two key registers of citizenship produced for young queers. First, that of formal/legal citizenship which as a result of age and incarceration is rendered remote, contested and emergent; and second, that of affective belonging which can be shaped by particular social and political projects offering emancipatory potential.

Thrivings and resistances

Many queer young people are not waiting for the police to reform, or for laws and policies to shift. In the USA, Groups like *Breakout! Streetwise and Safe, FIERCE!* and *Black Youth Project 100 (BYP 100)* (as well as now defunct groups such as *Gender JUST* and *Young Women's Empowerment Project*) – all initiated and led by queer youth of colour – have pushed back on the policing of non-white and queer young people. Grass-roots organising in Australia is more intergenerational, yet with the consistent and prevalent involvement of students and other young people. Groups such as *CAAH, Inside Out, #JustJustice, Unharm* and *NSW Beats Project* were all created to draw attention to, and end, the policing, criminalisation and/ or incarceration of queers, young people, and/or Aboriginal and Torres Strait Islander people.

Rather than demanding inclusion and 'belonging' within the carceral logics of policing and surveillance, these mobilisations are imagining and practising forms of safety, belonging and community in spite of, and outside of, carceral logics. Incidents such as Mardi Gras and Boystown, are flashpoints that illustrate how queer youth are organising and pushing back. Other examples from grass-roots and informal campaigns continue to emerge.

In New York, groups including *Streetwise and Safe* and *FIERCE!* ran a successful campaign to ensure that New York City police do not use condom possession as evidence to detain or arrest queer youth of colour on the charge of 'intent to solicit or engage in prostitution'. As policy, police interpreted the possession of a condom by some, particularly young people of colour, as evidence of sex work until young activists publicly organised to challenge this practice in 2013 (Dank et al. 2015). Condom possession is not a universal marker of sex work that justified arrest for all, stated adult ally and lawyer with *Streetwise and* Safe, Andrea Ritchie: 'If you're a student carrying condoms, you're practicing good public health; if you're a transgendered person of colour, you're a prostitute' (Bellafante 2013). Through know-your-rights campaigns, creative forms of direct action and political education, young queers have pushed back on this policy and highlighted how policing impacts their lives and does little to facilitate safety.[6] Not only have they raised awareness of biased policing practices, and demonstrated that safe communities are not produced via policing, but they have illustrated what an intersectional response might look like in practice.

Created in part to push back on the relentless police violence targeting Black communities, the *Black Youth Project 100* (*BYP 100*), a national organisation with a home in Chicago that was founded in 2013, always identifies as operating through a Black, queer, feminist and abolitionist lens. One of its explicit goals has been to demand that the state Fund Black Futures – funding public K-16 education, for example, and divesting from, and shrinking, the footprint of policing and prisons. These young queer Black activists know that having more Black, queer or female police or prison guards will not create safer communities. Research by *BYP 100* and associated organisations shows that approximately 40% of Chicago's general operating fund is allocated for policing (similar to many large US cities), and *BYP 100*'s direct action, political education and public events push us to imagine not only how to make a city without police but also how to spend Chicago's $1.4 billion police budget for ends that genuinely produce public safety (Hamaji et al. 2017).

In Sydney, *CAAH* through its collaborative history with the *Indigenous Social Justice Association* in Sydney (*ISJA Sydney*) maintains an intersectional focus in its work. It drew widespread attention to the death in custody in NSW of sister-girl Veronica (Paris) Baxter, and advocated for independent and Senate inquiries into her death (Jackson 2011). The campaign helped to raise questions about access to hormone replacement medication while in custody, and about the well-being of trans people in state detention. *CAAH* and *ISJA Sydney* were also active in organising the response to the regulation and brutality on queers by police at the 2013 Mardi Gras. Also adopting an intersectional approach, led by emerging Aboriginal leaders, *#JustJustice* has highlighted, through more than 90 publications, the health impacts of, and solutions to, the over-incarceration upon Aboriginal and Torres Strait Islander peoples and their communities, and has raised questions about Aboriginal and Torres Strait Islander queers in the criminal legal system (Bonson 2016 cited in Finlay et al. 2016). *#JustJustice* takes a strengths-based approach to identifying and profiling solutions to over-incarceration. One of its goals is to 'change the dominant narrative around incarceration, and to enable new connections and collaborations for change' (Croakey n.d.).

Unharm promotes alternatives to policing drug users and 'cultures of care' (Unharm n.d.), and has grown to include a queer contingent and a University of NSW student contingent. The queer contingent draws from Sydney's various queer activist histories that built cultures of care (for example, histories of HIV and AIDS, sex work and drug use activism), and links to a wider mainstream movement contesting the criminalisation of queers, youth and drug users. *Unharm* has organised community events and parties to build affective belonging and raise funds for a number of advocacy campaigns, including the decriminalisation of both drug use and personal possession; 'ditching the dogs' (ending police drug detection dog searches in NSW public places); and 'tests, not arrests' (to ensure that young people can engage in pill testing to minimise drug-related harms at parties and festivals). The more recently formed *Inside Out* initiative, based in

Melbourne, is 'building a network of support and solidarity amongst LGBTIQ+ people both inside and outside prisons' by distributing publications containing 'artwork, poetry, letters and articles by prisoners and former prisoners, as well as news from the LGBTIQ+ rights movement' (Inside Out n.d.).

What all of these groups share is an expressly abolitionist politic, with a vision and associated organising that expressly rejects the carceral state's attempts to shape sexual citizenship and belonging. A US-based organisation *Critical Resistance* offers a working definition of abolition as 'the creation of genuinely safe, healthy communities that respond to harm without relying on prisons and punishment' (Critical Resistance 2017). Abolition does not mean that there will be no violence. Rather, it acknowledges that policing and prisons do not provide a just, efficient or moral solution to the problems that shape violence and lack in our communities. Instead, these carceral institutions and logics create vulnerability and harm for many, do not produce public safety, and definitively mark who is not fully human – and who does not belong. Inclusion in the status quo of an over-policed, under-resourced and hyper criminalised state is not the goal. Rather, by chipping away at the carceral regime, these *ad hoc* and formal groups demand and make possible other forms of belonging.

Against the absence of clear and direct data on young queers in the criminal legal system, these thrivings and resistances, together with the various literature and data presented, indicate an over-representation and uneven surveillance and policing, particularly of queer youth of colour. Bodies that disrupt 'normal life' (Spade 2011) – or dominant white, middle-class and/or heteronormative spaces and practices – become most vulnerable within this landscape. For many, the carceral logics outlined not only facilitate a queer criminal career trajectory but also shape young people's forms of belonging. By drawing attention to evidence of the violence of policing and incarceration, particularly experienced by queer youth of colour, our aim is to support social and political projects and movements led by those affected which name and challenge the myth of a 'fair' criminal legal system.

Recognition of the intersecting factors that contribute to developing the sexual citizenship and belonging of queer young people is a vital step in understanding how investments in punitive systems bankrupt the advancement of social equality, community safety and full social belonging and citizenship. This outlining and visibility, we hope, make some, albeit modest, headway into dismantling the myth of a 'fair' criminal legal system – a myth that helps sustain acquiescence and investment in criminalisation and punishment systems that ensure that queer youth are marked as disposable, not full citizens.

Notes

1 Throughout this chapter, the term 'queer' refers to all sexualities and gender identities that are outside and challenging of normative, binary categories. We use the term queer as a replacement for the letters. And, in both Australia and the USA the legal and developmental category of 'youth' is, at best, both vague and flexible. In the criminal justice system, a matrix of laws and administrative regulations – shaped by

race, class, ability, gender and other factors – mark the uneven boundaries between child, youth and adult. While these boundaries may appear fixed and static, they are not. For example, in the USA, while 15-year-olds can be charged as adults, they are also denied the right to consent to sexual activity.

2 The legal theorist Kimberlé Crenshaw developed the term intersectionality to refer to the multiple ways that power and privilege intersect (Crenshaw 1994). An intersectional lens works to name how social positions and identities – ethnicity, gender, sexuality, ability, race, class and others – are mutually constitutive.

3 Many Aboriginal and Torres Strait Islander persons assigned one sex at birth but who identify as a gender that diverges from their designated sex prefer the term 'sister-girl' or 'brother-boy' over trans. The terms brother-boy and sister-girl have diverse meanings and uses in different social contexts and to different people, families and communities. For example, in Indigenous communities sister-girl can include gay men ('sisters') (Costell and Nannup 1999).

4 Descriptive cross-tab analysis conducted on the 2008 SHAAP database by author Paul Simpson.

5 'Beats' (Australian term) or 'cottages' (UK term) are typically public 'spaces where gay men "cruise" other men in the pursuit of desirous encounters' (Dalton 2007, pp. 375–376).

6 For example, see the toolkit *Get YR Rights!* http://getyrrights.org/wp-content/uploads/2015/02/GYR-Toolkit-FINAL-02-05-2015.pdf

References

AAP, 2014a. Accord Signed for Sydney Mardi Gras. *The Australian*, 14 February. Available from: www.theaustralian.com.au/news/latest-news/accord-signed-for-sydney-mardi-gras/news-story/f6ff662bee1e2160a68e9cc051d84a0d [Accessed 1 July 2017].

AAP, 2014b. Mardi Gras Teen May Sue Police Over Arrest After Charges Thrown Out. *The Guardian*, 6 February. Available from: www.theguardian.com/world/2014/feb/06/mardi-gras-teen-may-sue-police-over-arrest-charges-thrown-out [Accessed 1 July 2017].

AAP, 2017. Don Dale Guard Asked Boy for Fellatio as a "Joke", Urged Child to eat Faeces for Snapchat. *SBS News*, 20 March. Available from: www.sbs.com.au/news/article/2017/03/20/don-dale-guard-asked-boy-fellatio-joke-urged-child-eat-faeces-snapchat [Accessed 1 July 2017].

Aboriginal and Torres Strait Islander Social Justice Commissioner, 1996. *Indigenous Deaths in Custody: 1989 to 1996*. Sydney, NSW: Australian Human Rights Commission. Available from: www.humanrights.gov.au/publications/indigenous-deaths-custody-chapter-6-police-practices [Accessed 1 July 2017].

Aharonson, E., 2010. 'Pro-Minority' Criminalization and the Transformation of Visions of Citizenship in Contemporary Liberal Democracies: A Critique. *New Criminal Law Review*, 13 (2), 286–308.

Annie E. Casey Foundation, 2013. *Reducing Youth Incarceration in the United States: A KIDS COUNT Data Snapshot*. Available from: www.aecf.org/resources/reducing-youth-incarceration-in-the-united-states/ [Accessed 1 July 2017].

Asquith, N. L., Dwyer, A., and Simpson, P. L., 2017. A Queer Criminal Career. *Current Issues in Criminal Justice -Sydney-*, 29(2), 167–180.

Australian Bureau of Statistics (ABS), 2014. *General Social Survey Cat. No. 4159.0*. Canberra: Australian Bureau of Statistics.

Australian Institute of Health and Welfare (AIHW), 2016. *Youth Detention Population in Australia 2016.* AIHW Bulletin No. 138. Canberra: Australian Institute of Health and Welfare.

Beck, A. J., et al., 2013. *Sexual Victimization in Prisons and Jails Reported by Inmates, 2011–12.* Washington, DC: U.S. Department of Justice, Bureau of Justice Statistics.

Becker, H., 1963. *Outsiders: Studies in the Sociology of Deviance.* New York, NY: The Free Press.

Belknap, J., Holsinger, K., and Little, J. S., 2013. Lesbian, Gay and Bisexual Youth Incarcerated in Delinquent Facilities. In: D. Peterson and V. R. Panfil, eds. *Handbook of LGBT Communities, Crime, and Justice.* Dordrecht: Springer, 207–228.

Bellafante, G., 2013. Arrests by the Fashion Police. *The New York Times*, 15 April. Available from: www.nytimes.com/2013/04/07/nyregion/arrests-by-the-fashion-police.html [Accessed 1 July 2017].

Bernstein, N., 2014. *Burning Down the House: The End of Juvenile Prison.* New York, NY: New Press.

Butler, T., et al., 2010. *Sexual Health and Behaviour of Queensland Prisoners: with Queensland and New South Wales Comparisons.* Perth, WA and Sydney, NSW: National Drug Research Institute, Curtin University, and School of Public Health and Community Medicine, University of New South Wales.

Butler, T., et al., 2013. Sexual Behaviour and Sexual Health of Australian Prisoners. *Sexual Health*, 10 (1), 64–73.

Coalition for Juvenile Justice and Tribal Law and Policy Institute, 2015. *American Indian/Alaska Native Youth and Status Offense Disparities: A Call for Tribal Initiatives, Coordination and Federal Funding.* Brief. Coalition for Juvenile Justice. Available from: https://turtletalk.files.wordpress.com/2015/06/5e0511a9-1707-4ffa-83d0-082b339f9ad4.pdf [Accessed 1 July 2017].

Costell, M. and Nannup, R., 1999. *Report of the National Indigenous Sistergirl Forum.* Queensland: Australian Federation of AIDS Organisations.

Crenshaw, K. W., 1994. Mapping the Margins: Intersectionality, Identity Politics, and Violence Against Women of Color. In: M. A. Fineman and R. Mykituk, eds. *The Public Nature of Private Violence.* New York, NY: Routledge, 93–118.

Critical Resistance, 2017. *What Is the PIC? What Is Abolition?* [online]. Available from: http://criticalresistance.org/about/not-so-common-language/ [Accessed 15 July 2017].

Croakey, n.d. *#JustJustice – Tackling the Over-Incarceration of Aboriginal and Torres Strait Islander Peoples* [online]. Available from: https://croakey.org/justjustice-tackling-the-over-incarceration-of-aboriginal-and-torres-strait-islander-peoples/ [Accessed 15 July 2017].

Cunneen, C., Goldson, B., and Russell, S., 2016. Juvenile Justice, Young People and Human Rights in Australia. *Current Issues in Criminal Justice*, 28 (2), 173–189.

Cutcher, Z., et al., 2014. Poor Health and Social Outcomes for Ex-prisoners with a History of Mental Disorder: A Longitudinal Study. *Australian and New Zealand Journal of Public Health*, 38, 424–429.

Dalton, D., 2007. Policing Outlawed Desire: "Homocriminality" in Beat Spaces in Australia. *Law and Critique*, 18, 375–405.

Daniel-McCarter, O., Meiners, E., and Noll, R., 2017. Queer Disavowel: "Controversial Crimes" and Building Abolition. In: T. Hoppe and D. Halpernin, eds. *War on Sex.* Durham, NC: Duke University Press, 174–190.

Dank, M., et al., 2015. *Locked In: Interactions with the Criminal Justice and Child Welfare Systems for LGBTQ Youth, YMSM, and YWSW Who Engage in Survival Sex.* Washington, DC: Urban

Institute. Available from: http://streetwiseandsafe.org/wp-content/uploads/2015/09/Locked-In-FINAL-REPORT.pdf [Accessed 1 July 2017].

Dwyer, A., 2008. Policing Queer Bodies: Focusing on Queer Embodiment in Policing Research as an Ethical Question. *QUT Law and Justice Journal*, 8 (2), 414–428.

Dwyer, A., 2011. 'It's Not Like We're Going to Jump Them': How Transgressing Heteronormativity Shapes Police Interactions with LGBT Young People. *Youth Justice*, 11 (3), 203–220.

Dwyer, A., 2012. Policing Visible Sexual/Gender Diversity as a Program of Governance. *International Journal for Crime and Justice*, 1 (1), 14–26.

Dwyer, A. and Tomsen, S., 2016. The Past is the Past? The Impossibility of Erasure of Historical LGBTIQ Policing. In: A. Dwyer, M. Ball, and T. Crofts, eds. *Queering Criminology*. Basingstoke: Palgrave Macmillan.

Finlay, S. M., et al., 2016. *#JustJustice: Tackling the Over-Incarceration of Aboriginal and Torres Strait Islander People* (2nd ed.). New South Wales: Croakey.

Gilmore, R. W., 2007. *Golden Gulag: Prisons, Surplus, Crisis, and Opposition in Globalizing California*. Berkeley, CA: University of California Press.

GoPride.com News Staff, 2012. Private Security Patrol Hired for Boystown. *ChicagoPride.com*, 24, July. Available from: http://chicago.gopride.com/news/article.cfm/articleid/31472404 [Accessed 1 July 2017].

Gorner, J., 2015. Spike in "Contact Cards" from Street Stops Raises Legal, Strategic Concerns. *Chicago Tribune*, 23 March. Available from: www.chicagotribune.com/chi-contact-cards-20150323-story.html [Accessed 1 July 2017].

Grant, J., Mottet, L., and Tanis, J., 2011. *Injustice at Every Turn: A Report of the National Transgender Discrimination Survey*. Washington, DC: National Center for Transgender Equality and National Gay and Lesbian Task Force. Available from: www.thetaskforce.org/static_html/downloads/reports/reports/ntds_full.pdf [Accessed 1 July 2017].

Hamaji, K., et al., 2017. *Freedom to Thrive: Reimagining Safety & Security in Our Communities*. Center for Popular Democracy, Law for Black Lives, Black Youth Project 100. Available from: http://agendatobuildblackfutures.org/wp-content/uploads/2017/07/FreedomtoThriveWeb.pdf [Accessed 14 July 2017].

Hepworth, K., 2015. *At the Edges of Citizenship: Security and the Constitution of Non-Citizen Subjects*. Farnham: Ashgate.

Inside Out, n.d. *About – Inside Out Australia* [online]. Available from: https://insideoutaustralia.org/about/ [Accessed 15 July 2017].

Irvine, A. and Canfield, A. M., 2016. The Overrepresentation of Lesbian, Gay, Bisexual, Questioning, Gender Nonconforming and Transgender Youth Within the Child Welfare to Juvenile Justice Crossover Population. *Journal of Gender, Social Policy & the Law*, 24 (2), 243–261.

Jackson, R., 2011. *Why No Justice for Veronica Baxter? Why Did Paris Die?* [online]. Available from: http://indymedia.org.au/2011/04/08/why-no-justice-for-veronica-baxter-why-did-paris-die.html [Accessed 15 July 2017].

Kennelly, J., 2011. Policing Young People as Citizens-In-Waiting: Legitimacy, Spatiality and Governance. *British Journal of Criminology*, 51, 336–354.

Kunzel, R., 2008. *Criminal Intimacy: Prison and the Uneven History of Modern American Sexuality*. Chicago, IL: University of Chicago Press.

Lamble, S., 2013. Queer Necropolitics and the Expanding Carceral State: Interrogating Sexual Investments in Punishment. *Law and Critique*, 24 (3), 229–253.

Lister, R., 2002. Sexual Citizenship. In: E. F. Isin and B. S. Turner, eds. *Handbook of Citizenship Studies*. London: SAGE, 191–208.

Mardi Gras, et al., 2013. *Policing at NSW Lesbian, Gay, Bisexual, Transgender, Intersex and Queer (LGBTIQ) Events and Venues*. Sydney, NSW: Gay and Lesbian Rights Lobby, Sydney Gay and Lesbian Mardi Gras, Inner City Legal Centre and ACON. Available from: www.acon.org.au/wp-content/uploads/2015/04/Policing-Advocacy-document.pdf [Accessed 1 July 2017].

Mauer, M. and Chesney-Lind, M., eds., 2003. *Invisible Punishment: The Collateral Consequences of Mass Imprisonment*. New York, NY: New Press.

Mendel, R., 2011. *No Place for Kids: The Case for Reducing Juvenile Incarceration*. Baltimore, MD: Annie E. Casey Foundation. Available from: www.aecf.org/m/resourcedoc/aecf-NoPlaceForKidsFullReport-2011.pdf#page=4 [Accessed 30 May 2014].

Mogul, J., Ritchie, A., and Whitlock, K., 2011. *Queer (In)justice: The Criminalization of LGBT People in the United States*. Boston, MA: Beacon Press.

Morgensen, S. L., 2012. Queer Settler Colonialism in Canada and Israel: Articulating Two-spirit and Palestinian Queer Critiques. *Settler Colonial Studies*, 2 (2), 167–190.

Northern Territory, *Estimates*, Legislative Assembly, 20 June 2018, 64 (Jeanette Kerr).

NSW Ombudsman, 1999. *Policing Public Safety Report Under Section 6 of the Crimes Legislation Amendment (Police and Public Safety) Act*. Sydney, NSW: NSW Ombudsman.

Page, J., 2004. Eliminating the Enemy: The Import of Denying Prisoners Access to Higher Education in Clinton's America. *Punishment and Society*, 6 (4), 357–378.

Puar, J. K., 2013. Homonationalism as Assemblage: Viral Travels, Affective Sexualities. *Jindal Global Law Review*, 4 (2), 23–43.

Richardson, D., 2000. Constructing Sexual Citizenship: Theorizing Sexual Rights. *Critical Social Policy*, 20 (1), 105–135.

Richters, J., et al., 2014. Sexual Identity, Sexual Attraction and Sexual Experience: The Second Australian Study of Health and Relationships. *Sexual Health*, 11, 451–460.

Robinson, R. K., 2011. Masculinity as Prison: Sexual Identity, Race, and Incarceration. *California Law Review*, 99, 1309–1408.

Rodgers, J., Asquith, N., and Dwyer, A., 2017. *Cisnormativity, Criminalisation, Vulnerability: Transgender People in Prisons*. Hobart, TAS: Tasmanian Institute of Law Enforcement Studies, University of Tasmania.

Rose, C., 2013. Protesting Police Brutality at Mardi Gras. *National Union of Students Queer Department Blog*, 23 March. Available from: https://nusqueer.wordpress.com/2013/03/23/91/ [Accessed 1 July 2017].

Rubinsztein-Dunlop, S., 2013. Police Investigate Mardi Gras Brutality Claims. *ABC News*, 6 March. Available from: www.abc.net.au/news/2013-03-06/claims-of-police-brutality-at-mardi-gras-parade/4554958 [Accessed 1 July 2017].

Russell, E., 2017. A "Fair Cop": Queer Histories, Affect and Police Image Work in Pride March. *Crime, Media, Culture*, 13 (3), 277–293.

Smith, N. and Stanley, E., eds., 2011. *Captive Genders: Trans Embodiment and the Prison Industrial Complex*. Oakland, CA: AK Press.

Sosin, K., 2011. Hundreds Pack into Boystown Violence Forum. *Windy City Times*, 7 July. Available from: www.windycitymediagroup.com/lgbt/Hundreds-pack-into-Boystown-violence-forum/32676.html [Accessed 1 July 2017].

Spade, D., 2011. *Normal Life: Administrative Violence, Critical Trans Politics, and the Limits of Law*. Brooklyn, NY: South End Press.

Sydney's Pride History Group, 2015. *Chronology: 1978 Events*. Available from: http://camp. org.au/70s/20-1978 [Accessed 1 July 2017].

Taylor, I., Young, J., and Walton, P., 1973. *The New Criminology: For a Social Theory of Deviance*. London: Routledge.

Uggen, C., Shannon, S., and Manza, J., 2012. *State-Level Estimates of Felon Disenfranchisement in the United States, 2010*. Washington, DC: The Sentencing Project. Available from: http://sentencingproject.org/doc/publications/fd_State_Level_Estimates_of_Felon_ Disen_2010.pdf [Accessed 1 July 2017].

Unharm, n.d. *People Promoting Wellbeing in a World with Drugs* [online]. Available from: www.unharm.org/ [Accessed 15 July 2017].

Valverde, M., 2010. Practices of Citizenship and Scales of Governance. *New Criminal Law Review*, 13 (2), 216–240.

Vita, M., 2015. *Review of the Northern Territory Youth Detention System Report*. Available from: www.nt.gov.au/__data/assets/pdf_file/0004/238198/Review-of-the-Northern- Territory-Youth-Detention-System-January-2015.pdf [Accessed 1 July 2017].

Yuval-Davis, N., 2006. Belonging and the Politics of Belonging. *Patterns of Prejudice*, 40 (3), 197–214.

Yuval-Davis, N., 2016. Power, Intersectionality and the Politics of Belonging. In: W. Harcourt, ed. *The Palgrave Handbook of Gender and Development*. Palgrave, 367–381. Available from: www.palgrave.com/us/book/9781137382726#aboutAuthors [Accessed 1 July 2017].

Chapter 3

Reimagining, reclaiming, renaming

Samia Goudie

I respect and acknowledge our Ancestors, Elders and Traditional owners throughout Australia, past, present, and into the future, and our continuing connection to land, culture and community.

Being Aboriginal is one thing to deal with; identity is a constant issue, defined by the narrative of those who see us as other. Racism is passed down through the legacy of invasion and colonisation and continues to have impacts on our everyday lives.

Kinship from an Aboriginal perspective is to relate to one another within culturally informed protocols and to understand your personal connections to the lands one comes from and the lands one lives on. Relationships are central to our ways of knowing of being and doing (Martin and Mirraboopa 2003). Our well-being is intimately linked to this world view.

However, this is not straightforward; being Aboriginal in an invaded and colonised country that has systematically sought to destroy the fabric of Aboriginal lives has created huge displacements and schisms. This has resulted in the passing on of transgenerational traumas (Parker and Milroy 2014), which often underpin the serious burden of disease that we see reflected in statistics. In pretty much every data collection exercise to capture these issues we are faced with a tragic picture of our health and well-being.

Australian Aboriginal people have some of the highest rates in the world for suicide (Reser 1989, Tatz 2005, Priest et al. 2011, Australian Health Policy Collaboration 2016), cardiovascular problems, mental health issues, child health problems and incarceration (Vos et al. 2009). Researchers over the last decade have also found strong evidence that revealing there are direct links between racism and negative impacts that affect our well-being – physically, socially, psychologically, culturally and spiritually (Paradies 2006, Purdie et al. 2010).

There is very little research in Australia, much more in the USA and Canada that is specifically about the impacts of homophobia on Aboriginal and Torres Strait Islander people. However this is a growing field of research and early data indicates that homophobia also has a direct correlation to levels of distress, low access to medical support, high rates of suicide, sexual health problems and self-medication as it impacts the health and well-being of Aboriginal people who identify as gay, lesbian, bisexual, queer, trans and intersex (GLBQTI) (Fieland et al. 2007, Cruz 2015, Mooney-Somers et al. 2015).

Add to this the impact of the ideological colonisation that Western religions brought and the genocidal dictate of the Christian missions (Gaita 1997, Atkinson 2002, Tatz 2011) to wipe out any cultural understandings and/or traditional stories that included reference to what is now named in Contemporary Australia as GLBQTI, and the sense of marginality and isolation can become deafening.

In the culture and stories of other Indigenous nations, we see past and current reference to gendered roles other than those prescribed by heterosexuality, and these often include the possibility of healer and leadership roles within the culture of communities. This is evidenced in the Pacific, the Torres Strait and the Americas (Jacobs et al. 1997), despite these lands and their peoples' having experienced similar processes of colonisation. These histories and tensions live alongside the experience in contemporary Australian society of being seen as the other, as invisible or as a member of a 'high-risk population'. The effect is often confusing and isolating.

By shifting the conversation and focus onto the protective factors of culture, connection and creativity, we can start to support the reimagining of our identities and claim our place and space outside of a deficit colonised narrative (Fforde et al. 2013). As part of this work, it is important to continue the process of reclaiming stories about who we are.

Where this is absent, we must be proactive in creating new narratives and languages that describe us in the ways we choose. In doing this, it is imperative that we remember to focus on our strengths as Aboriginal people. We need to enlist allies to stand with us and together attend to altering the deficit marginalised positions we have often found ourselves in. By contesting the negative descriptors of our identities and using creative responses to racism, homophobia and class, we can create safer places to live in and play an important role as citizens within the greater community of people worldwide who identify as GLBQTI people.

Skin Names

My skin is ambiguous
To you
But not to me

My roots lie deep
Drawn like blood sap from trees
Painted on my skin to remind me of this fact

A map in the sky of stars
Woven with stories passed on and on

Our Elders sit around campfires
Wrapped in possum skins
Stories live in their words

We listen and they become medicine
Eucalyptus and Tea tree
Flooding the air with smoke
AND
All along I wonder at MY connection
My place
This two spirited Queer land
That I inhabit
Am I alone here, silently waiting to find a voice?
When all along I have been screaming

I ask

What name will you call me?
When I travel to that map in the sky
Will you call me Black and Queer?
Will it be another name?

Will you see me as I am?

My outer story is like the possum skin
Familiar and maybe to some exotic
Safe, warm and embracing

But on the inside close to my skin is my inside story
Inside the possum skin cloak, drawn like a tattoo
A story traced sinking deep inside
Like ochre, white, yellow, red as blood
A ceremony

A blak rainbow story

I am claiming myself back
And have been for a very long time
Retrieving the dream and truths
The ones the missions stole and threw away

I will pass down these stories

My life
Our lives
Our loving

The longing for the love of community
And how we made it strong
A bond that keeps us safe

These truths cannot be broken though others try

Despite our pain and loneliness
Despite those we have lost

We know what keeps us strong

Our cultures keep us strong
Our stories keep us strong
Our connections keep us strong
Our creativity keeps us strong

Our fires keep us strong

We are making new stories now
Reclaiming and retrieving
Like an archaeological dig

We are weaving strong baskets
Strand by strand
Each strand important to the whole
These baskets will hold our truths

So that those who come after
Will know
Who we have always been
And how we have dared to love

Samia Goudie, 2017

References

Atkinson, J., 2002. *Trauma Trails, Recreating Song Lines: The Transgenerational Effects of Trauma in Indigenous Australia*. North Melbourne: Spinifex Press.

Australian Health Policy Collaboration, 2016. *Australia's Health Tracker 2016: A Report Card on Preventable Chronic Diseases, Conditions and Their Risk Factors: Tracking Progress for a Healthier Australia by 2025*. Available at: www.vu.edu.au/sites/default/files/AHPC/pdfs/australias-health-tracker.pdf

Cruz, G., 2015. Systematic Review of Studies Measuring the Impact of Educational Programs Against Homophobia, Transphobia and Queerophobia in Secondary Schools of North America, Western Europe and Australia. *Psychology*, 6, 1879–1887.

Fforde, C., et al., 2013. Discourse, Deficit and Identity: Aboriginality, the Race Paradigm and the Language of Representation in Contemporary Australia. *Media International Australia*, 149 (1), 162–173.

Fieland, K., Walters, K., and Simoni, J., 2007. Determinants of Health Among Two-Spirit American Indians and Alaska Natives. In: I. Meyer and M. Northridge, eds. *The Health of Sexual Minorities: Public Health Perspectives on Lesbian, Gay, Bisexual and Transgender Populations.* New York, NY: Springer, 268–300.

Gaita, R., 1997. Genocide: The Holocaust and the Aborigines. *Quadrant*, 41 (11), 17–22.

Jacobs, S-E., Thomas, W., and Lang, S., eds., 1997. *Two-spirit People: Native American Gender Identity, Sexuality, and Spirituality.* Champaign, IL: University of Illinois Press.

Martin, K. and Mirraboopa, B., 2003. Ways of Knowing, Being and Doing: A Theoretical Framework and Methods for Indigenous and Indigenist Re‑search. *Journal of Australian Studies*, 76, 203–214.

Mooney-Somers, J., et al., 2015. *Women in Contact with the Gay and Lesbian Community in Sydney: Report of the Sydney Women and Sexual Health (SWASH) Survey 2006, 2008, 2010, 2012, 2014.* Sydney, NSW: ACON & VELiM, University of Sydney.

Paradies, Y., 2006. A Systematic Review of Empirical Research on Self-reported Racism and Health. *International Journal of Epidemiology*, 35 (4), 888–901.

Parker, R. and Milroy, H., 2014. Aboriginal and Torres Strait Islander Mental Health: An Overview. In: P. Dudgeon, H. Milroy, and R. Walker, eds. *Working Together: Aboriginal and Torres Strait Islander Mental Health and Wellbeing Principles and Practice.* Subiaco, WA: Telethon Kids Institute, 25–38. Available at: https://www.telethonkids.org.au/our-research/early-environment/developmental-origins-of-child-health/aboriginal-maternal-health-and-child-development/working-together-second-edition/

Priest, N., et al., 2011. Racism and Health among Urban Aboriginal Young People. *BMC Public Health*, 11, 568. doi: 10.1186/1471-2458-11-568.

Purdie, N., Dudgeon, P., and Walker, R., 2010. *Working Together: Aboriginal and Torres Strait Islander Mental Health and Wellbeing Principles and Practice.* Canberra: Australian Government Department of Health and Ageing.

Reser, J., 1989. Aboriginal Deaths in Custody and Social Construction: A Response to the View that There Is No Such Thing as Aboriginal Suicide. *Australian Aboriginal Studies*, 2, 43–50.

Tatz, C., 2005. *Aboriginal Suicide Is Different: A Portrait of Life and Self-destruction* (2nd ed.). Canberra: Aboriginal Studies Press.

Tatz, C., 2011. *Genocide in Australia: By Accident or Design? Indigenous Human Rights and History: Occasional Papers 1.* Clayton, VIC: Monash University.

Vos, T., et al., 2009. Burden of Disease and Injury in Aboriginal and Torres Strait Islander Peoples: The Indigenous Health Gap. *International Journal of Epidemiology*, 38 (2), 470–477.

Section 2

Schooling and education

Chapter 4

Lawrence 'Larry' King and too muchness

Complicating sexual citizenship through the embodied practices of a queer/trans student of colour

Ricky Gutierrez-Maldonado

In February 2008 Lawrence 'Larry' King, a student at E.O. Green Junior High School in Oxnard, California,

> was playing [a game] with a group of his[1] girlfriends in the outdoor quad. The idea was you had to go up to your crush and ask them to be your Valentine. Several girls named boys they liked then marched off to complete the mission. When it was Larry's turn, he named Brandon, who happened to be playing basketball nearby. Larry marched right on to the court in the middle of the game and asked Brandon to be his Valentine
>
> (Setoodeh 2008)

Two days after Larry asked Brandon to be his valentine, Brandon brought a gun to school and shot Larry twice at point-blank range. Larry was admitted to a hospital, declared brain dead the following day and later taken off life support. The murder appeared across national news stories and was described by Ramin Setoodeh (2008) from *Newsweek* as 'the most prominent gay-bias crime since the 1998 murder of Matthew Shepard'.

The murder gained broad news coverage, investigative stories and became the focus of a documentary, *Valentine Road* (2013), which premiered at the Sundance Film Festival and was picked up by HBO. Initial news coverage painted Larry as a victim to horrific violence and prompted US lesbian, gay, bisexual, transgender and queer (LGBTQ) advocacy organisations like the Gay, Lesbian & Straight Education Network (GLSEN) to underscore the rights of LGBTQ students and the need for schools to create inclusive environments. Secondary schools, colleges and universities organised vigils and Day of Silence events to remember Larry and draw much needed attention to the harassment LGBTQ students face in schools. Larry became stapled into the memory of the LGBTQ community and the case served as an important reminder about the role schools play in anti-LGBTQ violence.

The sympathetic response was quickly muddled with investigative stories detailing Larry's flamboyance and flirtations with boys at school, including Brandon. These stories reanimated the predictably racist, homophobic and transmisogynistic rhetoric condemning minoritised identities as disruptive and antagonistic, wildly sexual, and altogether too much. The conservative rhetoric, which was eventually adopted by Brandon's defence team, held Larry accountable for their own death. A subtle feature of this debate was the sexual citizenship of Larry that hinged on their right to be protected from harm. The protectionist discourse and the initial image of Larry as innocent victim were met with rhetoric that highlighted Larry's over-the-top and flamboyant demeanour.

Now, some 10 years later, this chapter remembers Larry and sifts through the archive of news coverage, investigative stories, responses from advocacy organisations like GLSEN, and the documentary, *Valentine Road* (2013), which provide accounts of Larry's life through interviews with teachers, friends and those involved in the subsequent murder trial of Brandon. This archive illustrates the life of a young, biracial, Black, trans, femme, gay student who moved through her school with uninhibited joy. I read Larry's life and sense of being through a mode of what Kathryn Bond Stockton (2009) calls *growing sideways* or what I name here as *too muchness*. Growing sideways signals modes of irregular growth that defy a linear trajectory towards full stature and citizenship. Larry's unrestrained sense of themselves, in all their subjectivities, defied social expectations of how a queer kid may live their life. Importantly for the chapter, Larry's too muchness is situated within and against the metanarrative of sexual citizenship grounded in discourses of protection and inclusion.

In the first section of this chapter, I trace the two discursive renderings of Larry as either victim or instigator of violence that demarcate and contain the race, gender and sexuality of young people like Larry. Advocating for sexual citizenship/rights of LBGTQ students from organisations like GLSEN relied on an image of Larry as victim that effaced the racialised characteristics involved in both Brandon's motive for murdering Larry and within Larry's own embodied subjectivities. The protectionist discourse propping up the image of Larry as victim reprised pleas for inclusion for LGBTQ youth, but at the expense of Larry's Black feminine sexuality.

Ironically, the predictably racist, homophobic, and transmisogynistic rhetoric condemning Larry as too disruptive and antagonistic, is precisely the language this chapter makes use of. Rather than dismiss descriptions of Larry as unruly and irreverent, I seek to appropriate and dislodge these characterisations from oppressive discourse and rework them in favour of a queer and trans of colour politics. Reading Larry's sense of being with Stockton's (2009) growing sideways shapes the theoretical framing of 'too muchness' that speaks back to the well-intended protectionist discourse and the overtly oppressive rhetoric blaming Larry for their own murder. My repurposing and framing of too muchness tells an altogether different story about Larry and of queer and trans of colour life in schools more broadly. This story contributes to the growing queer of colour literature in education and what Ed Brockenbrough (2015, p. 32) outlines as the 'expanded research agenda that explores and learns from the agentive practices of queers of color in educational spaces'. The attention given to agentive practices echoes

Cris Mayo's (2014, p. 54) suggestion for researchers and practitioners to strongly consider the ways youth 'are actively and creatively involved in making their lives and communities'. My writing aims to be attentive to Larry's life, particularly the unabashed style through which Larry expressed their young, biracial, Black, trans, femme and gay sense of himself – their sense of too muchness.

Sexual citizenship and protecting Larry's rights

LGBTQ advocacy organisations mourned Larry's death and called on schools to do more to protect LGBTQ students from harassment and violence. Carolyn Laub, the former executive director of the Gay-Straight Alliance (GSA) Network called 'The tragic death of Larry King…a wake-up call for our schools to better protect students from harassment at school' (NBC News 2008). GLSEN's 2008 Day of Silence dedication to Larry was joined with vigils organised by the GSA Network to memorialise Larry. Larry became an example of the extremes of anti-LGBTQ youth harassment, and the continued failure of schools to intervene. Larry's story was indicative of the alarming data emphasising the problems of harassment, mental health issues, drug abuse, dropout rates, depression and suicide among LGBTQ youth, and particularly among LGBTQ young people of colour (Human Rights Campaign 2012). The national attention to the murder rendered Larry's death a catalyst for change and reminded school administrators, policymakers and teachers to protect students against anti-LGBTQ violence.

GLSEN's viewing guide (2013, p. 4) for the documentary, *Valentine Road* (2013), urges educators to 'use the film and the ensuing discussion to increase awareness, examine your school climate and create safe and affirming learning environments for all students'. Their guide encourages educators to adopt predictable strategies like Safe Spaces, No Name Calling Week and sensitivity training in the name of protecting all students from harassment and violence. The recurring language of making schools safer for *all* students reproduced an inclusive equal treatment argument from a rights-based discourse of sexual citizenship, urging schools to treat LGBTQ students the same as heterosexual and cisgender students. GLSEN's response to the murder of Larry echoed the social movements of the 1980s that were, as Diane Richardson (2005, p. 64) describes, couched in the terms of lesbian and gay rights and increasingly used the language of citizenship. GLSEN advocated for LGBTQ students' basic civil right of protection against abuse and violence underpinning a right to an equal education for LGBTQ youth.

Richardson (2000) describes identity-based strategies as moving away from conduct-based arguments that advocate for free expression and behaviour, particularly sexual behaviour. Whereas conduct-based sexual citizenship fights against restrictive laws, an identity-based strategy argues for inclusion based on a sexual or gender identity. GLSEN's response, along with other advocacy organisations, was set within the limits of an identity-based and inclusion-driven sexual citizenship – limits defined by the focus on protection and safety of identities rather than behaviours and actions.

The narrative of Larry as victim to violence and martyr for social change firmly situated her within the 'martyr-target-victim' narrative Eric Rofes (2004) describes. As martyrs, LGBTQ youth come into meaning solely through the spectacle of their deaths or hyper-visible suffering. Without diminishing how homophobia and transphobia matter to the composition of a school or classroom, Rofes critiques the singular emphasis given to the suffering of LGBTQ youth. The martyr-target-victim narrative describes the totality of LGBTQ youth through an especially bleak story at the expense of young people's relationship with agency, desire and pleasure. Since Rofes's (2004) initial criticism, queer youth studies has increasingly shifted its focus from the figure of the victim to that of a resistant LGBTQ young person. Many have echoed Rofes's (2004) initial writing and insist researchers and educators take seriously the ways young people 'are actively and creatively involved in making their lives and communities' (Mayo 2014, p. 54).

This shift from victim to agent, however, is not seamless or simple. In prompting his students to recognise their own agency in the creation of their identities, Rofes (2004) suggested their sexualities along with their victimisations were a result of conscious decisions. His students instead understood their sexualities as something beyond conscious choice. For the students their sexuality and gender was not a matter of agency but of an embodiment that overflowed and spilled into the norms of gender and sexuality where they were met with ridicule or persecution.

For Larry, the question of agency is similarly entangled within discourses of embodiment and conscious choice. The narrative holding Larry accountable for his own death underscored Larry's irreverent actions, especially as Larry disobeyed suggestions from teachers to restrain his flamboyance and flirtation. Too muchness speaks directly to those features of gender and sexuality Rofes's students referenced as uncontrollable and beyond conscious choice. They are features of race, gender and sexuality that are disobedient and unruly, and rooted in Larry's everyday performative play. Too muchness offers a direct counter to the identity-based strategy that has used the image of the LGBTQ victim by highlighting the joys and pleasures of queer and trans of colour life. These joys and pleasures highlight Larry's race, gender and sexuality as actions, demeanours and behaviours that trouble inclusive-based sexual citizenship reliant on stable identities. They are, however, precisely the targets of Brandon's violent white hetero-masculinity.

Chasing boys in stilettoes

> [Larry] started to show up for class at Oxnard, Calif.'s E. O. Green Junior High School decked out in women's accessories…He bought a pair of stilettos at Target, and he couldn't have been prouder if he had on a varsity football jersey. He thought nothing of chasing the boys around the school in them, teetering as he ran.
>
> (Setoodeh 2008)

In addition to the enjoyment he gained from chasing boys, Larry would often tell them they 'looked hot', expressing his desire towards the boys at school. Larry defied teachers' suggestions to minimise his flamboyance and flirtations. When Larry told his teacher, Shirley Brown, he was gay she advised him to keep his feelings private, but Larry had '…progressed day by day in his outward appearance as a girl' (*Valentine Road* 2013). Even with all the cautionary advice, Larry continued to parade through the playgrounds, halls and classrooms of E.O. Green – disobeying mandates to limit his expression.

Teachers raised concerns to school administrators about Larry's modifications to her school uniform and behaviour. Larry's hair, use of makeup and femininity were viewed as excessive. Teachers routinely advised Larry to contain both his look and behaviour in the name of his own safety. Shirley Brown expressed her understanding of Brandon's actions, describing the possibility of her having a similar reaction to Larry's effeminacy, 'I don't know if I would've taken a gun. But a good swift kick in the butt might work well' (*Valentine Road* 2013). Sue Crowley, the special needs teacher, oversaw Larry's Individualised Education Program (IEP) and set a goal for Larry to 'extinguish' his behaviour, but Larry refused (*Valentine Road* 2013). *Newsweek* reported Larry's transgressions had become so pronounced that even teachers who wanted to support Larry were not sure how they could, concerned about the balance between the right of self-expression and the disruption to other students. Dawn Boldrin, Larry's English teacher, who had often advocated on his behalf, gave Larry her daughter's used, glittery homecoming dress. In an interview with *20/20* she admitted giving Larry the dress may have been a mistake and only encouraged Larry's disruptive behaviour and unintentionally accelerated an already dangerous situation (ABC News 2011).

Larry's bodily ornamentation and exaggeration had irritated Brandon, 'Whenever Brandon talked about Larry, it was about what Larry was wearing', says Samantha, Brandon's girlfriend. 'I think Larry was kinda shoving it in everyone's face. For you to come to school dressed like that, you're making a big statement' (*Valentine Road* 2013). Larry made their presence known at school, coming 'to school in makeup, high heels and earrings. And when the other boys made fun of him, he would boldly tease them right back by flirting with them. That may have been what got him killed' (NBC News 2008). As students harassed Larry, he deflected the bullying, wielding his gender and sexuality as both shield and weapon.

Larry's flirtations, chasing the boys in his stilettos and marching onto the basketball court to ask Brandon to be his valentine were recounted by teachers in the subsequent murder trial of Brandon, replacing the initial representation of Larry as an innocent victim with an image of Larry as an instigator. As the *LA Times* reported, 'One teacher after another […] testified in the murder trial about their deep worries that King's feminine attire and taunting behaviour could provoke problems — and that E.O. Green Junior High administrators ignored them' (Saillant 2011). The assistant principal, Joy Epstein, sent a memo to all staff regarding Larry's right to wear makeup and girl's clothes but her action was interpreted by news outlets and Brandon's defence team as dismissive of teacher concerns and warning signs. While LGBTQ advocacy organisations held the school accountable for not protecting Larry, Brandon's defence case presented the school as unwilling to restrain Larry's actions. Larry's choices were deemed so harmful during Brandon's trial that the defence team succeeded in flipping the script, resulting in a mistrial.

Even though Brandon brought a gun to school with the intent of shooting Larry, defence lawyers conveyed an image of Brandon as tormented and used an expert witness to speak on behalf of Brandon's mental state before the shooting. Dr Donald Hoagland, a forensic psychologist, told the jury that Brandon had decided to abandon his original plan to shoot Larry, but 'the ultimate trigger was Larry saying "I'm changing my name to Leticia"', a name and identity Larry embraced, an alternative persona another student described as indicative of a trans identity (*Valentine Road* 2013).

Larry's Black femininity

Leticia was importantly a name Larry often used to signal both his female and Black identity. *Newsweek* (Setoodeh 2008) reported Larry once called his foster mother and told her he wanted a sex change operation 'and he told a teacher that he wanted to be called Leticia, since no one at school knew he was half African American'. Averi, a friend of Larry, describes Larry's identification with Black female personas, 'One day [they] would be Laquisha and the next day Latonya but it always started with La-. Everyone knew that Larry was part Black. So it was kind of generic kind of Black name' (*Valentine Road* 2013). Larry's play with identity involved the creation of alternative personas of sassy Black female figures. Latoya and Leticia were confident and defiant personas that paraded through the halls and classrooms of E.O. Green and helped to deflect the bullying Larry received. As Averi states, 'You don't mess with Latoya or Latonya' (*Valentine Road* 2013).

Larry's Blackness had been central to their feminine sexuality and was a large factor in Brandon's motivation for murder. The documentary, *Valentine Road* (2013), unpacks several details about Brandon's racist motivations. The film includes interviews from Brandon's family that spoke to Brandon's links with white supremacy, although not described as such within the film. Samantha, Brandon's girlfriend, claimed 'white is a minority now. Like fully white people like me...or like Brandon' are disappearing and is cause for concern (*Valentine Road* 2013). Brandon's brother rationalised Brandon's mentorship from a known white supremacist who preached the separation of races and repudiated interracial relationships, which stood in direct opposition to Larry's Black, biracial identity (*Valentine Road* 2013). These interviews with Brandon's family and friends, Brandon's own beliefs of white superiority, and Dr Donald Hoagland's testimony all helped to shape Larry's Black femininity and sexuality as hostile and redrew associations between 'Blackness with an imagined uncivilized, wild sexuality'

(Collins 2004, p. 27). Leticia and Latonya entered into the white imaginary of the defence and jury, recapitulating the relationship of a wild Black femininity and an innocent whiteness. *Valentine Road* (2013) provides a haunting scene of three jurors gathering in one of their homes in the affluent white community of Chatsworth, sharply different from the predominately Latino working-class community of Oxnard where Larry attended school. The three white women drink wine and bond over their sympathetic feelings towards Brandon and their perception of him as one of their own, a kid who could have been their child or grandchild (*Valentine Road* 2013). Their condemnation of Larry, and Larry's Black femininity and sexuality, authorises the violence of white masculinity.

While the documentary itself spoke to Larry's biracial identity, Blackness, and Brandon's whiteness, GLSEN failed to acknowledge race as a significant factor. GLSEN's viewing guide for *Valentine Road* adamantly states, 'Five years later, the central facts of this story remain the same: homophobia is at the core of what killed Larry King and destroyed Brandon McInerney's life' (Gay Lesbian Straight Education Network 2013, p. 1), eschewing any link the murder had to white supremacy. GLSEN advocated for a set of sexual rights but determined those rights in response to homophobia, without considering the racialised features that had been so central to Larry's subjectivity and subjugation.

The erasure of Blackness is perhaps a strategy conscious of the cultural associations made between Blackness and criminality. A recent study from the University of Iowa shows white participants maintain a racial bias in assuming young Black men and boys to be more violent and criminal (Todd et al. 2016). Such studies speak to the cultural assumptions of Blackness as 'bad' or criminal and exclude Black people from the protection that comes with a presumption of innocence. By erasing Larry's Blackness and underlining his victimhood, perhaps GLSEN hoped to secure Larry's innocence by propping up an image of Larry victim to only homophobia. But it was clear that Larry's assertive Black femininity and sexuality were already presumed guilty; as one of the three jurors asks while being filmed for *Valentine Road*, 'Where are the civil rights of the one being taunted by another person who is cross dressing?' The three jurors continue to presume Brandon's innocence and describe Brandon's associations with white supremacy as the innocent curiosity of a kid (*Valentine Road* 2013).

Larry's embodiment and too muchness

My shift here seeks to untie Larry's Black femininity and sexuality from the oppressive discourse of culpability. Rather than condemn descriptions of Larry as one extreme conservative blogger wrote, 'erotic provocateur' (Clough 2008), I want to take up and repurpose Larry's characterisations as exaggerated and undisciplined to provide a theorisation of too muchness. I understand the risk of reproducing the same predictable clichés from anti-Black racism that describe Black bodies as wild and uncivilised but answer these concerns by suggesting that it is not so much that Black queer and trans bodies are too much but that schools do not offer enough. I dislodge the characterisations of Larry's unruliness and excessiveness from the grips of hateful discourse. And rather than insisting on Larry's innocent victimhood within an argument of rights-based sexual citizenship, I interpret Larry's unyielding sense of being as moving the language of sexual citizenship or public life beyond requests or pleas for protection.

Too muchness borrows from Lee Airton's (2013 p. 534) description of 'queerness as the possibilities and excesses of sexuality, where sexuality is the unstructured flow of desire that tends to organise and become identifiable as *sexualities*', but never simply as non-heterosexuality. As an unstructured flow that pushes and exceeds the discursive boundaries of sexuality, queerness is located perhaps in a place of unintelligibility. I understand the contradiction in naming embodied performances that may seek to escape that very designation. Yet, I have settled on the imperfect term of too muchness to talk about Black and Brown queer lives that are full of life, overflowing and bigger than any word or set of words could fully describe. Like others, I will forever face misrepresenting Larry because I simply do not have access to a language that could be enough to completely capture the multiplicity and vitality of their life. For this reason, too muchness is not a catchall term for queer and trans youth of colour; rather, it describes a mode of being that pushes against the discursive and material boundaries policing these young people's lives.

I want to extend the thinking of 'unstructured flows' to embodiments of race and gender that cannot be reduced to 'intersecting identities'. Race and gender operate in similar ways described by Airton, as bodies of colour and gendered bodies contextually determined, and travelling through and within each other. The metaphor of intersectionality, however, is perhaps too spatially rigid. Sandra K. Soto (2010, p. 3) argues

> race, sexuality, and gender are much too complex, unsettled, porous (and I do mean to be wordy here), mutually constitutive, unpredictable, incommensurable, and dynamic, certainly too spatially and temporally contingent, *ever* (even if only for an instant) to travel independently of one another.

In rethinking intersectionality, Cris Mayo (2015b, p. 246) urges us to develop 'processes that would not make connections and complexities easier, but would remind us of the difficulties of the work we try to do when advocating for education and justice…'. Too muchness keeps with this unsettled and overly complicated work of identity via what Deborah Britzman et al. (1993, p. 188) has called the 'embodied politics of identity' that speaks to the differences, ambiguities and multiplicities of LGBTQ people and LGBTQ people of colour.

Too muchness also signals this mode of identity and experience as multiple, unyielding, messy, anarchistic and overwhelming. For Larry, too muchness speaks to a mode of over identification, or an abundance of identity when and where a body is in relationship with multiple signifiers and categorical markings. Larry's Blackness and transness were compounded with the various social locations through which Larry moved, travelling in and out of various identities, unapologetically Black, coming out as gay and trans, and adopting racial and gender markings the school was unfit to understand or even imagine. While Aliyah, a seventh grader at the time of Larry's murder, insisted on Larry's transgender identity rather than Larry's being gay, Larry's gender identity remains largely uncertain. As Melinda D. Anderson from *The Atlantic* writes (2015), 'History will remember Larry as Larry. Although, given what we know, we are left to ask if perhaps in that name—"Larry"—the tragedy and denial of Leticia is lived over and over again, like looping trauma'. But trans and gay identity are not mutually exclusive, nor does memory need to be limited to honouring Larry or Leticia. Too muchness lies precisely within this multiple identifications and uncertainty. Larry was boy, girl, trans, genderqueer, Black, white, etc. all of the above, and none of the above. Larry's multiplicity resists the consolidation towards a singularity and allows for identity to remain open.

Within this multiplicity lies the indeterminacy of queerness, its openness and ability to be shaped and reshaped. Mary Lou Rasmussen (2006, p. 31) describes this as 'the process of continuously becoming subjects, a process that may involve not only the struggle but also creativity in the reinscription of subjectivities and identities'. Larry reinscribed historic tropes about Black women onto his body, adopting both the sassy Black woman and the jezebel, impudent and excessively sexual and using the stereotype for the purposes of survival and to express his Black femininity and sexuality. Rather than being the simple reproduction of racist tropes, these performances were an explicit embrace of Larry's Blackness and became a point of Black joy and pleasure. While the continual invention and negotiation of identity works against the tendency to stabilise the subject within discourses of sexuality, gender, race and schooling, more importantly it adopts the task of creating something distinctive. The impossibility of accommodating a Black female sexuality within a middle school like E.O. Green is pushed upon the school through Larry's irreverent demeanour, forcing students and staff to contend with new and unexpected subjectivities. As a form of critique, the inability for the school to contain Larry 'indicates not only adult insufficiency of understanding but also perhaps adult lack of control of young people's identities' (Mayo 2015a, p. 38).

'Larry, being Larry, pushed his rights as far as he could'

The moves in subjectivity point to what Kathryn Bond Stockton (2009) has named growing sideways. This mode of growth resists a specified trajectory of 'growing up' that describes the 'supposed gradual growth, their suggested slow unfolding, which unhelpfully, has been relentlessly figured as vertical movement upward (hence, "growing up") toward full stature' and subjecthood (Stockton 2009, p. 4). The process of growing up reproduces the typical developmental narratives that structure and regulate young people's growth and learning.

Sideways growth on the other hand signals a horizontal shift away from the expected ways in which young people are meant to develop into full participating citizens. The possibilities of too muchness reside within this indeterminate trajectory and suggest growing sideways eludes adult agendas in regulating young people's growth.

I reimagine this sideways growth to signal Larry's horizontal sprawl across the school, as his transgressions became widely known among students and staff, soliciting the school-wide memo from the assistant principal, Joy Epstein. Too muchness as a mode of sideways growth signals subjectivities as expanding and overflowing beyond the contours of the body. Larry's body was too much to the point of affecting school culture and the everyday happening of classrooms and schoolyards. Revisiting and re-reading Larry's march onto the basketball court to ask Brandon to be his valentine, Larry intrudes on a scene of normalised masculinity by making public his desire for Brandon. The same-sex and interracial desire toward Brandon spurred a very different relationship from the typical romantic relationship the question of 'Will you be my valentine?' would initiate. The question, reminiscent of childhood crushes and normal heterosexual childhood coupling, is thrown off course. Larry's intrusion had reshaped the question to one saturated with homosexual and interracial desire, threatening both Brandon and the school's investment in whiteness and normative gender expectations. The innocence of the question would be stripped away, forcing educators to reconsider a seemingly normal interaction between two schoolyard children during Valentine's Day.

Larry's actions would typically do this, intrude onto scenes of normativity and push teachers and administrators to rethink everyday practices of the school. The everyday dress code of the school was challenged with Larry's ornamentations, pressuring administrators to familiarise themselves with school dress codes and legal protections of gender expression and identity. Assistant principal Joy Epstein had informed Larry of his right to wear makeup and the high-heeled shoes he started to wear to school. But 'Larry, being Larry, pushed his rights as far as he could', wearing a Playboy bunny necklace and approaching the most popular boys' table at lunch, asking in a high-pitched voice, 'mind if I sit here?' (Setoodeh 2008). Larry relished in the ways she interrupted and disturbed the students and teachers, and refused to minimise her Black femininity and flirtations.

The act of *pushing his rights* adds to arguments of sexual citizenship that unsettle the private-public division of sexuality, particularly as Larry disobeyed requests to minimise his Black femininity and sexuality. Larry's exceedingly public life worked beyond the identity-based strategies of acceptance or inclusion that typically are okay with students being gay, but not acting gay. Larry's Black femininity and sexuality was an engrossing and occupying force, unsettling even those teachers who were sympathetic to Larry's subjectivities. Larry's overly sexual, gender-transgressing, and disobedient Blackness on a child's body complicates the citizen subject when arguing on behalf of Larry's rights. Whereas GLSEN's guide argues for creating welcoming spaces in which students like Larry might feel included, too muchness demands more than this of schools.

Larry's creative unruliness undermined and altered the dynamics of traditional school space, as Larry paraded through the school swerving his hips and blowing kisses to the boys. Larry's subjectivities reached beyond to influence the cultural and social space offered by the school. Hallways became runways and classrooms became stages. His march onto the basketball court could be read as a precursor to his tragic murder, but can also be read as an act exposing the violent white hetero-masculinity the school continued to defend even after the shooting. At the time of the documentary, *Valentine Road* (2013), the school would not allow a permanent memorial on school grounds.

Ultimately, Larry's identifications pushed against the material and discursive boundaries of E.O. Green. While teachers may have felt inadequately trained or prepared to respond appropriately to Larry, it would be wrong to suggest we need better preparation for teachers to more accurately and precisely recognise emerging modes of racial, gendered or sexual being. Instead, educators might better engage with the embodied politics of subjectivity while resisting minimising identifications and bodily displays. Changing a school's coercive practices requires the continuous work of educators and policymakers to allow too muchness, the multiplicities of their students, to change them and their schools.

While education has done well in providing tools for affirming identity, too muchness lends itself more readily to the task of what Cris Mayo (2014) has suggested by creating practices and policies allowing for new modes of being and subjectivities to emerge. Pedagogies and policies should remain open – allowing kids like Larry to express new and sometimes surprising modes of expressing identities of race, gender and sexuality. Gender non-conforming Black children and youth may express Blackness in ways teachers consider incorrect or inauthentic. Larry's use of the sassy Black woman archetype serves as an example to the ways young people may repurpose codes of Blackness. Leticia and Laquisha were powerful women who deflected the harassment Larry received at school. Larry reworked the figure for his survival and joy.

Carrying Larry forward and educational implications

I recognise the danger in moving the memory of Larry forward to current educational contexts. This removes Larry from the conditions in which they lived in E.O. Green and Oxnard, California and decontexualises Larry. But the context in which Larry was killed, that of trans misogyny and white supremacy constitutes the structures, both material and discursive, in which queer and trans of colour youth find themselves today. While these contexts manifest themselves differently across schools, their consequences are strikingly similar. A 2014 report from the GSA Network 'shows that LGBTQ youth of colour face persistent and frequent harassment and bias-based bullying from peers and school staff as well as increased surveillance and policing, relatively greater incidents of harsh school discipline, and consistent blame for their own victimization' (Burdge et al. 2014). The implication lies within the ability for Larry's life to reverberate and affect change, to have too muchness spill over onto education today, both in research and in practice.

This is not to argue for a sweeping radical change but more a response to Ed Brockenbrough's (2015) recent call for researchers to begin exploring and sharing stories of agency from queer and trans youth of colour. In documenting the agentive practices of queer and trans youth of colour, however, we should not rely on what Cris Mayo (2007, p. 82) describes as a trend within queer research in education to centre 'the most easily identified members of sexual minorities [who] are "out", that is, they self-consciously and publicly identify as a member of a sexual minority group and thus can be contacted, observed, and collaborated with on research projects'. By looking to those students who are 'out' and identify with a sexual or gender identity, we lose the features of too muchness explored in this chapter. We lose the embodiments of race, gender and sexuality that simultaneously complicate efforts of inclusion-based sexual citizenship and highlight the beauty of queer and trans life.

Larry's most provocative subjectivities and interruptions did not emerge from a state of systematised political consciousness but from feelings of joy and pleasure. Too muchness serves as a reminder to privilege those emotional registers queer and trans of colour youth experience and spread throughout their schools, much like the horizontal orientation of sideways growth (Stockton 2009). This is perhaps connected to the concept within queer of colour vernacular of *giving life*, which describes aesthetics, art and attitudes that evoke delight and excitement. This requires the excavation of joy from stories that emerge from tragedy and which are typically found in memory, memoirs, media, etc., while simultaneously extending the viable spaces through which queerness and transness of colour are shaped and reinvented.

Too muchness may open possibilities for more imaginative ways of practising education that respond creatively to the queer growing of young people. Where securing rights and protection from violence is necessary, so should be the promise of joy and pleasure. So in standing side by side with LGBTQ youth we should be cautious that our strategies of sexual citizenship do not seek to name all that is, or all that could be. Instead, by allowing too muchness to overwhelm us, we may begin to reimagine our classrooms and schools as places of queer and trans of colour passion and pleasure.

Note

1 Gender pronouns are used interchangeably throughout this chapter to illustrate the shifting gendered identities Larry played with while at school. Larry was boy, girl, trans, non-binary, etc., and played with several selves that resist a singular gender identity or expression. Throughout this chapter, the gender pronouns he/him and she/her, and the neutral pronoun they/them are used in reference to Larry.

References

ABC News, 2011. Shots in a Classroom [online]. *ABC News*, 7 October. Available from: http://abcnews.go.com/2020/video/shots-classroom-14694384 [Accessed 19 January 2015].

Airton, L., 2013. Leave 'Those Kids' Alone: On the Conflation of School Homophobia and Suffering Queers. *Curriculum Inquiry*, 43 (5), 532–562.

Anderson, M. D., 2015. To Be Black and Transgender in Junior High [online]. *The Atlantic*, 16 November. Available from: www.theatlantic.com/education/archive/2015/11/the-denial-of-leticia/415968/ [Accessed 3 March 2016].

Britzman, D., et al., 1993. Slips that Show and Tell: Fashioning Multiculture as a Problem of Representation. In: C. McCarthy and W. Crichlow, eds. *Race, Identity, and Representation in Education*. New York, NY: Routledge, 188–200.

Brockenbrough, E., 2015. Queer of Color Agency in Educational Contexts: Analytical Frameworks from a Queer of Color Critique. *Educational Studies*, 51 (1), 28–44.

Burdge, H., Licona, A. C., and Hyemingway, Z. T., 2014. *LGBTQ Youth of Color: Discipline Disparities, School Push-Out, and the School-to-Prison Pipeline*. Gay-Straight Alliance Network and Crossroads Collaborative, University of Arizona. San Francisco, CA.

Clough, T., 2008. On the Killing of Larry King [online]. *Weird Republic*, 24 April. Available from: www.weirdrepublic.com/episode87.htm [Accessed 19 January 2015].

Collins, P. H., 2004. *Black Sexual Politics: African Americans, Gender, and the New Racism*. New York, NY: Routledge.

Gay Lesbian Straight Education Network, 2013. *Valentine Road Viewing Guide*. New York, NY: Gay Lesbian Straight Education Network.

Human Rights Campaign, 2012. *Growing Up LGBT in America*. Available from: www.hrc.org/youth-report/about-the-survey

Mayo, C., 2007. Queering Foundation: Queer and Lesbian, Gay, Bisexual, and Transgender Educational Research. *Review of Research in Education*, 31 (1), 78–94.

Mayo, C., 2014. Excessive Gesture and Equitable Access: Tensions in Queer Education. *American Education Research Association Annual Meeting*, 3–7 April 2014, Philadelphia, PA.

Mayo, C., 2015a. *LGBTQ Youth & Education: Policies & Practices*. New York, NY: Teachers College Press.

Mayo, C., 2015b. Unexpected Generosity and Inevitable Trespass: Rethinking Intersectionality. *Educational Studies*, 51 (3), 244–251.

NBC News, 2008. Gay California Student's Slaying Sparks Outrage [online]. *NBC News*, 28 March. Available from: www.nbcnews.com/id/23847511/ns/us_news-education/t/gay-california-students-slaying-sparks-outcry/#.WMxovWQrJhB [Accessed 19 January 2015].

Rasmussen, M. L., 2006. *Becoming Subjects: Sexualities and Secondary Schooling*. New York, NY: Routledge.

Richardson, D., 2000. Constructing Sexual Citizenship: Theorizing Sexual Rights. *Critical Social Policy*, 20 (1), 105–135.

Richardson, D., 2005. Claiming Citizenship? Sexuality, Citizenship, and Lesbian Feminist Theory. In: C. Ingraham, ed. *Thinking Straight: The Power, Promise and Paradox of Heterosexuality*. New York, NY: Routledge, 63–84.

Rofes, E., 2004. Martyr-target-victim: Interrogating Narratives of Persecution and Suffering Among Queer Youth. In: M. L. Rasmussen, E. Rofes, and S. Talburt, eds.

Youth and Sexualities: Pleasure, Subversion, and Insubordination In and Out of School. New York, NY: Palgrave Macmillan, 41–62.

Saillant, C., 2011. Oxnard School's Handling of Gay Student's Behavior Comes Under Scrutiny [online]. *Los Angeles Times*, 11 April. Available from: http://articles.latimes.com/2011/aug/11/local/la-me-0811-gay-student-20110811 [Accessed 19 January 2015].

Setoodeh, R., 2008. Young, Gay and Murdered in Junior High [online]. *Newsweek*, July. Available from: www.newsweek.com/young-gay-and-murdered-junior-high-92787

Soto, S. K., 2010. Introduction: Chican@ Literary and Cultural Studies, Queer Theory, and the Challenge of Racialized Sexuality. In: S. K. Soto, ed. *Reading Chican@ like a Queer: The De-mastery of Desire.* Austin, TX: University of Texas Press, 1–14.

Stockton, K. B., 2009. *The Queer Child: Or Growing Sideways in the Twentieth Century.* Durham, NC: Duke University Press.

Todd, A., et al., 2016. The Generalization of Implicit Racial Bias to Young Black Boys: Automatic Stereotyping or Automatic Prejudice? *Social Cognition*, 34 (4), 306–323.

Valentine Road, 2013. Film. Directed by Marta Cunningham. USA: Home Box Office.

Chapter 5

Beyond cultural racism

Challenges for an anti-racist sexual education for youth

Anna Bredström and Eva Bolander

Official sexual educational materials reflect the context in which they were written. They come with contemporary styling and address the challenges facing society at the time they were produced, as imagined by those in power. Thus, in the early days, sexual education in Sweden reflected eugenic notions of racial purity and the supremacy of white Nordics (Svendsen 2017), intertwined with the sexual hygiene beliefs of left-wing socialists (Lennerhed 2002). With the advent of HIV, there was an upsurge of new material deeply entrenched in risk discourses, reflecting – at least at the beginning of the pandemic – moral assumptions about sexual identities, stigma and blame (Henriksson 1995, Bredström 2008). Today, the most manifest message is that migration seemingly challenges the current state of affairs regarding sexuality, which corresponds to a shift in migration policy towards a neo-assimilatory discourse in which gender and sexual values are put forward as pivotal (Bredström 2008, 2016). This has resulted in the development of numerous programmes and a variety of educational materials specifically targeting newly arrived migrants.

The overall purpose of this chapter is to query deeper into this nexus of migration and sexual education. To do so, we have singled out one piece of sexual educational material that we will read closely through a hermeneutic lens. Our choice of empirical material is not made on representative grounds. Rather, in Sweden, most initiatives aiming to address the needs of newly arrived migrants tend to reproduce what Michael Billig (1995) has conceptualised as a *banal nationalism*. That is to say, they explicitly or implicitly refer to notions of Swedishness as both different from, and superior to, the characteristics of other nations and ethnicities. For instance, Swedishness is produced by informing migrants about 'Swedish' ways of living, loving and having sex, often with an emphasis on how 'Swedes' generally embrace gender equality and liberal views on LGBTQ-people's rights (Bredström 2008, Rosén 2013, see for example Saleh 2017, pp. 26–27).

In sharp contrast to the sexual exceptionalism (Puar 2007) of much mainstream material, the resource we will analyse in this chapter refute such a normative and nationalist stance. Instead, it positions itself as anti-discriminatory and critical of the dominant norms of society. It is particularly careful not to reproduce notions of 'us' and 'them' based on racialised apprehensions of immutable cultural differences, and seeks instead to offer an anti-racist position that moves beyond what critical race scholars would conceptualise as cultural racism or culturalist neo-racism (Jonsson 2003). The material in question is called *Sexual Education in Easy Swedish (Sexualundervisning på lättare svenska)*.[1] It comprises two books: a teacher's manual (RFSU 2013a) and a class book (RFSU 2013b). The teacher's manual includes in-depth discussions on perspectives, theories and methods, while the class book is filled with colourful drawings and easy-to-read sentences to be used in a classroom setting. *Sexual Education in Easy Swedish* was first published by the Swedish Association for Sexuality Education (RFSU) in 2013. Updated editions are available online,[2] and to our knowledge,[3] the material is used both in education and in in-service teacher training.

The material targets students taking introductory Swedish language classes, which comprise both so-called Swedish for immigrant classes, i.e. introductory language education for adults, and introductory language programmes for 16- to 20-year-olds. The latter is the preparatory education provided to newly arrived migrant youth, making them eligible for entry into national programmes in upper secondary schools and the equivalent. Following the recent increase of refugee minors coming to Sweden, as many as 10% of all 16- to 20-year-olds in Sweden are currently attending a language introductory programme (Swedish National Agency for Education 2017, p. 6).

Sexual Education in Easy Swedish thus potentially reaches a large number of young people. Young people in general are also subjected to intervention by a range of public health institutions as they are considered a vulnerable group in relation to HIV and sexually transmitted infections (Proposition 2005/06:60). In line with this, from time to time Swedish authorities map sexual behaviours and attitudes among youth. The most recent report published by the Public Health Agency of Sweden (2017) emphasises health disparities in relation to gender and transgender identities. It also points to ethnic discrimination as having a negative impact on young people's sexual well-being. To combat such inequalities, the Agency highlights the importance of promoting sexual and reproductive human rights.

Promoting sexual rights is also highlighted as an important strategy in *Sexual Education in Easy Swedish*, and in this chapter we will query its potential drawbacks, in particular its promotion at a time of neo-assimilatory, universal racism (Jonsson 2003). In doing so, we aim to reveal current challenges in developing an anti-racist sexual education. Before doing this, however, we will describe the background and context in which all of this takes place, and flesh out the RFSU's norm-critical agenda.

The RFSU and norm-critical sexual education

Sexual education played a pivotal role in the formation of the Swedish welfare state. The idea was that officially sanctioned information on sexuality would serve to create a prosperous population and counteract religious as well as commercial influences (Seifarth 2005). As part of this social project, statutory directives have been accompanied by initiatives from prominent non-governmental organisations, in particular the RFSU. The RFSU was established by their well-known spokesperson Elise Ottesen-Jensen in 1933 and ever since the organisation has been a key voice in public debate about sexuality in general, and sexual education in particular (Lennerhed 2002). The RFSU sees young people as a key target group and produces a range of sexual educational materials targeting both youth in general, as well as specific groups of young people, such as migrant youth, which is the focus of this chapter.

The RFSU's work includes local, national and international activities. At a local level, members organise public lectures, workshops and film screenings. They also visit schools, organise youth activities, distribute information and materials at festivals and so on. At a national level, the RFSU employs sex educators, experts, communicators, lobbyists and lawyers to pursue its goals of a sexual politics based on the individual 'freedom to choose, enjoy and be oneself'.[4] The RFSU also run a clinic, the quarterly magazine *Ottar*, and a company, RFSU Inc., that develops and sells products such as condoms, lubricants, pregnancy tests and sexual aids. Internationally, the RFSU runs different development projects in among other countries, Bangladesh, Cambodia, Georgia, Ghana and Tanzania, promoting gender equality, sexual health and sexual education.

The RFSU is thus no minor player when it comes to sex and sexual education, yet the organisation stands out as controversial at times, most often being perceived as too liberal and sex positive. The RFSU is also cautiously critical of mainstream sexual education. For instance, in the teacher manual of *Sexual Education in Easy Swedish* it says that, historically, sexual education has been a central tool for equality, but that it also often invokes 'problematic viewpoints' (RFSU 2013a, p. 15). As an example of such a problematic viewpoint, the manual highlights the historical connection between sexual education and eugenics. It also references studies of more recent mainstream sexual education that have revealed misconceptions, such as that girls lack sex drive or that homosexuality would be dangerous to boys.

The teacher manual also repeatedly refers to several scholars who have been engaged in critically analysing how gendered, sexual and racialised norms are reproduced in mainstream sexual education (e.g. Reimers 2007, Bredström 2008, Bolander 2009, see also Bolander 2015, Bredström et al. forthcoming). *Sexual Education in Easy Swedish* seeks to follow the same path. To be norm-critical and anti-discriminatory is emphasised as a way of being inclusive and reaching people. However, knowledge about 'norms, values, equality, mutuality, identity and rights' is also emphasised as relevant in itself; it is 'just as relevant as factual knowledge' (about the body, safer sex and reproduction) (RFSU 2013a, p. 9) for example. That is to say, the RFSU also has the ambition of teaching norm-critical perspectives to their presumptive audience. To do so, they argue, is a way to prevent discrimination and contribute to greater equality with regards to people's sexual and reproductive rights (RFSU 2013a, p. 16).

This norm-critical perspective was developed by a queer pedagogical network of researchers, practitioners and activists that sought to be more inclusive and intersectional in their feminist critique of gender and sexuality (Bromseth and Darj 2010). The approach draws in particular on Kevin Kumashiro's (2002) *Anti-Oppressive Pedagogy*, which, in turn, seeks to combine liberatory education with poststructuralist (queer feminist) views on power and identity. In short, Kumashiro calls for an increased focus on exposing norms themselves and the privileges they entail, rather than focussing on those being marginalised.

The RFSU's norm-critical ambition is in line with current school policy. A norm-critical perspective became mainstreamed in sexual education through national guidelines published in 2013 (Swedish National Agency for Education 2013a, b). These guidelines also emphasise the importance of equality and stress that sexual education should be integrated into all school subjects in order to provide students with a broad view on sexual matters.

Kumashiro's ideas about centring the norm itself permeate *Sexual Education in Easy Swedish*, and underline the needs to elucidate what is being taken for granted in society. The teacher manual describes the RFSU's understanding of norms in the following way:

> Norms can be unwritten rules, ideal values, and expectations on what's desirable. Simply stated; what is considered normal in a specific context or society? The norm is visible everywhere, on TV, in school books, in everyday conversations and so on, while other ways to live are made invisible. The norm to live in a nuclear family is, for instance, strong in our society, despite the fact that many people live in other family constellations. We are often unaware of norms, they are simply taken for granted. It is only when someone disobeys the norm, and if the surrounding community reacts, that they become visible.
>
> (RFSU 2013a, p. 17)[5]

It is further explained how norms are linked to power and that power is everywhere; 'in what we say, and what we do, in how we divide people into groups that we then have different ideas about and expectations of' (RFSU 2013a, p. 17). It is also stressed that power is shifting and that norms may change if challenged.

The chapter then goes on to highlight norms of particular importance to the RFSU's anti-discriminatory approach. Regarding gender and sexuality, it describes heteronormativity and its importance for norms concerning sexual identity, masculinity and femininity, as well as trans and cis identities. Further norms of importance for sexual education, the RFSU states, are those concerning love, twoness/monogamy and intercourse. Norms concerning Swedishness and whiteness are dealt with under a separate heading, and we will return to them shortly. First though, let us say something about how *Sexual Education in Easy Swedish* translates their theoretical perspectives into practice.

Basically, two main strategies are suggested. First, the material encourages self-reflection as an important pedagogic method (see Bredström et al. 2018).

This is developed particularly in the teacher manual, which also contains several exercises in which the educators are to reflect on their own privileges and normative understandings. These exercises include questionnaires listing sexual experiences and activities that aim to open up educators' views in different ways. They are urged to draw (separate) timelines detailing their personal experiences of love and sex throughout life (RFSU 2013a, p. 41) and are reminded that most people have experience of being marginalised to some extent (RFSU 2013a, p. 19) (i.e. as a woman, as having a working-class background or as a LGBTQ-person).

However, the manual strongly advises against having students talk about personal experiences in a similar self-reflective way. Thus in class, educators are urged to rephrase questions and comments so that they become more general, and to speak about people in the third person (e.g. 'if you had a friend who…', 'this is the experience of Abel, what do you think Abel should do…' *etc.*). With respect to students, the manual underlines that to be norm-critical does not mean being critical of those who live according to the norm; but to be critical of the system that construes some practices and identities as normal and not others. The goal, thus, is to be as inclusive as possible by constantly addressing many different sexual identities and practices. By doing so, everybody can recognise themselves and feel that this is something that concerns them. As the manual explains:

> An inclusive spirit of conversation is created if we, as impartial as possible, try to *meet the person* by always reminding ourselves of that, in every group, there are numerous different opinions and experiences. […] Always refer to several different ways to be and act and present them as equally available options, avoid making those who do not fit the norm into *others*. […] To teach in an inclusive way can be as simple as saying partner instead of boyfriend/husband or girlfriend/wife, and avoid words such as 'normal' and 'natural', as they present certain ways of living as more desirable than others. Another tip is to give a wider answer than the question suggests.
>
> (RFSU 2013a, p. 19)

This encompassing approach is also reflected in the pictures of the class book which include bodies of various sizes and colours. In order to decentre the norm of vaginal intercourse, the book always describes numerous different sexual practices, using both words and pictures of the body parts and arrows as illustrations. In addition, most people are given gender neutral names. Thus, for instance, a picture aiming to encourage students to talk about sexual preferences depicts two persons on top of one another. They are called Gabi and Kit, and by the images in their respective dream bubbles we are informed that one has a penis, and the other has a vagina, but we do not know who has what. The teacher manual points out that some students might be provoked or confused by the gender neutrality. 'If so, you may suggest that they choose a gender for each character' (RFSU 2013a, p. 104). Then you may also 'discuss why they feel gender is important' (RFSU 2013a, p. 104). Instead of taking gender for granted, gender is thus made a topic of discussion.

Sexual education beyond the norm of Swedishness

This way of problematising gender and sexual norms fits well into the queer feminist theoretical framework from which norm-critical pedagogy was developed. In the past decade, the RFSU has produced several educational materials with similar messages. However, *Sexual Education in Easy Swedish* is one of the few norm-critical materials that explicitly addresses race and ethnicity. The intention is to avoid reproducing norms of Swedishness, and, more generally, refrain from using problematic notions of 'us' and 'them'. Accordingly, the manual states that it only uses the word 'Swede' when it aims to problematise different perceptions, or to show how people's living conditions are affected by whether they are categorised as Swedes or as non-Swedes (RFSU 2013a, p. 13). Elaborating on its views on 'Whiteness and Swedishness as norms', the manual explains that it is a norm to be 'Swedish' in our society, and that this norm stems from 'an understanding [in society] of culture and religion as something neatly defined, static and uniform, and that it determines people's behaviours' (RFSU 2013a, p. 32).

While mentioned in the heading, whiteness is not further discussed in either of the two books except in the glossary at the end of the manual where it is explained that 'whiteness as a norm implies that it [in society] is seen as desirable and positive to be white'. It is also indicated that there is an increased risk of discrimination if you are not perceived of as white, and that in Sweden, 'whiteness is strongly connected to ideas about Swedishness' (RFSU 2013a, p. 223).

The manual further clarifies how norms of Swedishness relate to norms of gender and sexuality. Here, it is highlighted that gender and sexuality are often at the centre of discussion concerning belonging, culture and religion, and that:

> 'Swedishness' is, in these contexts, linked to more attractive values such as openness, tolerance, and equality, and liberal views on sexuality. People from other, in particular non-western, countries are presumed to be unequal, homophobic, narrow, and governed by taboos around sexuality.
>
> (RFSU 2013a, p. 33)

This division between 'us and them', the manual states, has major consequences for society: When people are presumed to be or think in certain ways depending upon their cultural background, they become reduced to their ethnic identity. Thus, for instance, as Swedishness is associated with positive virtues such as gender equality, any expression of gender equality among 'other' cultures is interpreted as an exception that proves the rule. Correspondingly, negative expressions – such as gender violence – are individualised if they concern a 'Swede', whereas the same phenomena among those seen as 'others' is explained with reference to 'their' culture. This articulation of otherness as a problem to society, the RFSU argues, is key to understanding how discriminatory social structures function. Also, the racialisation of gender and sexuality makes it more difficult to expose inequalities in Swedish majority society.

In order *not* to reproduce norms of Swedishness, the RFSU argues that it is crucial to have 'an open mind'. To acquire this, educators are encouraged to reflect upon their own biases, for instance, by problematising who they perceive their students to be in terms of their experiences and opinions. They are also to think carefully about how they treat others and be particularly careful not to treat people in a condescending way: for instance by infantilising migrant students. Most importantly, the RFSU argues that educators should be careful not to ascribe a particular experience or value to a person's ethnicity, culture or religion. On the contrary, they should always 'be open to participants who may have different views on gender and sexuality, even when they do not follow prevailing understandings of culture and religion' (RFSU 2013a, p. 44). Neither should they see 'students or yourself as representatives of a particular culture' (RFSU 2013a, p. 44).

A similar approach extends teaching the Swedish law. Here, the RFSU encourages teachers to highlight that laws are not static or indisputable, but subject to change (RFSU 2013a, p. 174). The manual also points out that Swedish law is not always necessarily 'better' when it comes to sexual rights. While some people may receive rights that they did not have in their countries of origin, the opposite is equally true, i.e. some people may lose rights they used to have, such as having a neutral gender in their passport or being able to marry more than one partner (RFSU 2013a, p. 175).

Thus educators are repeatedly encouraged to take an open view, and to be open to encountering experiences and views that are different from those of the majority society; but at the same time as they should not presume people to be different. Let us now see how such an approach may play out in practice by looking closely at two particular phenomena that *Sexual Education in Easy Swedish* seeks to address: circumcision and honour-related violence, topics that appear regularly in mainstream discourse on Swedishness and non-Swedishness (Bredström 2014).

Anti-discriminatory sexual education in practice

Both 'female genital mutilation' and 'honour-related violence' are nodal points in mainstream sexual exceptionalist discourse (Bredström 2014), and it is thus interesting to see how these topics are dealt with in *Sexual Education in Easy Swedish*. Interestingly, they turn out to be illustrative of both the RFSU's approach to a norm-critical inclusiveness and its limits.

Regarding genital cutting of the penis and vulva, the RFSU sees these as important issues to address in order for sex education to be inclusive. Thus the manual stresses that educators should always bring up circumcision practices in their teaching. They should also always include, or preferably start out from, pictures of circumcised genitals. By doing so, the RFSU argues, everyone can 'recognise themselves' and 'feel that this is something that concerns me' (RFSU 2013a, p. 92). Students are also to be informed about different varieties of circumcision practices, and educators should avoid generalised explanations or references to particular cultures.

As seen, the RFSU avoids turning circumcision into a gendered practice. Instead of speaking about 'female' and 'male' circumcision, the materials refer to a circumcised vulva and penis. The RFSU does, however, also bring up the alternative concept of *genital mutilation*, which is sometimes preferred to capture the circumcision, as some of these procedures entail greater health risks. The manual also alerts readers to the Swedish law that forbids female genital mutilation (SFS 1982:316). However, the RFSU argues that in order to reach out to and avoid stigmatising people, using the less charged concept of circumcision may be the better choice within the classroom.

The RFSU's approach is noteworthy given that one of the organisation's principles is to be against *any* procedure on children's genitals that is not medically motivated, regardless of sex (2013a, p. 80). To be inclusive thus implies accepting values that diverge from one's own. Furthermore, while it is seen as important to address possible health concerns relating to different circumcision practices, the RFSU argues that it is equally important to bring up issues relating to sexual pleasure. Focussing on pleasure, it is claimed, is a good way to encourage people to explore their own sexuality (RFSU 2013a, pp. 81–82). Educators are thus to point out that although sensitivity in the penis and vulva may be affected by some of the different procedures, sexual pleasure is still possible. The body or shaft of the clitoris, for instance, lies inside the body and can be felt 'though massaging the vulva alongside the edge of the pubis' (RFSU 2013a, p. 79). It is also stressed that touching other body parts and use of the imagination may be equally useful. As a possible study question on the topic, to be used in class, *Sexual Education in Easy Swedish* thus suggests:

How can you masturbate if you are circumcised?

When Yaasmiin was young they took away a piece of her clitoris. She has heard that many people think that it feels nice to touch the area around the clitoral glans. Yaasmiin wants to have sex with her self. She wants to know what she can do to make it feel nice. What do you want to say to Yaasmiin?

(RFSU 2013a, p. 94)

By being inclusive and focussing on pleasure, *Sexual Education in Easy Swedish* departs from the more problem-oriented discourse that otherwise surrounds this topic. As we will see, however, this accepting outlook is more difficult to achieve when we turn to the other topic, honour-related violence.

Just as female genital mutilation, honour-related violence is also highly topical in everyday discourse. In fact, one could argue, it serves as a trope for most discussions about migration, gender and sexuality in Sweden today (Carbin 2010).[6] For the RFSU, honour-related violence seems to be more difficult than circumcision to approach norm-critically, at least the options to be inclusive and open are fewer. The teacher manual brings up the topic of honour in a specific chapter on sexuality, relationships and society. The chapter includes Swedish laws and rights concerning sexuality and includes discussion of harassment and violence. Honour-related violence is not mentioned under any separate heading, but is dealt with in relation to 'violence and control in the family'. Here, we are told that young people may be subjected to control and violence by their families and relatives with reference to sexual behaviours that are said to bring shame on the family. It is also pointed out that these negative responses mostly affect girls and LGBTQ-people, and that they derive from heteronormativity and narrow norms regarding female sexuality. Rumours about bad behaviour are often what ignite the violence, and young people are said to bring shame on their families and therefore need to be controlled or punished.

So far, the RFSU's depiction corresponds well to the general accounts of honour-related violence prevalent in mainstream Swedish society. However, in order to pursue a norm-critical logic the resources argue *against* linking this kind of control and violence to any specific culture, religion or ethnicity. They also point out that, while the concept of honour may have the advantage of capturing the specificities of this particular kind of violence, in everyday life it is too intimately linked to certain migrant cultures and religions. Thus, using the concept of honour may miss out on how similar processes also occur in so-called Swedish families, particularly in relation to LGBTQ-youth. The manual also states that other problems in migrant families may be interpreted as honour-related even when they are not (RFSU 2013a, pp. 178–179).

To avoid *culturalising* the problem, the RFSU urges educators to shift focus, and address the issue in terms of sexual rights:

> You need to address different forms of control and violence and, at the same time, have a broad approach to equal rights in preventive work. Using *rights* as a starting point will enable you to bring up these difficult questions in a positive way. It concerns the right to choose your own life, and the rights to express gender and sexuality in ways that make you feel good about yourself.
> (RFSU 2013a, p. 168)

This in our view is a far from adequate response; we will use the remaining part of this chapter to argue why, and to point to some possible alternatives.

Colour blindness?

To recapitulate, we have identified three main strategies that the RFSU utilises in order not to reproduce norms of Swedishness. First, it aims to be as inclusive as possible by always referring to a wide variety of practices and bodies, and addressing issues in a non-pejorative mode. Secondly, it seeks to detach the linkage of specific phenomena or practices to a particular ethnicity, culture or religion. And finally, it seeks to use a rights-based discourse to transcend certain conflictual values. We will deal with the last two of these strategies first.

In contrast to much mainstream material, *Sexual Education in Easy Swedish*, as seen earlier, denies any clear-cut connection between a particular practice or sexual value and a particular ethnicity, nation or culture. This also includes those norms that the RFSU considers 'positive norms', such as *mutuality* and *equality*. The key here, the RFSU argues, is to avoid presenting these norms as 'Swedish' (RFSU 2013a, pp. 34–35). While we agree that there is value in recognising the heterogeneity of any ethnicity, and reminding ourselves of the many people who are, for instance, both Muslim and feminist there is, we argue, an inherent paradox in the way the RFSU reasons. On the one hand, their norm-critical approach leads them to refute culture as relevant to sexuality. On the other, their understanding of norms draws heavily upon a perspective that sees identities and practices as social and cultural constructions. To pose the problem differently, what are norms, if not culture? Seeing sexuality as inherently cultural rather than biological has been central to critical theories of sexuality for quite some time (Parker and Aggleton 2007). Leaving culture out of the picture thus seems to be a counterproductive strategy.

Entering into a similar discussion on religion, Mary Lou Rasmussen (2012, 2016) criticises progressive sexual education for relying on a secular logic that separates culture and religion from sexuality. She writes:

> There is a focus on reason and education as central to helping young people develop as sexual subjects. While I am compelled by this argument, I am concerned that such an approach often fails to see value in other aspects of young people's lives that may influence their sexual decision making. Here, I am thinking of kinship networks, culture and religion, spirituality and ethics – how these are integrated (or not) into young people's decision making. I am also concerned that culture, religion and morality are often constructed as somehow outside reason and, therefore, always something that diffuses rather than reinforces young people's capacity to act as agentic subjects.
>
> (Rasmussen 2012, p. 477)

Following her logic, by neglecting the importance of culture, the RFSU obfuscates the ways in which our choices are always already shaped by culture. Ironically then, despite its intentions, and despite its many efforts to be inclusive, the RFSU's strategy appears just as 'colour blind' as those that refuse to acknowledge that racism still permeates Western societies (Lentin and Titley 2011). However, what the RFSU aims to contest is not that sexuality is shaped by culture; rather, their critique focusses on the racialised use of culture that frequent mainstream discourse on migrant integration employs, whereby culture is portrayed as a problematic trait that lingers on for generations. The RFSU also quotes critical scholars in the field (including ourselves) and highlights how present-day racisms rely more upon notions of immutable cultural differences than biology (RFSU 2013a, pp. 34–35).

Yet, by not providing a clear alternative perspective on culture, the RFSU reinforces the liberal notion of an 'abstract, genderless, colorless sovereign subject' who is able to choose freely and independently (Samuels 1999, Rasmussen 2012). This also fits well with the turn towards universal rights. Critical scholars have problematised the human rights discourse from numerous perspectives, highlighting that universal values are only universal in the abstract. As Stefan Jonsson (2010, p. 118, italics in original) phrases it: 'Inevitably, every coding of universality is a *particular* representation'. Most relevant for our argument, however, is the timing of the RFSU's reference to universal rights. Because, while *Sexual Education in Easy Swedish* underscores the social construction, and historicity, of ethnic and racial boundary-making, and theorises cultural racism accordingly, their model does not adequately take into account recent shifts from a multicultural ideology established in the early 80s to a neo-assimilatory outlook emerging around the millennium.

The main difference in this shift is that neo-assimilatory discourse does not only centre on cultural differences, but also proposes universal values as a key doctrine through which racial differences are established and sustained (Jonsson 2003). In sexual education, the shift was obvious. In the early 1980s, migrants were to be treated with cultural sensitivity and respect for difference (Bredström 2008). Back then, culture was seen as essential to identity, as well as society at large. People 'losing their culture' – or being 'squeezed between cultures' – was understood as detrimental to social stability (Ålund and Schierup 1991). It was within this context that critics argued that policy reflected cultural neo-racism; i.e. culture was portrayed as an immutable difference and used to conceal problems of social and economic origins (Ålund and Schierup 1991, Jonsson 2003).

In line with a broader 'securitization of migration' in the 1990s (Guild 2009), by which migration increasingly became articulated in terms of 'risks' to society, migrant integration policy increasingly shifted towards an assimilatory discourse which portrayed migrant cultures as a problem for society. Following this trend, cultural differences gradually became a major difficulty for sexual education whereby migrant sexuality came to be associated with a range of social problems such as honour-related violence, virginity/hymen issues and female genital mutilation (Bredström 2008). As a consequence, earlier discourse on cultural sensitivity and tolerance faded away. Instead, more and more voices were raised in favour of defending certain values, representing these values as universal and thus unchallenged.

A quote by the then director general of the National Board of Health and Welfare, Claes Örtendahl, where he talks about why he dislikes a multicultural approach to sexual education, is telling:

> To say that we should refrain from interfering when it comes to their views on sexual relations as a way of showing respect for their culture is, I believe, in fact a way of not showing respect. Following such reasoning, the work that we do here in Sweden would only be an expression of some provincial idea of

different human values, which I do not consider our view on sexual relations to be. As I see it, the right to love, lust and community forms part of universal values rather than of something 'culturally specific' in need of respect.

(Claes Örthendahl, in Mossberg 1996)

Thus, while the RFSU manages to defy the banal nationalism and the cultural racisms of mainstream discourse, the aspirations to universal rights in *Sexual Education in Easy Swedish*, as we see it, feeds all too well into a neo-assimilatory framework, and as such they cannot fully manage to escape the racism they seek to challenge.

Concluding remarks

As has been suggested in recent scholarship on sexual citizenship, the promotion of sexual rights in general, and LGBTQ-rights in particular, has increasingly been absorbed into nationalist rhetoric, leading to what Puar (2007) conceptualises as a form of 'homonationalism' and the sexual exceptionalism of many Western nations described earlier. This makes sexual politics a highly charged terrain, especially if one shares the RFSU's ambition of developing a sexual politics that is equally antiracist and anti-discriminatory, given that the very articulation of sexual values might, in itself, be experienced as racist. To put it simply, if discourses on racial difference are articulated through discourses about sexual values, then the reverse is also true: *any* talk about sexual values will inevitably partake in the production of racial inequality (Bredström 2016).

But, how then, could one act otherwise when it comes to promoting sexual recognition and citizenship? That is to say, how can one *not* be in favour of the values that the RFSU proposes: namely, mutuality and equality and the right to define one's own sexual needs and pleasures (without violating anyone else's rights). A more beneficial approach may be to target the issue from another angle. The chief deficiency in RFSU's approach is the way it constantly tries to avoid the heat of the moment. None of the resources we have examined go in-depth into how to deal with conflicting values. Despite how *Sexual Education in Easy Swedish* suggests several strategies for being inclusive and addressing heterogeneity, it only touches upon potential disagreements on a few occasions. At these times, in addition to not culturalising specific groups, the RFSU emphasises the need to defend mutuality and equality, and protect those that might be hurt by discriminatory views. To put it slightly differently, the only strategy that the RFSU seemingly has is to argue for the possibility of everyone sharing the same 'open views'.

If the RFSU materials were to acknowledge the centrality that universal values play in present-day racisms, then it would also be clear that one needs to do more than avoid casual reference to Swedishness. And it is this potentially irresolvable conflict that constitutes the main challenge for an anti-racist sexual education that seeks to move beyond cultural racism and norms that the concept of Swedishness brings with it. We suggest that we take this conflict seriously.

That is to say, instead of trying to undo existing tensions, a more fruitful strategy would be to seek alternative ways to live with difference.

One way of doing this could be to start from the RFSU's model of inclusivity. Indeed, the multiplicity of identities, bodies and practices that *Sexual Education in Easy Swedish* presents has the potential to address a heterogeneous audience, as has the way in which the RFSU approaches different values in a non-condescending way. What could be added to these strategies, we suggest, is a model of dialogue that does not require tensions to be solved, such as the transversal politics promoted by scholars engaged in intersectionality theory (Yuval-Davis 2011). Central to transversal politics is a standpoint epistemology that sees people's different ideas on life as equally true. This also requires a dynamic concept of culture that treats culture in an anti-essentialist way, focussing on the ways in which people negotiate meanings and recreate cultural identities (Kirmayer 2006).

Drawing upon the many years of fieldwork we have conducted with young people in Sweden – including an ongoing project examining sexual education in Swedish schools[7] – we remain hopeful about the possibilities of developing an anti-racist sexual education with this ambition. Indeed, while policy insists on portraying multiculturalism in endless negative ways, we agree with Paul Gilroy (2016) that critical scholars need to recognise the everyday meetings and dialogues – and the simply 'living together' (conviviality) – that takes place despite the deep ruptures that racism causes in society. It is within young people's everyday lives that we may find inspiration on how to take the norm-critical agenda one step further.

Notes

1 With reference to the material under study in this chapter, we use the concept of Sexual Education. However, the RFSU uses this concept interchangeably with that of Sex and Relationship Education (Sex- och samlevnadsundervisning) which is the concept used in school curricula in Sweden.

2 www.rfsu.se/sv/Sexualundervisning/Sexualundervisning-pa-lattare-svenska/

3 This chapter draws on findings from a research project conducted by Anna Bredström (PI), Eva Bolander and Jenny Bengtsson and funded by the Swedish Research Council (2011-5850). Research for the chapter has also benefited from Bredström's stay as a visiting scholar at the Swedish School of Social Science in Helsinki in March 2017.

4 www.rfsu.se/en/Engelska/About-rfsu/Organization/RFSU---Association/

5 All quotes from *Sexual Education in Easy Swedish* are originally in Swedish and have been translated by the authors.

6 Public debate on honour-related violence has been ongoing since the early 2000s, following the murder of a young Kurdish girl who was killed by her father. The act was said to be in defence of family honour and reached massive media attention. As of then, numerous policies and action plans on all levels of society – including school, healthcare, police, social work – have been issued to tackle honour-related violence (Carbin 2010). For critical race scholars, the widespread attention given to honour-related violence is interpreted as part of the larger neo-assimilatory discourse mentioned earlier, which constructs 'other cultures' as intolerably patriarchal and violent (Jonsson 2003).

7 See Note 3.

References

Ålund, A. and Schierup, C-U., 1991. *Paradoxes of Multiculturalism: Essays on Swedish Society*. Aldershot: Avebury.

Billig, M., 1995. *Banal Nationalism*. London: Sage.

Bolander, E., 2009. *Risk och bejakande: sexualitet och genus i sexualupplysning och sexualundervisning i TV*. Linköping: Linköpings universitet.

Bolander, E., 2015. The Condom Works in All Situations? Paradoxical Messages in Mainstream Sex Education in Sweden. *Sex Education*, 15 (3), 289–302.

Bredström, A., 2008. *Safe Sex, Unsafe Identities: Intersections of 'Race', Gender and Sexuality in Swedish HIV/AIDS Policy*. Linköping: Linköpings universitet.

Bredström, A., 2014. Sex på kartan? Om tonårssexualitet, rasism och sexualupplysning i Sverige. In: K. Sandell, M. Sager, and N. Räthzel, eds. *Kritiska gemenskaper: att skriva feministisk och postkolonial vetenskap*. Lund: Lunds universitet, 125–133.

Bredström, A., 2016. Normkritik, rasism och rättigheter: en svårvandrad terräng. *Ikaros: tidskrift om människan och vetenskapen*, 13 (1–2), 31–33.

Bredström, A., Bolander, E., and Bengtsson J., forthcoming. Norm Critical Sex Education in Sweden: Tensions within a Progressive Approach. In: J. Gilbert and S. Lamb, eds. *The Cambridge Handbook of Child and Adolescent Sexual Development*. Cambridge: Cambridge University Press.

Bromseth, J. and Darj, F., eds., 2010. *Normkritisk pedagogik: makt, lärande och strategier för förändring*. Uppsala: Centrum för genusvetenskap, Uppsala universitet.

Carbin, M., 2010. *Mellan tystnad och tal: flickor och hedersvåld i svensk offentlig politik*. Stockholm: Stockholms universitet.

Gilroy, P., 2016. Humanism till havs. Om att rädda flyktingar och oss själva. *Ord och Bild*, 5, 10–29.

Guild, E., 2009. *Security and Migration in the 21st Century*. Cambridge: Polity.

Henriksson, B., 1995. *Risk Factor Love: Homosexuality, Sexual Interaction and HIV Prevention*. Göteborg: Göteborgs universitet.

Jonsson, S., 2003. Rasism och nyrasism i Sverige 1993–2003. In: K. Mattsson and I. Lindberg, eds. *Rasismer i Europa: kontinuitet och förändring*. Stockholm: Agora, 45–77.

Jonsson, S., 2010. The Ideology of Universalism. *New Left Review*, 63, 115–128.

Kirmayer, L. J., 2006. Beyond the 'New Cross-Cultural Psychiatry': Cultural Biology, Discursive Psychology and the Ironies of Globalization. *Transcultural Psychiatry*, 43 (1), 126–144.

Kumashiro, K. K., 2002. *Troubling Education: Queer Activism and Antioppressive Pedagogy*. New York, NY: Routledge Falmer.

Lennerhed, L., 2002. *Sex i folkhemmet: RFSU:s tidiga historia*. Hedemora: Gidlund.

Lentin, A. and Titley, G., 2011. *The Crises of Multiculturalism: Racism in a Neoliberal Age*. London: Zed.

Mossberg, M-B., 1996. *Det mest privata i det svenska folkhälsoarbetet: Sex, samlevnad och hiv/aids i ett mångkulturellt samhälle*. Stockholm: Folkhälsoinstitutet.

Parker, R. and Aggleton, P., eds., 2007. *Culture, Society and Sexuality: A Reader*. London: Routledge.

Proposition, 2005/06:60. Nationell strategi mot hiv/aids och vissa andra smittsamma sjukdomar.

Puar, J. K., 2007. *Terrorist Assemblages: Homonationalism in Queer Times*. Durham: Duke University Press.

Public Health Agency of Sweden, 2017. *Sexualitet och hälsa bland unga i Sverige. UngKAB15 – en studie om kunskap, attityder och beteende bland unga 16–29 år.* Stockholm: Folkhälsomyndigheten.

Rasmussen, M. L., 2012. Pleasure/Desire, Sexularism and Sexuality Education. *Sex Education,* 12 (4), 469–481.

Rasmussen, M. L., 2016. *Progressive Sexuality Education: The Conceits of Secularism.* New York, NY: Routledge.

Reimers, E., 2007. Always Somewhere Else – Heteronormativity in Swedish Teacher Training. In: L. Martinsson et al., eds. *Norms at Work: Challenging Homophobia and Heteronormativity.* Stockholm: Transnational cooperation for equality.

RFSU, 2013a. *Sexualundervisning på lättare svenska. Lärarhandledning och metoder.* Stockholm: Riksförbundet för sexuell upplysning (RFSU).

RFSU, 2013b. *Sexualundervisning på lättare svenska. Lektionsunderlag.* Stockholm: Riksförbundet för sexuell upplysning (RFSU).

Rosén, J., 2013. *Svenska för invandrarskap?: språk, kategorisering och identitet inom utbildningsformen Svenska för invandrare.* (diss.). Örebro: Örebro universitet.

Saleh, D., 2017. *Sex och samlevnad för nyanlända.* Stockholm: Gothia fortbildning.

Samuels, J., 1999. Dangerous Liaisons: Queer Subjectivity, Liberalism and Race. *Cultural Studies,* 13 (1), 91–109.

Seifarth, S., 2005. Från desarmering till utlösning under ansvar: sex- och samlevnadsundervisning i skolradion 1954–1974. In: M. Kylhammar and M. Godhe, eds. *Frigörare?: moderna svenska samhällsdrömmar.* Stockholm: Carlsson, 221–250.

SFS, 1982:316. *Lag med förbud mot könsstympning av kvinnor.*

Swedish National Agency for Education, 2013a. *Sex- och samlevnadsundervisning i grundskolans senare år: jämställdhet, sexualitet och relationer i ämnesundervisningen: årskurserna 7–9.* Stockholm: Swedish National Agency for Education.

Swedish National Agency for Education, 2013b. *Sex- och samlevnadsundervisning i gymnasieskolan.* Stockholm: Skolverket.

Swedish National Agency for Education, 2017. *Uppföljning av språkintroduktion.* Rapport 454. Stockholm: Skolverket.

Svendsen, S. H. B., 2017. The Cultural Politics of Sex Education in the Nordics. In: L. Allen and M. L. Rasmussen, eds. *The Palgrave Handbook of Sexuality Education.* Basingstoke: Palgrave Macmillan, 137–153.

Yuval-Davis, N., 2011. *The Politics of Belonging: Intersectional Contestations.* Los Angeles, CA: Sage.

Chapter 6

Regulating sexual morality

The stigmatisation of LGB youth in Hong Kong

Adrian Kin Cheung Yan and Denise Tse-Shang Tang

Introduction

In this chapter, we aim to provide an overview of how sexual morality, cultural traditions and religious conservatism shape the educational system and its institutions in Hong Kong, resulting in a prevailing social discourse that stigmatises marginalised youth. We will first outline the sociopolitical landscape of lesbian, gay, bisexual and transgender (LGBT) visibility in recent years by pinpointing the key debates for and against the advancement of equal rights for lesbian, gay and bisexual (LGB) youth in Hong Kong.[1] Then, we will illustrate how the government, religious sponsoring bodies of education and social services, along with evangelical activists, have formed a 'trinity of governance' that dominates sexual morality in Hong Kong society, asserting a particular set of views about sexuality while marginalising and seeking to deny other expressions of sexuality (Kong et al. 2015). Finally, we will discuss how LGB youth manage their everyday lives inside and outside of school settings within the city.

Fighting for LGBT rights

Hong Kong is often perceived as a cosmopolitan city that celebrates a free-market economy, cultural diversity and plurality of values, but in terms of sex education and sexual rights the city has been trailing behind many of its counterparts in the East Asian region (Sanders 2015, Suen et al. 2016). Sex education in schools focusses primarily on biological sex criteria and seldom addresses issues of sexualities (Tang 2014). Anti-discrimination legislation protecting the rights of LGBT persons is absent in Hong Kong.

It was only after a decade of public and legal debate that male homosexuality was eventually decriminalised in Hong Kong in 1991 under the Crimes Amendment Ordinance. Since then, Hong Kong gay and lesbian community groups have begun to emerge with different purposes ranging from social and cultural activities to advocacy and education. On the legal front, there has been very limited progress in enacting protection on the grounds of sexual orientation and gender identity. Since 1994, repeated attempts by lawmakers to ensure the inclusion of sexuality in discrimination ordinances have been met with resistance from the Hong Kong government, citing public education on sexual orientation as more important than legislation protecting the rights of sexual minorities. In 2012, the Equal Opportunities Commission (EOC) initiated a motion to invite public consultation on the prohibition of discrimination based on sexual orientation in the workplace. This motion triggered considerable resistance from conservative religious groups and affiliated organisations, such as The Society for Truth & Light and Hong Kong Alliance for Family (Yau 2016). Established in 1997, the former of these organisations is an evangelical Christian group, which employs traditional family values as a platform on which to educate the public on issues ranging from gambling to homosexuality and pornography. The Hong Kong Alliance for Family set up in 2003 as an affiliate organisation with the explicit purpose of defending heterosexual marriage. Both organisations belong to larger global evangelical churches, namely the Baptist Convention and the Christian and Missionary Alliance.

On the issue of workplace discrimination, both organisations have promoted the view that the introduction of legislation to prevent discrimination against LGB individuals could lead to reverse discrimination – namely people facing criminal liabilities for criticising homosexuality. The issue thus became a battleground between the progressive liberals and conservative groups, which have led government officials to delay the timing of the proposed legislation, claiming it 'will only lead to arguments, divisions and conflicts' (Carney 2013, n.p.). A recently commissioned EOC report, entitled a 'Study on Legislation against Discrimination on the Grounds of Sexual Orientation, Gender Identity and Intersex Status', also concluded with the key recommendation to conduct a public consultation on the scope of anti-discrimination legislation rather than the need to establish such legislation (Suen et al. 2016).

Whereas there have been obstacles to enactment of anti-discrimination legislation and legal recognition of same-sex marriages or civil unions, court challenges have recently been launched to address discriminatory state practices. A judicial review in 2005 resulted in Court of First Instance and the Court of Final Appeal judgements that the age of consent for sexual behaviour between men should be lowered from 21 to 16 on par with that for heterosexuals. First filed in 2009, the case of W v Registrar of Marriages saw a transgender woman who has undergone sex reassignment surgery finally winning the right to marry her boyfriend five years later after filing an appeal against the Court of First Instance. In 2015, senior immigration officer Leung Chun-kwong launched a court challenge against the secretary for civil service and the commissioner of the Inland Revenue Department arguing for entitlement of benefits be awarded to his husband Scott Adams. Two years later, Leung won his case against the secretary for civil service but lost to the Inland Revenue Department as tax laws state that marriage is a union between a man and a woman whereas the term spouse is used under civil service regulations. In the same year, a British lesbian expatriate known as QT won an appeal against the Immigration Department's decision to reject her application for a spousal visa. QT had been in a civil partnership with her partner SS when they both relocated to Hong Kong for SS's job offer in 2011. Yet within months of both court victories, the Department of Justice applied to appeal against the entitlement of civil servant benefits to Leung's husband and the Hong Kong Immigration Department followed suit to appeal over the Court of Appeal's decision to grant QT a spousal visa.

Regulating sexual morality: trinity of governance

Sexual beliefs and practices are regulated by powerful mechanisms of social control (Delamater 1981) operating in various aspects of social life and present at different levels of institutional arrangement. In both sexuality studies and educational research it is recognised that individual choices are profoundly influenced by the norms and values imposed by wider social structures (Walker and Barton 2013).

As argued by Ho (2004), the British colonial government adopted a largely depoliticised approach towards governing the local population through its emphasis on laissez-faire economics since 1842. Hong Kong residents quickly learned that market rights were easier to attain than the political right to participate in the government (So 2004). The Bill of Rights was only established in 1991 and takes into account the provisions of the International Covenant on Civil and Political Rights for Hong Kong people. Media representations of same-sex sexualities and portrayal of transgender persons are widely found in popular culture but at times depicting negative and stereotypical representations. The decriminalisation of homosexuality in 1991 marked a watershed for increased social recognition of same-sex relationships in the territory, facilitating the emergence of lesbian and gay communities. Sexual citizenship in terms of public recognition of LGBT persons and the fight for the advancement of LGBT rights has also begun to emerge in wider society.

Yet the handover of Hong Kong to China in 1997 has seen a shift in local identity politics. Under Beijing's rule, the new Hong Kong government has been actively instilling a strong sense of patriotism among Hong Kong citizens, notably in the form of emphasising Chinese values such as harmony and moderation to ensure the smooth transition of sovereignty and the cultivation of a Chinese national identity (Ma and Fung 2007). The return of Hong Kong to China in 1997 was accompanied by a strong dose of re-Sinicisation (Ma and Fung 2007), with an emphasis on Chinese values so as to ensure the smooth transition of sovereignty. Consequently, the emergence of sexual minority voices has been systematically offset by the political discussion on the status of Hong Kong as part of China and the economic concerns of the city as an international financial centre. This explains in part why LGBT communities in Hong Kong in the post-colonial period have largely eschewed a confrontational politics when it comes to advocating for the rights for sexual minorities. Even if demands for LGBT rights cause social controversy, these claims are often subsumed under the rhetoric of broader human rights and freedom of expression (Wong 2004).

According to Lau (1978), traditional Chinese values and beliefs are by and large underpinned by Confucian philosophy and have a relatively strong influence on the ethos of the local population. Confucianism promotes the image of a harmonious society and provides a powerful framework for the social conduct and expectations for individuals. Every individual has a social role (or *fen*) in social life and people are expected to behave according to their role so as to contribute to the well-being of the society. As traditional Chinese culture places high value on authority as the basis of social order, obedience and respect are highly valued within the family where they are seen as indications of filial piety. Being openly out as a person with same-sex desires would jeopardise the harmonious makeup of a family in Confucianist terms. Having a gay son or a lesbian daughter amounts to the losing of 'face' for many Chinese families (Chou 2000).

In a Chinese family, parenting is often oriented towards the achievement of success in society and ensuring the continuity of the paternal family lineage, thus bringing honour to the family. In the school context, teachers are often perceived as authority figures with high moral standards. Students generally do not challenge teachers' judgements in the course of learning.

Against this backdrop, we will examine the contemporary position of LGB youth in Hong Kong. By untangling the complex relationships between government, evangelical activists and schools, we will seek to explore the 'trinity of governance', as Kong et al. (2015) assert it in their analysis of mechanisms of social control over sexual morality in contemporary Hong Kong society.

Governmentality – family planning and sexual conjugal familism

The emergence of family planning in Hong Kong is closely related to the British colonial government's approach to population policy in the 1960s. Back then, the influx of refugees escaping from political instability in mainland China led to a rapid growth of the city. The colonial government expanded its services to cope with issues arising from changes in the population composition (Chan 2007). The Family Planning Association of Hong Kong (FPAHK), formerly known as the Hong Kong Eugenics League in 1936, received substantial support from the government to develop policies to control the local population. Borrowing models of family planning from England, the services provided by FPAHK included regular medical check-ups, the supply of contraceptives and the dissemination of sex-related information to the general public during the 1950s and 1960s. As argued by Cho (2013), the FPAHK played an instrumental role in constructing the nuclear family model as the norm for local families in Hong Kong. The emergence of a focus on 'sexual conjugal familism' (Cho 2013) or monogamous heterosexual marriage took place in several stages. First, concubinage was criminalised as the result of repeal of the Chinese Marriage Preservation Ordinance, and its replacement by the Marriage Ordinance in October Executive 1971 (Hong Kong Executive Council 1970). Second, the nuclear family model was promoted by the

FPAHK in the 1970s as the most desirable family configuration both to ensure lineage through procreative sex and to lead towards overall life satisfaction.

Parallel to a growing focus on the nuclear family model in the 1970s and 1980s was an apparent increase in the prevalence of pornography, and an upsurge in sex crimes and teenage pregnancy, all of which were regarded by the colonial government as well as the general public as symptoms of moral decline (Chou and Chiu 1992). Parents' groups and school associations expressed growing concern over the need to instil appropriate attitudes towards sex in young people, advocating for things like chastity before marriage. They also urged the government to impose stricter regulations on the dissemination of obscene materials and to address the sexuality of adolescents in the face of an increasingly explicit sexual climate. However, as indicated by Cho (2013), sex education initiatives at the time showed a paradoxical recognition of young people as sexual beings. On the one hand, the *Guidelines on Sex Education in Secondary Schools* (Education Department 1986) sought to address the physiological and biological aspects of male and female sexuality; on the other hand, the document's undertone implied that sex should only be discussed within the context of adult (heterosexual) marriage. Since young people had yet to achieve adulthood, they were advised to focus on their academic studies instead and to channel their 'surplus energy' into sports and extra-curricular activities. In these ways, the prevailing discourse of sexual conjugal familism and initiatives in sex education curriculum colluded to exclude alternative forms of sexuality and denied the erotic desires of young people (Ho and Tsang 2012).

School management and curriculum: heterosexism

According to the Education Bureau (2016), about 52% of public and directly subsidised secondary schools in Hong Kong are affiliated Christian churches including both Protestant congregations and Roman Catholic diocese. These missionary-sponsored schools, with their mode of subsidy, enjoy a relatively higher level of autonomy when it comes to implementing the school curriculum. This enables them to incorporate Christian teaching and conservative gender ideals into the formal curriculum, which are then disseminated through the very fabric of school life (Ng and Ma 2001). As part of a larger study on everyday experiences of Hong Kong *tongzhi* students, Kwok et al. (2012) conducted a study on the experiences of secondary school counselling services by interviewing nine *tongzhi* students aged between 14 and 18.[2] They found an entrenched notion of heterosexism inherent within the counselling sessions through the narrative accounts of Chinese *tongzhi* students, alluding to the prevalent view that heterosexuality is the only legitimate type of sexuality.

These findings echo the results of recent research commissioned by the Equal Opportunities Commission and conducted by the Hong Kong Institute of Education (now the Education University of Hong Kong), which documented the perception that 'homosexuality is immoral' in many of these religious-affiliated schools (Kwok 2015). Heterosexism and the stigmatisation of LGB youth in schools are contributing factors to poor mental health, declining school performance, poor sexual health, substance abuse and increased suicidal ideation among LGB youth (Tang 2014).

Heterosexism and homophobia in Hong Kong schools is also facilitated by the lack of a formal curriculum for sex and sexuality education (Kwok 2016). Although the Education Department updated the *Guidelines on Sex Education in Schools* in 1997, the content of the guidelines is heavily tilted towards conservatism (Education Department 1997). Long-time advocate for positive sex education, Ng (1998) regards these guidelines as a depiction of basic sexual anatomy and physiology representations with the intent to indoctrinate youth on proper sexual morals by neglecting discussion on diverse sexualities or controversial issues such as pornography and prostitution. Ho and Tsang (2012), in a study of university students' responses to a human sexuality course, note the extent to which sex education based solely on heterosexuality provides students with a limited view of the body and the articulation of their sexual experiences. Their findings also show how female university students view sex and sexuality as only involving heterosexual couples. Conservative cultural notions of how a good woman should always resist men's sexual advances, how the loss of virginity will reduce a woman's 'market value' in marriage, and how sexual desire and pleasure are relevant only in marriage were also reported by the study's participants. As a result, safer sex practices and sex before marriage are often neglected in the school curriculum, not to mention a lack of discussion on same-sex sexualities. The dual influence of Confucianism and Judeo-Christianity affects how the notion of proper sexuality is taught and constructed in schools. The absence of an inclusive sex education curriculum in schools limits the potential for other issues to be explored as in the formation of sexual identities and communities for young people. Positive support for LGB youth in schools remains as individual cases rather than institutional policies.

In the absence of a good quality sex education curriculum, the dissemination of sex- and sexuality-related knowledge to a large extent hinges on the teaching style of individual teachers. Tong (2008), in her study of tomboys in local secondary schools, describes a conservative image of school teachers who rely heavily on regulatory practices to discipline students' sexual activities. Teachers with conservative views about morality tend to perceive LGB students as 'abnormal' and rebellious for their refusal to conform to conventional notions of masculinity and femininity. Teachers' punitive responses, along with the malicious gossip of other students often contribute to the negative stigmatisation of sexual and gender minorities (Touch Project of The Boys' and Girls' Clubs Association of Hong Kong 2009).

Although teachers' attitudes towards the teaching of sex education is lukewarm, Fok's (2005) study of the implementation of sex education in Hong Kong secondary schools points to an array of pedagogical approaches used by some school teachers, including open forums and video programme analysis, both of which facilitate critical discussion of issues such as homosexuality and abortion, and promote greater understanding of sexual and gender diversity among students.

However, Fok also notes that the religious ethos of schools, the lack of qualified teaching staff and a shortage of teaching resources continue to be significant barriers against the implementation of more inclusive forms of sex and sexuality education. Sex education in Hong Kong often takes the form of patronising advice; LGBT issues, though occasionally discussed, remain a peripheral component of the curriculum.

The Code for the Education Profession of Hong Kong cum Practical Guidelines makes no reference to sexual orientation as a basis for discrimination, meaning that there are currently no ethical guidelines for school teachers to tackle the issue of homophobia and solicit assistance on behalf of gender and sexual minorities (Council on Professional Conduct in Education 2017). Moreover, because their job security is largely dependent on the decisions of school management, teachers often remain silent on controversial issues such as LGB rights and refrain from discussing same-sex relationships in education contexts. Their task is made more difficult by the stresses imposed by education reform, including associated new professional development programmes and accountability measures. Coupled with the administrative work, frontline teachers often become the prime victims of 'curriculum reform syndrome' (Cheng 2009). Studies of teachers' psychological well-being (Leung et al. 2009, Pattie 2009) highlight how distress, depression and burnout are common among teachers, leaving little space for teachers to help LGB students. School-based social workers, in particular, have been regarded as a possible source of positive rapport for these sexual minorities owing to their professional training in coping with youth issues and their critical understanding of social policies. However, as To (2009) indicates, social workers in Hong Kong are generally regarded as auxiliary services within the education sector. Their performance and job security often hinge on the evaluation by school management, which, to a large extent, discourages them to be outspoken when it comes to advocating inclusive practices in schools.

Religion – LGB youth marginalisation by evangelical activists

Sexual life in Hong Kong as well as life in general are regulated by two major cultural systems, namely Confucianism and Judeo-Christianity, which share a common concern for family values and heterosexual relationships. While for a time the British government sought to address population growth and development through its support for the work of the Family Planning Association of Hong Kong and the expansion of municipal services, living conditions for the majority of the residents remain generally poor. As a result, Catholic and Protestant missionary groups[3] have become major providers of social, medical and educational services to the more socially marginal parts of the population. As suggested by Li et al. (1998), their emerging role in this respect was the result of both humanitarian and strategic considerations. By settling in Hong Kong, missionaries were able to anchor themselves on the peripheral regions of China in preparation for their goal of spreading Christianity to the mainland; they could also secure their existence by collaborating with the colonial government in restoring social order and helping the needy from the 1950s to the 1970s.

The establishment of missionary-sponsored schools facilitated the growth of religious teaching amidst increasing demands for mass education in the 1970s. However, the signing of the Sino-British Joint Declaration in 1984 posed a challenge to the partnership between the government and the Catholic and the Christian churches. Religious groups which had hitherto enjoyed a stable relationship with the colonial government, wished to retain their social status upon the transfer of sovereignty to China in 1997 (Chan 2007). This compelled them to rethink their role in Hong Kong society, given uncertainties concerning freedom of religion under the 'One Country Two Systems' rhetoric. Wong (2013) has noted that the churches' role changed from being the providers of services to advocacy in the 1980s. She further asserts that changes in the churches role were carefully calibrated between the need to restore social order and accepted means of political participation. For instance, in July 2004, a statement signed by 179 evangelical Protestants on political reform in Hong Kong, stated that controversies about the political system would only further divide the people. At the same time, it called for a clearer focus on spirituality and a greater tolerance of diverse views (Chan 2007). Capitalising on their pre-existing relationships with the colonial government and their pragmatic support for the new Hong Kong Special Administrative Region (HKSAR) Government, missionary groups managed to construct themselves as credible and reliable sources of moral authority in a predominantly Chinese society, securing their continued influence in the social service and education sectors.

Although Catholic and Protestant missionary groups have become outspoken figures on sociopolitical issues since the handover, they have been largely negative with respect to the issue of sexual diversity despite their call for a greater acceptance of diverse views (Li et al. 1998). This is most evident in the extensive media campaigns initiated by evangelical activists and conservative organisations – especially missionary groups and interest parties upholding traditional family values – surrounding the proposed Legislative Council motion to launch the public consultation on a proposed Sexual Orientation Discrimination Ordinance in 2012.[4] The evangelical activist organisation The Society for Truth and Light highlighted the issue of reverse discrimination in its media campaigns. Along with other religious bodies that claimed that homosexuality is immoral in religious terms, the organisation feared that open discussion of human sexuality would arouse inappropriate desires and tempt some students to become homosexual. As for the Hong Kong Alliance for Family (HKAF), which was founded in 2003 and maintains that family is the most fundamental unit of human societies and the key to the protection of children's well-being, it perceived the growth of the LGBT movements as a threat to the institutions of family and marriage. In line with a procreative rhetoric, the association asserted that marriage is the union of one man and one woman, fearing new legislation might lead to advocacy for same-sex marriage, raising further controversies such as adoption rights and housing benefits. With their membership comprised largely of social welfare non-governmental organisations and Protestant evangelicals, family-value-centred groups and evangelical organisations constitute a significant opposition to the advancement of the Hong Kong LGBT rights movement (Tang 2014).

In line with a 'hydraulic' model of sexuality, the Alliance also maintains that homosexuality is tantamount to hedonism and promiscuity, conflicting with Confucian ethics that stress the importance of restraining one's desires and acting according to social roles. In consequence, sexual orientation therapy has emerged as a means to 're-direct' individuals with non-heterosexual orientations to heterosexual ones. For instance, the New Creation Association Hong Kong, a Christian-faith-based non-profit organisation, has offered counselling services to lesbian and gay individuals on a voluntary basis, in the belief that a homosexual identity can be corrected through therapy. Their framing of sexual difference implies a strong heterosexual configuration, by persuading counsellees that a homosexual 'lifestyle' is destructive and that heterosexuality provides the authentic source of happiness and life satisfaction.

Despite religious conservatism and cultural stigmatisation, non-governmental groups and community organisation have been established to provide social spaces and support services for LGBT communities. In particular, Christian-affiliated LGBT organisations have emerged to counter the homophobic and transphobic discourse propagated by the evangelical groups. The Hong Kong Christian Institute, founded in 1988 by a group of Christian priests and followers, adopts a more liberal stance towards sexual minorities and has shown keen concern for human rights issues in the city over the past few decades. The Blessed Minority Christian Fellowship was established in 1992 as an offshoot group from a larger gay and lesbian organisation in the 1990s, the Hong Kong Ten Percent Club. The Queer Theology Academy is the most recent addition to the spectrum of Christian-affiliated LGBT groups, advocating for gender justice and equal rights through education and publications. The practice of queer theology is a key tenet for the Queer Theology Academy through the provision of pastoral counselling. These groups remain marginalised, however, in the larger context of Christian communities in Hong Kong. In summary, the historical Christian dominance in social services and educational institutions forms one of the major reasons for its influence in limiting open discussion of positive LGBT issues. Conservative religious values combined with traditional Confucian values form the majority views on sexualities in primary and secondary schools, thereby limiting opportunities to enact a sex education curriculum that speaks to diverse sexualities. Abstinence from any form of sexual activity is still promoted in sex education, with no mention of young people's access to condoms or contraceptives in school clinics.

Resisting heteronormativity and conditional spaces

Given lack of support within educational institutions, young people often go on the Internet to explore issues of sex and sexuality. Exposure to pornography, in particular, has been facilitated by advances in communication technology and social media, allowing young people to gain access to a range of virtual platforms on which to express their views. The rise of new social media also signals a departure from the previous assumption that young people as the major recipients of Internet information are passive consumers receiving content without criticality; rather, they are perhaps best understood as prosumers who possess the agency to appropriate various cultural artefacts and construct their sexual identities accordingly (Gauntlett 2008).[5]

Aside from the virtual world, some physical settings in urban areas also provide a relatively safe space for young LGBT community members. In an ethnographic study of Hong Kong lesbians, Tang argues that there exist conditional spaces 'within a global city where lesbian desires are often articulated through everyday existence' (Tang 2015, p. 220). These may take the form of social support groups, film festivals, lesbian cafes and bookstores. These social and cultural spaces are of particular importance to young lesbians who live with their families and are not out to their family members.

A study by Tong (2008) illustrates how secondary school students who identified themselves as tomboys sustained their sexual and gender identities through practices such as heavy smoking and the use of bawdy language which transgresses the image of a feminine, obedient and hard-working Hong Kong schoolgirl. Although they were subjected to mockery and discrimination by their counterparts, young women in Tong's study formed informal support groups in which to share their grievances and affirm their own sexual and gender identity as tomboys.

However, the general atmosphere in Hong Kong society remains sceptical and, arguably, hostile towards non-heterosexual modes of identity, expression and being – with its relatively firm grip on gender and sexual identity being underpinned by Confucian-family values and conservative Judeo-Christian ethics (Tsang 1987). Nevertheless, this does not necessarily mean that young people will be dogmatically accepting of these values and beliefs. Given rising awareness of sexual minority rights, the availability of social media for individuals to express their identities and the several victories in court cases concerning same-sex relationships, LBG youth in Hong Kong are beginning to find positive rapport to affirm their alternative sexual orientations in these conditional spaces and to advocate social change through engaging in public intellectual debates on gender and sexuality. Such trends are likely to serve as the major propellant for transforming understanding of sexual citizenship from exclusive, conservative terms to a more diversified and tolerant perspective.

Conclusion

This chapter provides discussion on the relationship between schooling and sexualities, with a specific focus on sexual minority youth in Hong Kong. By describing experiences of marginalisation and stigmatisation both within and beyond school settings and the factors causing these, structural obstacles preventing LGB youth from seeking support and assistance have been identified.

The Family Planning Association of Hong Kong, being a quasi-governmental organisation, has had a powerful role to play in constructing a normative family model and limiting discussion of sexual desire to within the framework of monogamous marriage during the British colonial era. Although the Association is not solely responsible for establishing the existing sex education curriculum, it is influential through its strong ties with the Department of Education. Along with the evangelical activists who uphold conservative interpretations of love, marriage and family, and the HKSAR Government with its desire for social stability, these three stakeholders constitute a trinity of governance which dominates sexual morality in Hong Kong society. The ongoing experiences of LGB youth in Hong Kong thus provide a glimpse into how reluctant government authorities and schools have been in responding to changing social norms and the evolving needs of contemporary societies.

As the political visibility of LGBT communities gain currency across the globe, key stakeholders in world cities such as Hong Kong need to rethink the configuration of values and practices that best promotes a sexual citizenship that is inclusive of all. Sex and sexuality education in Hong Kong should no longer be oriented towards shielding young people from discussion of gender and sexuality but should aim to recognise the diversity of human sexual and gender desire. Recognising and responding to sexual and gender differences should be actualised in pedagogical practices, in the teaching curriculum and at the policy level.

Notes

1 We focus on LGB youth with a survey of literature addressing the needs of LGB youth. We recognise transgender youth as a highly stigmatised group that has been absent in discussion on sex education in schools and faces complex issues often extending beyond same-sex desires. Instead of simply including the 'T' in 'LGBT', we opt to first focus on LGB youth in this chapter.

2 The term *tongzhi* is commonly used in Chinese societies to denote persons with same-sex attraction.

3 According to Chan (2007), Protestant communities in Hong Kong can be classified into four major groups: mainline, evangelical, fundamentalist and charismatic. Despite their differences in interpreting Christian faith, Wong (2013) suggests that there is no clear distinction among their stance with respect to the LGBT community. Given that Catholic- and Protestant-sponsored schools are the majority (Education Bureau 2016), this article will focus its discussion on these two religious groups.

4 On 7 November 2012, legislator Cyd Ho raised a motion urging the Hong Kong government to launch a public consultation on enacting legislation to protect sexual minorities from discrimination based on sexual orientation. While the public opinion survey conducted by the Social Science Research Centre at the University of Hong Kong revealed greater acceptance of the LGBT community compared to previous years, the motion was passed by a majority of members in the geographical

constituency, but was vetoed members in the functional constituency. The geographical constituency voting members are elected by all eligible Hong Kong voters according to districts. Whereas the functional constituency members are elected by
professional interest groups such as accountants and lawyers.
5 Prosumers as digital citizens actively participate in social media by voicing their
opinions on social and political issues, therefore making an impact in both online
and offline social worlds.

References

Carney, J., 2013. Police Inspector John MacLennan Was 'Hounded' into Suicide over
Homosexuality. Hong Kong, *South China Morning Post*, 2 June.

Chan, S., 2007. Christian Social Discourse in Postcolonial Hong Kong. *Postcolonial
Studies*, 10 (4), 447–466.

Cheng, Y., 2009. Hong Kong Educational Reforms in the Last Decade: Reform Syndrome
and New Developments. *International Journal of Educational Management*, 23 (1), 65–86.

Cho, M. K., 2013. *Mapping the Sexual Landscape: A Study of the Family Planning Association of
Hong Kong (1950s–1980s)*. Unpublished PhD Thesis. Hong Kong: Chinese University
of Hong Kong.

Chou, W. S. 2000. *Tongzhi: Politics of Same-sex Eroticism in Chinese Societies*. New York, NY:
Haworth Press.

Chou, W. S. and Chiu, M. C., 1992. *Pornographic Phenomenon: I am Looking at Porn Looking At
Me*. Hong Kong: Subculture Publishing. (in Chinese).

Council on the Professional Conduct in Education, 2017. *Code for the Education Profession
of Hong Kong cum Practical Guidelines (Consultation Draft)*. Hong Kong: Education Bureau,
The Hong Kong Special Administrative Region.

Delamater, J., 1981. The Social Control of Sexuality. *Annual Review of Sociology*, 7, 263–290.

Education Bureau, 2016. *Student Enrolment Statistics, 2015/16 (Kindergarten, Primary and
Secondary Levels)*. School Education Statistics Section. Education Bureau: Hong Kong
Special Administrative Region Government.

Education Department, 1986. *Guidelines on Sex Education in Secondary Schools*. Hong Kong:
Government Printer.

Education Department, 1997. *Guidelines on Sex Education in Schools*. Hong Kong:
Government Printer.

Fok, S. C., 2005. A Study of the Implementation of Sex Education in Hong Kong
Secondary Schools. *Sex Education*, 5 (3), 281–294.

Gauntlett, D., 2008. *Media, Gender and Identity: An Introduction*. London and New York, NY:
Routledge.

Ho, D. K. L., 2004. Citizenship as a Form of Governance. In: A. S. Ku and P. Ngai, eds.
Remaking Citizenship in Hong Kong: Community, Nation and the Global City. Oxford: RoutledgeCurzon, 18–33.

Ho, S. and Tsang, K., 2012. *Sex and Desire in Hong Kong*. Hong Kong: Hong Kong University
Press.

Hong Kong Executive Council, 1970. *Memorandum for Executive Council, Marriage Reform
Bill*. Hong Kong: Government Records Service.

Kong, T. S., Lau, H. L., and Li, C. Y., 2015. The Fourth Wave? A Critical Reflection on
Tongzhi Movement in Hong Kong. In: M. McLelland and V. Mackie, eds. *Routledge
Handbook of Sexuality Studies in East Asia*. London: Routledge, 188–201.

Kwok, D. K., 2015. *Research Report on the Experiences of Harassment and Discrimination Among Same-sex / Bisexual and Transsexual Secondary School Students* (In Chinese). Funded by the Equal Opportunities Commission. Hong Kong: The Hong Kong Institute of Education.

Kwok, D. K., 2016. School Experience of Chinese Sexual Minority Students in Hong Kong. *Journal of LGBT Youth*, 13 (4), 387–396.

Kwok, D. K., Winter, S., and Yuen, M., 2012. Heterosexism in School: The Counseling Experience of Chinese Tongzhi Students in Hong Kong. *British Journal of Guidance & Counselling*, 40 (5), 561–575.

Lau, S., 1978. *Utilitarian Familism: The Basis of Political Stability in Hong Kong*. Hong Kong: Chinese University of Hong Kong, Social Research Centre, Occasional Paper.

Leung, S. S., et al., 2009. Occupational Stress, Mental Health Status and Stress Management Behaviors Among Secondary School Teachers in Hong Kong. *Health Education Journal*, 68 (4), 328–343.

Li, K., Cheung, K., and Chan, K., 1998. The Social Role of Catholics in Hong Kong Society. *Social Compass*, 45 (4), 513–531.

Ma, E. K. and Fung, A. Y., 2007. Negotiating Local and National Identifications: Hong Kong Identity Surveys 1996–2006. *Asian Journal of Communication*, 17 (2), 172–185.

Ng, M. L., 1998. School and Public Sexuality Education in Hong Kong. *Journal of Asian Sexology*, 1, 32–35.

Ng, M. L. and Ma, J. L. C., 2001. Sexuality in Hong Kong Special Administrative Region of the People's Republic of China. In: B. Francoeur and R. J. Noonan, eds. *The Continuum Complete International Encyclopedia of Sexuality*. New York, NY: Continuum.

Pattie, L. F. Y. Y., 2009. Teachers' Stress and a Teachers' Development Course in Hong Kong: Turning 'Deficits' into 'Opportunities'. *Professional Development in Education*, 35 (4), 613–634.

Sanders, D., 2015. What's Law Got to Do with It? Sex and Gender Diversity in East Asia. In: M. McLelland and V. Mackie, eds. *Routledge Handbook of Sexuality Studies in East Asia*. London: Routledge, 127–149.

So, A. Y., 2004. One Country, Three Systems? State, Nation, and Civil Society in the Making of Citizenship in the Chinese Triangle of Mainland-Taiwan-Hong Kong. In: A. S. Ku and P. Ngai, eds. *Remaking Citizenship in Hong Kong*. Oxford: RoutledgeCurzon, 235–253.

Suen, Y. T., et al., 2016. *Study on Legislation against Discrimination on the Grounds of Sexual Orientation, Gender Identity and Intersex Status*. Hong Kong: Equal Opportunities Commission, Gender Research Centre, Hong Kong Institute of Asia-Pacific Studies, The Chinese University of Hong Kong.

Tang, D., 2014. Perspectives on Same-sex Sexualities and Self-harm Amongst Service Providers and Teachers in Hong Kong. *Sex Education*, 14 (4), 444–456.

Tang, D. T., 2015. Lesbian Spaces in Hong Kong. In: M. McLelland and V. Mackie, eds. *Routledge Handbook of Sexuality Studies in East Asia*. London: Routledge, 218–229.

To, S. M., 2009. Empowering School Personnel for Positive Youth Development: The Case of Hong Kong School Social Workers. *Adolescence*, 44 (174), 465–477.

Tong, C., 2008. Being a Young Tomboy in Hong Kong – The Life and Identity Construction of Lesbian Schoolgirls. In: F. Martin et al., eds. *AsiaPacifiQueer: Rethinking Genders and Sexualities*. Urbana, IL: University of Illinois Press, 117–130.

Touch Project of The Boys' and Girls' Clubs Association of Hong Kong, 2009. *A Report on the Situations of Tongzhi students in Secondary Schools*. Hong Kong: Touch Project of The Boys' and Girls' Clubs Association of Hong Kong.

Tsang, A. K. T., 1987. Sexuality: The Chinese and the Judeo-Christian Traditions in Hong Kong. *Bulletin of the Hong Kong Psychological Society*, 19 (20), 19–28.

Walker, S. and Barton, L., 2013. *Gender, Class and Education (Routledge Revivals)*. UK: Routledge.

Wong, D., 2004. (Post-)identity Politics and Anti-normalization: (Homo) Sexual Rights Movement. In: A. S. Ku and N. Pun, eds. *Remaking Citizenship in Hong Kong: Community, Nation and the Global City*. Abingdon: RoutledgeCurzon, 174–190.

Wong, W. C. A., 2013. The Politics of Sexual Morality and Evangelical Activism in Hong Kong. *Inter-Asia Cultural Studies*, 14 (3), 340–360.

Yau, C., 2016. Family Concern Groups to Protest After Hong Kong's Equalities Chief Claims Consensus on Law to Protect Sexual Minorities. Hong Kong: *South China Morning Post*.

Section 3

Well-being and health

Chapter 7

Divergent pathways to inclusion for transgender and intersex youth

Tiffany Jones

Introduction

Concepts of sexual citizenship have been applied broadly to lesbian, gay, bisexual, transgender and intersex (LGBTI) people in social research (Plummer 2003) and social policy (Brandzel 2005) – however, until recently much of this work has overlooked or conflated the experiences of transgender and intersex youth. Some writers have noted how ideas about sexual citizenship create a schism between heterosexual citizenships and other citizenship types (Brandzel 2005); other writers view sexual citizenship in terms of the 'opportunities' it provides for a wide range of groups to redefine themselves and their relations in the personal and political realms (Richardson 2000, Plummer 2003).

Richardson has defined sexual citizenship as 'a status entailing a number of different rights claims, some of which are recognized as legitimate by the state' (2000, p. 107). She describes three types of sexual citizenship claims: those that are conduct-based, those that are relationship-based and those linked to identity. Identity-based sexual citizenship rights claims are strongly influenced by the terminologies used in making a claim. In the LGBTI acronym, for example, the 'T' for transgender and the 'I' for intersex appear at the end of the list for several reasons. First, the acronym (originally GLB or LGB) used initially in the 1980s referred only to lesbian, gay and bisexual individuals and alliances, with other letters being added from the end of that decade onwards (Gunderloy 1989). Second, whilst the first three letters (LGB) describe different kinds of sexual orientation, the last two (T and I) do not define sexualities. Clarifying exactly what they *do* define has been a source of debate for the last three decades (Davis 2011), visible in the shifting terminologies and activism foci used.

Against this background this chapter compares the rights claims made by transgender and intersex youth in the decades of the 1990s and the 2010s thus far, two periods selected for their striking contrast with respect to the issues concerned. The chapter draws on secondary data from the literature on transgender and intersex youth generally and primary data from several recently conducted Australian studies including the following:

- *Writing Themselves in 3*: a Buckland Foundation-funded comparative survey of 3043 same-sex-attracted youth and 91 trans-spectrum youth aged 14–21 years (Jones and Hillier 2013).
- *From Blues to Rainbows*: a Beyondblue-funded survey of 189 transgender and gender-diverse youth aged 14–25 years (Smith et al. 2014, Jones, Smith et al. 2016).
- *E-males'*: a University of New England-Partnerships-funded survey of 273 female-to-male (FtM) transgender Australians aged 16–64 years (Jones et al. 2015).
- *National Intersex Survey*: a University of New England-Partnerships-funded of 273 intersex Australians aged 16–68 years (Jones 2016, Jones, Hart et al. 2016).

All of these surveys were completed anonymously, and the pseudonyms given to participants in the original reports are used here.

The 1990s: medical and gender aberrations

Medical and psychological intervention: one sex or the other

Until relatively recently, transgender and intersex variance were understood in terms of their potential to violate male-female social roles and norms of heterosexual marriageability (DeFranza 2015). In the early part of the twentieth century, however, Freudian psychoanalytic frames re-cast this role violation as a confusion or failure of psychological and physical development, known then as 'inversion' (Freud 1961 [1905]). Psychoanalysis and later sexology linked cross-gender identification with aberrant sexual desire, and religious and social conservatives drew the link to social degeneration and a weakening of the gender roles, particularly during the First World War, when women took over traditionally 'male' jobs and responsibilities (Halberstam 2012). To distinguish inversion from more general social anxieties about female empowerment, theorists like Otto Weininger pushed for the liberation of the invert who was psychically and physically like the 'opposite sex', arguing that 'feminine' women belonged 'at home' whilst masculine female inverts (a concept combining both butch lesbians and female-to-male transgender people) should have the right to work, marry and engage in military roles – rights more akin to those of male citizens (Weininger 1906). Weininger's work advanced rudimentary notions of sexual citizenship tying invert identity to rights; however his medical definition of inversion offered minimal opportunity for the political self-definition central to Plummer and Richardson's later theories.

Later in the twentieth century, endocrinologists and geneticists such as Henry Turner conducted genetic and chromosomal studies of young people with anatomical and physiological sex differences – characterising a variety of syndromes by the physical features and chromosomal patterns involved (Turner et al. 1963). Studies of these variations were published in academic journals such as *The Lancet* and *British Medical Journal* accompanied by black and white pictures of naked individuals displaying these syndromes, sometimes with their eyes covered by a black bar in a poor attempt at making them de-identifiable.

In psychological and psychiatric research, inversion later developed into the concept of Gender Identity Disorder (GID) as cited in the American Psychiatric Association's *Diagnostic and Statistical Manual of Mental Disorders* (versions III and IV) published in the 1980s and 1990s (Newman 2002). At worst the dominant psycho-medical discourse of the period demanded that patients' bodies and minds be 'corrected' through hormonal treatment and surgery, so as to fit the two-sex model (taking the individual from male or intersex to female, or female or intersex to male). A rigidly gendered upbringing was recommended to fix what was seen as a sex-gender alignment aberration (Money and Ehrhardt 1996). This medical perspective did not question or challenge the two-sex model of biological health and normalcy but encouraged individuals to learn how to 'pass' as either female or male. It also had implications for participants in the Australian studies described earlier. For example, in the recent *E-males* study Jay (FtM transgender, 30s) explained how 1990s psychological intervention encouraged the attitude that he was now and had always 'really' been male: 'Even seeing the parts of my body that are not that typical of a natal born male, I still see myself as male because I don't see these parts as belonging to me' (Jones et al. 2015, p. 47).

At about the same time, there was growing anxiety that transgender and intersex young people might become 'homosexual'. Warnings that girls with large clitorises would likely become lesbian and boys with small penises would become gay goaded parents into approving surgical and hormonal interventions for their children – if indeed their consent was sought at all (Dreger 2015). Preventive psychological treatment for potential homosexuality was sometimes employed in countries including the USA, especially for girls with congenital adrenal hyperplasia (Turner 1999). At best, some level of choice in treatment types and access to clinician and parent-led services and social interaction (Chase 1997) was made available to young people, depending on their clinician. Therefore, only very basic sexual citizenship rights around medical choices were available to members of these groups if at all, and the notions of sexual citizenship until recently offered very limited opportunities for medical and political self-definition, limiting options for the material bodies and the lived realities of these groups.

Social activism: conflated spaces and limited funds

Up until the 1990s transgender and intersex youth were viewed as a threat to women's rights. Some radical feminists, for example, saw them as attempting to assume women's bodies using medical technology or, alternatively, attempting to access male privilege by becoming man-like in ways that reaffirmed patriarchal power (Raymond 1994). Members of this supposedly 'aberrant' group were often made to feel unwelcome at both feminist and LGB rallies and events. However, the feminist biologist Anne Fausto-Sterling (1993) argued for the inclusion and recognition of people who fitted neither traditional expectations of male nor female biology, claiming that intersex physiology demonstrated the equality of sexes by revealing how sex traits previously argued for as distinct, are more biologically similar than previously understood. Queer theory, popularised in the 1980s and 1990s by Judith Butler and others, took a similar approach by attacking essentialist and restrictive notions of gender- and sex-based identities such as male and female (Butler 2004).

Early queer theorising was, however, so focussed on disrupting the assumed relationships between gender and sex (the alignments of maleness with masculinity and femaleness with femininity, for example) that it often overlooked important differences in experience for transgender and intersex people (casting both statuses as disrupting these alignments in similar ways, with an inadequate understanding of their different contributions). Butler's work even inaccurately applied concepts of intersex and gender transgression to people who were neither intersex nor the transgressors of the gender norms assigned to them. In one notable example, she misapplied the concept of intersex to David Reimer (Butler 2004), who was not born with a congenital sex variation but was brought up as a girl following a botched circumcision causing the loss of his penis. Significantly, Reimer did not actively transgress gender norms (he never 'desired' to have a feminine female identity or expression). He was instead a cisgender man raised in a female identity, which he resisted, who ultimately committed suicide due to feeling inadequate in a husband role (Colpinto 2000). While Reimer's story thus remains relevant to queer perspectives (and Butler's deconstruction of gender) as an example of the costs of bodily and gender role normativity, conflating his experience with that of intersex or transgender youth creates a false equivalence between his and their bodies, identities and medical experiences.

Despite the creation of the Intersex Society of North America (ISNA), which held rallies at paediatric medicine conferences in the mid-1990s (Davis 2011), until recently there were few opportunities to publish the testimonials of intersex individuals. One exception to this was *Chrysalis* – a journal focussed on transgressive gender identities and transgender people (Chase 1997). Beyond this, there was little academic or activist space available for work by and for intersex people beyond those offered by medicine or notions of gender aberration. It therefore became necessary for intersex groups to work within these two conceptual confines (Stone 1991).

In the Australian *National Intersex Survey* cited earlier, participant Barbara (trans intersex female, 40s) described having engaged in activism 'at all levels' during the 1990s in Australia (Jones, Hart et al. 2016, p. 205), participating in both transgender and intersex peer groups. Transgender activism started to attract financial support, while intersex activism faced more difficult times. By the end of the 1990s, however, social activism for transgender and intersex youth had developed new descriptors such as 'sex and gender diverse (SGD) youth', and terms such as 'sex and gender diversity' were being used inclusively to cover a very diverse range of medical and social issues (Turner 1999). Problematically, the term 'sexual and gender minority youth' could be used interchangeably for intersex or transgender or same-sex-attracted youth, so that programmes of support became conflated for all groups or simply focussed on provision for lesbian, gay and bisexual youth (O'Brien et al. 2016). Intersex issues were often overlooked but occasionally tacked on to better funded or more strongly populated work on LGBT and SGD issues.

Family and social relationships: frictions and silences

For transgender and intersex youth in the 1990s, family relationships were often fraught. In the *E-males* study, transgender people growing up during this time reported that family relationships were difficult to negotiate (Jones et al. 2015). There could be awkward social interactions with family members distancing themselves from transgender relatives, refusing to use new pronouns and names, and trying to keep the trans-identity a secret. Some transgender people experienced violence from and broken contact with their families. Doc79 (FtM transgender, 30s), an *E-males* survey participant, explained that he actively hid his transition history from his child to prevent the negative consequences he personally had experienced being passed on:

> How much stigma, and isolation and rejection have you faced as a trans person? (...) All I can do is be the best parent I can, and right now I am CHOOSING not to tell my child, to protect my child from facing any of the crap I have had to face.
>
> (Jones et al. 2015, p. 111)

As for friendships, many transgender youth felt supported by a small community of close friends, after periods of difficulty at school. This could be because friends are often chosen and therefore were selected based on their ability to be accepting of a trans-identity. A few transgender youth in the *Writing Themselves in 3* study described having created their own 'extended family' or 'second family' out of friends who had cared for them when they come out as transgender (Jones and Hillier 2013, p. 297). This helped them weather ostracism by their natal families.

Intersex people in the *National Intersex Survey* who grew up during the 1990s also said they faced silence from their parents about their intersex variation, and that parents had colluded with enforced medical intervention and gender norm training (Jones 2016, Jones, Hart et al. 2016). For example, Jacky (intersex individual, 30s), a *National Intersex Survey* participant, had their gonads removed at birth and a vagina created as a child in the 1990s. Jacky described how relationships with doctors were strongly influenced by their parents and that although their doctor had wanted to explain to them that Jacky was intersex, 'this was blocked by my parents, who then also forced the doctors to put me on oestrogen. My parents have been in denial of this since, despite the intervention being recorded as such by my doctors' (Jones, Hart et al. 2016, p. 115). Jacky tried to stop taking the oestrogen therapy in their early years as a teenager, but had been told off by both parents and endocrinologists for 'failing' to take it.

In contrast, the *National Intersex Survey* featured a few intersex individuals who welcomed early intervention. Tina (intersex individual, 30s) was operated on as a child to create the aesthetics of clinically 'normative' genitalia and began hormone therapy in her teens. She commented, 'Of course, I could not 'consent' – my parents did that on my behalf and I'm very glad that they did' (Jones, Hart et al. 2016, p. 216).

If their variation was less visible, discrimination by strangers and peers was less frequently experienced by intersex people growing up in the 1990s (some variations only impact features largely hidden in daily life such as chromosomes and genitalia). Since at the time the term intersex was almost entirely unknown outside medical circles, those with less visible variations could even talk about the variation with relatively little backlash sometimes because people often misunderstood the topic. However, those participants in the *National Intersex Survey* who had noticeable physical differences did describe instances of bullying.

The 2010s: the emergence of distinct transgender and intersex concerns

Medical and psychological intervention: decreasing versus increasing barriers

The 2010s witnessed an increased politicisation of the medical and psychological treatment of transgender and intersex people. Both the idea that gender identity variance could be traced back to prenatal hormonal exposure in the brain and understandings of gender as socially constructed enabled advance in the ways in which transgender youth were understood by medicine and psychology – impacting the decision-making process of the DSM-5 Workgroup on Sexual and Gender Identity Disorders and the International Classification of Diseases Working Group (Drescher and Byne 2012), for example. To erase the idea that transgender was a 'disorder', the *DSM-5* diagnosis was changed from gender identity disorder to 'gender dysphoria' – signifying a marked difference between the individual's experienced gender and the gender others assign them, creating significant distress. A reduction in stigmatisation of transgender people prompted calls for the Australian court system to abandon the lengthy legal process minors had to undergo when seeking bodily interventions such as puberty blockers and surgery before the age of 16 – with cases to decrease barriers to intervention for transgender and gender-diverse youth being won for those as young as 11 years old (Bannerman 2014).

In educational psychology there has also been a shift to supporting transgender students gain access to specialist expertise, and creating a network of support without the requirement for 'full transition' (Jones and Lasser 2017). In line with this, while half of the *From Blues to Rainbows* study participants had MtF or FtM transgender identities and planned to have a medical transition, the other half had non-binary or genderqueer identities and did not plan to do so (Jones, Smith et al. 2016). One survey participant Shannon (trans*,[1] 25 years), explained that for many young people in the 2010s transitioning medically was unnecessary: 'I doubt I will ever go 'all the way' to 'male' from 'female' …my life just makes more sense now. I just want to be acknowledged for who I am' (Jones, Smith et al. 2016, p. 163). The increased availability of non-binary identities and growing critique of dominant ways of being male, female or transgender allowed increased opportunities for transgender and gender-diverse youth to engage in the kind of political self-definition that both Plummer and Richardson highlight as a prerequisite for sexual citizenship.

While activism has focussed on decreasing barriers to different forms of therapeutic intervention for transgender youth, in contrast intersex activists have wished to create protections against intervention. In 2005, US clinicians and a few members of ISNA declared at a Chicago medical conference that the clinical terminology for intersex should be changed to 'disorders of sex development' or DSD (Davis 2011). Intersex advocates explained that ISNA hoped this would open the doors to greater recognition of individual needs for bodily integrity and collaboration over treatment; instead they were to experience further pathologisation (Carpenter 2016). The International Intersex Organisation (OII), for example, officially objected to the application of terms such as DSD or gender dysphoria to intersex young people in psychological and legal texts (Kraus 2015). They argued that, unlike transgender people, intersex people who are unhappy with their bodies are often unhappy *as the result of* the surgical interventions often imposed on them without consent in their infancy or youth. Intersex organisations began to ground claims to intersex variance in terms of a natural diversity in congenital biological sex characteristics – whether chromosomal, hormonal and/ or anatomical. This represented an important turning point in their advocacy for self-definition which allowed the potential for the emergence of a fuller form of sexual citizenship (within Plummer and Richardson's definitions).

In late 2012 and early 2013, the Australian chapter of the International Intersex Organisation (OII Australia) determined that terms such as sex and gender diverse (SGD) and diversity in sexes and genders (DSG) were 'confusing the media, policy makers, and the public about intersex and intersex people' because they conflated gender identities with biology, and elided 'differences between intersex and trans groups' in ways that meant transgender people were often mistakenly called on to speak to intersex people's interests (OII Australia 2013, p. 1). Historically, this meant that school and educational psychologists encouraged gender normativity for intersex youth, fearing they might grow up to be transgender (Jones and Lasser 2017). The *National Intersex Survey* revealed that many intersex students believed their school psychologists still did not know what intersex variations were. Ruth (intersex female student, 18 years) said her school counsellor 'just said it was not his area' (Jones 2016, p. 13). Educating counsellors to get the support they needed was a key way intersex students were starting to engage in rights-based activism in their schools, and many intersex students showed an awareness that their right to better mental health support at school lay in developing ideas of sexual citizenship.

Social activism: separate arenas, separate backlash

Since 2011, a key arena for transgender and gender-diverse youth activism has been education, as international agencies have drawn attention to the problem of transphobic bullying in schools. The rights of transgender and gender-diverse students to equal access to education, and to meaningful forms of sexuality education, in particular, have been recognised at the global level (United Nations 2012). At a United Nations sponsored meeting in 2016, ministers from around the world released a Call to Action against transphobia in educational contexts (UNESCO 2016). In Australia, transgender and gender-diverse students correspondingly witnessed a growing level of visibility through the work of organisations such as the Safe Schools Coalition, Ygender and others. In 2013, Australia's Sex Discrimination Amendment Act provided protection against discrimination at school on the basis of students' gender identity and expression (with exemptions for religious schools), and all states and territories have prohibited discrimination in education related to transgender issues (Jones 2015).

Specific education policy guidelines now address equal access for transgender and gender-diverse students in South Australia (South Australia Department for Education and Child Development 2017), and Tasmania (Tasmanian Department of Education 2012). These guidelines focus not so much on 'managing' the student as on managing and guiding the educational context's support such that an individual's gender affirmation is facilitated in the most beneficial way (depending on the need for privacy, change of documentation, access to amenities and/or other adaptations). *The Australian Curriculum: Health and Physical Education (F–10)* provides a definition of the term gender-diverse in its glossary.[2] It is prefaced by a statement on student diversity which highlights 'same-sex attracted and gender-diverse students' for special consideration in inclusive classrooms and in sexuality education.[3]

However, across Australia backlash to inclusion efforts for transgender students was triggered by a 2016 conservative media campaign denouncing curriculum changes and the Safe Schools Coalition's gender resources and staff, with particularly frequent criticisms being published in the Murdoch-owned right-wing newspaper, *The Australian* (Urban 2016). Elsewhere in the world there has also been resistance to inclusion efforts for transgender students, including efforts to criminalise and ban so-called 'propaganda' promoting inclusion (for example Russia, Malkin 2014). In the USA, there have been legislative attacks on transgender students, including the repeal of North Carolina's 'Bathroom Bill' which had allowed transgender students from using toilets that align with their gender identity (Piltman 2017).

For students with intersex variations, there were lower levels of activism to enhance inclusion in schools. Where there is mention of intersex students in education policies, this is mainly through 'add-ons' to provision for transgender students (see, for example, South Australia Department for Education and Child Development 2017). Instead, the main arena for social activism for intersex youth is in the field of human rights where the right to freedom from torture and the move to greater concern for bodily autonomy have been tested in the courts. Representatives of intersex groups from around the world have worked with the UN on these issues, which now takes the clear position of protecting intersex infants against enforced medical correction, supporting intersex groups' push for the right to make decisions about surgical intervention only if it is chosen later in life (United Nations 2012). The 2013 United Nations' *Special Rapporteur on Torture and Other Cruel, Inhuman or Degrading Treatment* report, for example, called on member states to repeal laws allowing the intrusive and irreversible treatment of children with intersex variations (Office of the High Commissioner for Human Rights 2015). On Intersex Awareness Day 2016, a number of UN committees and experts released a joint statement making informed consent a requirement for any cosmetic intervention for people with intersex variations (United Nations 2016).

Actions by the European Commission have paralleled the UN's lead in promoting the right to non-discrimination for people with intersex variations (European Commission 2011). Australia has banned discrimination against intersex people (Australian Senate Community Affairs Reference Committee 2013), and the legality of infant genital surgery is being tested in a growing number of legal cases. In Germany and the USA, for example, damages have been awarded for cosmetic genital surgery conducted on individuals without their informed consent (Magaldi 2015). In Australia, despite government enquiries and efforts to overhaul medical interventions for intersex youth and the requirement that interventions need to be approved by courts (Australian Senate Community Affairs Reference Committee 2013), forced intervention still takes place. Media criticism of forced surgical intervention for intersex youth has been strong, coming somewhat paradoxically from the same conservative newspapers (e.g. *The Australian*) that have been responsible for the backlash against transgender youth (see Overington 2016). These responses show how different social activism has become for transgender and intersex youth.

Family and social relationships: disclosure differences

Compared to the 1990s, the overwhelming majority of transgender youth surveyed in 2010s have disclosed their transgender status to key people in their lives (Kosciw et al. 2017). This had had mixed impact. In the *From Blues to Rainbows* survey, two-thirds (63%) of 189 participants aged 14–25 years reported having received support from at least one parent or carer for their disclosure – which differs from those in previous decades where support was usually accessed outside the original family or context of care (Smith et al. 2014). However, in this same survey fully one-quarter of the transgender and gender-diverse young people reported having experienced abuse, discrimination or harassment at home. One gender questioning young person (18 years) described having been verbally abused by several family members; 'Mum said I'd look unattractive at formal, my sister said I'd be a virgin forever and my (...) aunties and grandma gathered around me and all shouted offensive things' (Smith et al. 2014, p. 59). About two-thirds (65%) of the transgender youth sample in this same survey reported having experienced verbal transphobic abuse, and 21% had experienced physical transphobic abuse (Jones, Smith et al. 2016). The most common location for such abuse was the street (40%), followed by the school (38%).

Transgender students aged 14–25 years with supportive classmates appear less likely to have experienced discrimination at school (Jones, Smith et al. 2016). Overall, 68% of *From Blues to Rainbows* survey participants without supportive classmates reported experiencing 'social exclusion', compared to 30% of those with supportive classmates. Transgender students without supportive classmates were also more likely to report rumours being spread about them (50% *vs* 36%); graffiti being written about them (27% *vs* 3%); being bullied via social media (47% *vs* 21%); being humiliated (53% *vs* 28%); and/or having people deliberately use incorrect pronouns (50% *vs* 26%). Robin, a 21-year-old genderqueer survey participant, had no supportive classmates and said, 'I'd get called dyke, fag, freak, shemale, shim' (Jones, Smith et al. 2016, p. 166).

Supportive family relationships are an important protective factor for transgender students' mental health: the 63% of transgender *From Blues to Rainbows* survey participants with parental support were half as likely to consider suicidal thoughts as those without parental support (30% compared to 58%), and twice as likely to report seeing a health professional if they did have suicidal thoughts (32% *vs* 16%). They were also significantly less likely to report abuse in the home (15% *vs* 40%), and only half as likely to report that they had experienced depression (30% *vs* 60%). Andy (genderqueer, 22 years) explained, 'there's a forest right near my house where I walk and I like to go with my dad to vent. Being able to talk to him and being in such a nice place always helps'. Being socially encouraged to define their own gender identity in the sense of Plummer and Richardson's ideas concerning the right to self-definition as part of sexual citizenship clearly enhanced the mental health of transgender youth.

Differences in social support for intersex youth between the 2010s and the 1990s were less dramatic than the significant differences seen for transgender youth. Part of the reason for this may be that people with intersex variations growing up in the 2010s were not more likely to 'come out' about their intersex variation to people in their lives than those who grew up in the 1990s. In the *National Intersex Survey*, there was no statistically significant difference in disclosure around hereditary family intersex variations between those who were adolescents in the 2010s compared to those who had been adolescents in the 1990s (Jones, Hart et al. 2016). On the one hand, the majority of members of both groups reported that their parents generally knew of their intersex variation, but both groups generally learned about their variation in negative terms and often went through a period of suicidal ideation (60% considered suicide and 19% attempted it). On the other hand, members of both groups kept their intersex variations hidden from school staff and other people in their lives, for example, by generally only telling a few friends.

Perhaps the main difference for intersex youth coming of age in the 2010s is the existence of the Internet which offers social networking opportunities and support not so easily accessed by their counterparts in the 1990s: fully 60% of the younger generation in the *National Intersex Survey* reported having accessed intersex social support groups via the Internet (Jones, Hart et al. 2016). Accessing social support groups carries emotional benefits; 65% of those who had done so from both groups said engaging with others had improved their sense of personal well-being. In particular, accessing intersex communities enabled young people in the 2010s to have more opportunity to identify as intersex and participate in defining this concept with peers online, in ways aligned to Plummer and Richardson's notions of political self-definition as key to sexual citizenship. This led these participants to have greater autonomy in decision-making about their bodies where this was possible, as they were able to consult with their peers about possible intervention outcomes.

Cary (intersex girl, 19 years), for example, said her doctor had recently recommended reducing the size of her clitoris. However, after researching the risks using online intersex social networks, Cary rejected the proposed procedure: 'If anything I feel a bigger clit would be more fun' (Jones, Hart et al. 2016, p. 109). The Internet also offers intersex youth positive images of intersex people. Gabriel (intersex boy, 19 years) reflected that intersex young people's self-representations online are often more positive than media stories about intersex athletes such as Caster Semenya. 'They represent themselves rather than be represented... [Semenya], is the only person people talked about on the news and that was really, really bad because she was being treated as a liar or a fake woman' (Jones, Hart et al. 2016, p. 200). This quotation illustrates why notions of self-identification are so central to sexual citizenship – in being able to (re)define oneself in positive ways, intersex youth move beyond definitions which trap them in 'illness', 'fakeness' or 'correction' requirements. The availability of opportunities for self-definition for transgender and intersex youth, then, impacts opportunities for asserting sexual citizenship rights to better treatment and bodily integrity.

Discussion and conclusion

This chapter has compared and contrasted the experiences of transgender and intersex youth in the 1990s and 2010s.

It has shown that while the two groups have often been understood as coterminous, theorisation concerning the social nature of gender and the biological nature of human sex characteristics has made it clear that their circumstances and needs are very different. With the passage of time, more opportunity (particularly online) has been created for transgender and intersex youth to engage in the political self-identification and self-definition work that is so central to sexual citizenship rights claims. This has led to a push to *decrease* the barriers to surgical and hormonal intervention for transgender youth on the basis of the right to mental health and well-being, alongside a parallel move to *increase* the barriers to surgical and hormonal intervention for intersex youth on the basis of bodily integrity rights claims. There has been a corresponding increase in the visibility of transgender people in the academic literature, in everyday life and in school, alongside growing effort to protect intersex people from premature psychological and medical labelling and to maintain their privacy.

As activism on the part of transgender youth and intersex youth becomes more divergent, contemporary constructions of each group through advocacy has allowed for more appropriately tailored human rights and polity group responses to the two youth groups, better supporting individual and personal well-being. Whilst more has been done for transgender youth in terms of improving social and emotional relationships and educational services, the struggles of intersex youth have garnered greater support from conservative quarters (including the mainstream media which has generally shown opposition to transgender student rights). In the 2020s, the two groups' advocacy efforts may necessarily become more distinctive due to their different sources of support, the ways in which conservative religious groups differentiate between what they perceive to be a 'chosen' difference (gender diversity) as opposed to a 'biological' difference (intersex variation), and the manner in which policy advocacy for transgender youth may deflect attention from the needs of intersex youth.

There is clearly a need for LGBTI activism to foreground both the 'T' and the 'I' contributions with respect to Richardson's (2000) notion of identity-based sexual citizenship rights claims. Sexual citizenship concepts, however, need to be expanded to embrace the right to gender identity and expression, and the medical technologies that may enable these (including for and beyond transgender youth), alongside the right to bodily autonomy and freedom from unnecessary enforced 'medical correction' (including for and beyond intersex youth). In thinking more carefully about identity-based rights claims, however, we should guard against the tendency to assume that transgender youth and intersex youth identities or community memberships are fixed and stable. Evidence from this chapter has shown how transgender and intersex youth identities and related rights issues can change significantly over time. Instead, it is important to recognise that current identities provide shifting conceptual 'sites' in which sexual citizenship rights-claims can be argued for, refuted and negotiated over time, with very 'real' impacts for young peoples' bodies, medical care, education, social inclusion and well-being. Importantly, this chapter has also highlighted instances in which rights to freedom of gender identity and expression, and bodily integrity, extend well beyond transgender and intersex experience in social, medical or other contexts. In planning for the future, it is important, therefore, to champion such rights in both identity-based and more general sexual citizenship terms.

Notes

1 The term trans* denotes only the transgender status of a group or individual; it does not specify their gender history, gender identity or gender stability (for reasons of inclusiveness, politics or privacy).
2 See for example http://v7-5.australiancurriculum.edu.au/health-and-physical-education/glossary accessed 4.1.17.
3 See for example http://v7-5.australiancurriculum.edu.au/health-and-physical-education/student-diversity accessed 23.8.17.

References

Australian Senate Community Affairs Reference Committee, 2013. *Involuntary or Coerced Sterilisation of Intersex People in Australia – Second Report*. Canberra: Australian Parliament.

Bannerman, M., 2014. Family Court Chief Justice Calls for Rethink on How High Court Handles Cases Involving Transgender Children. *ABC News*, 17 November. Retrieved from: www.abc.net.au/news/2014-11-17/chief-justice-calls-for-rethink-on-transgender-childrens-cases/5894698

Brandzel, A. L., 2005. Queering Citizenship? Same-Sex Marriage and the State. *GLQ: A Journal of Lesbian and Gay Studies*, 11 (2), 171–204.

Butler, J., 2004. *Undoing Gender*. New York, NY: Routledge.

Carpenter, M., 2016. The Human Rights of Intersex People: Addressing Harmful Practices and Rhetoric of Change. *Reproductive Health Matters*, 24 (47), 74–84.

Chase, C., 1997. Special Issue on Intersexuality. *Chrysalis: The Journal of Transgressive Gender Identities*, Fall/Winter, 2 (5), 1–57.

Colpinto, J., 2000. *As Nature Made Him: The Boy Who Was Raised as A Girl*. New York, NY: Deckle Edge.

Davis, G., 2011. DSD is a Perfectly Fine Term: Reasserting Medical Authority through a Shift in Intersex Terminology. In: P. McGann and D. Hutson, eds. *Advances in Medical Sociology*. Bingley: Emerald Group Publishing, 155–182.

DeFranza, M., 2015. *Sex Difference in Christian Theology: Male, Female, and Intersex in the Image of God*. Grand Rapids, MI: Eerdmans Publishing Co.

Dreger, A., 2015. *Galileo's Middle Finger: Heretics, Activists, and the Search for Justice in Science*. New York, NY: Penguin Press.

Drescher, J. and Byne, W., 2012. Gender Dysphoric/Gender Variant (GD/GV) Children and Adolescents: Summarizing What We Know and What We Have Yet to Learn. *Journal of Homosexuality*, 59 (3), 501–510.

European Commission, 2011. *Trans and Intersex People: Discrimination on the Grounds of Sex, Gender Identity and Gender Expression*. Luxemburg: European Union.

Fausto-Sterling, A., 1993. The Five Sexes: Why Male and Female Are Not Enough. *The Sciences*, 1 (March/April), 20–24.

Freud, S., 1961 [1905]. *Three Essays on the Theory of Sexuality*. Trans. J. Strachey, ed. Harmondsworth: Penguin.

Gunderloy, M., 1989. Acronyms, Initialisms & Abbreviations Dictionary. *Factsheet five*, 1 (1), 32–36.

Halberstam, J., 2012. Boys Will be… Bois? Or, Transgender Feminism and Forgetful Fish. In: D. Richardson, J. McLaughlin, and M. E. Casey eds. *Intersections Between Feminist and Queer Theory*. New York, NY: Palgrave MacMillan, 97–115.

Jones, T., 2015. *Policy and Gay, Lesbian, Bisexual, Transgender and Intersex Students*. Cham, Heidelberg, New York, NY, Dordrecht and London: Springer.

Jones, T., 2016. The Needs of Students with Intersex Variations. *Sex Education*, 16 (6), 602–618.

Jones, T., et al., 2015. *Female-to-Male (FtM) Transgender People's Experiences in Australia*. Cham, Heidelberg, New York, NY, Dordrecht and London: Springer.

Jones, T., Hart, B., et al., 2016. *Intersex: Stories and Statistics from Australia*. London: Open Book Publisher.

Jones, T. and Hillier, L., 2013. Comparing Trans-Spectrum and Same-sex Attracted Youth: Increased Risks, Increased Activisms. *LGBT Youth*, 10 (4), 287–307.

Jones, T. and Lasser, J., 2017. School Psychology with Gay, Lesbian, Bisexual, Transgender, Intersex, and Questioning (GLBTIQ) Youth. In: M. Thielking and M. Terjesen, eds. *Handbook on Australian School Psychology: Bridging the Gaps in International Research, Practice, and Policy*. Dordrecht: Springer, 595–612.

Jones, T., Smith, E., et al., 2016. School Experiences of Transgender and Gender Diverse Students in Australia. *Sex Education*, 16 (2), 156–171.

Kraus, C., 2015. Classifying Intersex in DSM-5: Critical Reflections on Gender Dysphoria. *Archives of Sexual Behavior*, 44 (5), 1147–1163.

Kosciw, J. G., et al., 2017. *The 2013 National School Climate Survey. The Experiences of Lesbian, gay, Bisexual, and Transgender Youth in our Nation's Schools*. New York, NY: The Gay, Lesbian, and Straight Education Network.

Malkin, B., 2014. Vladimir Putin Signs Anti-Gay Propaganda Bill. *The Telegraph*, 7 July. Retrieved from: www.telegraph.co.uk/news/worldnews/europe/russia/10151790/Vladimir-Putin-signs-anti-gay-propaganda-bill.html

Magaldi, K., 2015. Gender Reassignment Surgery: Parents Sue Doctors for Making Their Child a Girl, Claiming Genital Mutilation. *Medical Daily*, 13 August. Retrieved from: www.medicaldaily.com/gender-reassignment-surgery-parents-sue-doctors-making-their-intersex-child-girl-347804

Money, J. and Ehrhardt, A., 1996. *Man & Woman, Boy & Girl: Gender Identity from Conception to Maturity*. Northvale, NJ: Jason Aronson.

Newman, L. K., 2002. Sex, Gender and Culture: Issues in the Definition, Assessment and Treatment of Gender Identity Disorder. *Clinical Child Psychology and Psychiatry*, 7 (3), 352–359.

O'Brien, K., et al., 2016. Sexual and Gender Minority Youth Suicide: Understanding Subgroup Differences to Inform Interventions. *LGBT Health*, 3 (4), 248–251.

Office of the High Commissioner for Human Rights, 2015. *Intersex Fact Sheet*. Geneva: United Nations.

OII Australia, 2013. 'Sex and Gender Diverse' Discussion Paper on Terminology. Retrieved from: https://oii.org.au/21550/sex-and-gender-diverse-discussion-paper/

Overington, C., 2016. Carla's Case Ignites Firestorm Among Intersex Community on Need for Surgery. *The Australian*, 8 December. Retrieved from: www.theaustralian.com.au/national-affairs/health/carlas-case-ignites-firestorm-among-intersex-community-on-need-for-surgery/news-story/7b1d478b8c606eaa611471f70c458df0?csp=4f59d201ee2c7ae8983925404ca8ea97

Piltman, J., 2017. NCAA Should Stay Out of North Carolina Until 'HB2.0' is Repealed. *Huffington Post*, 31 March. Retrieved from: www.huffingtonpost.com/entry/im-a-tar-heel-and-im-urging-the-ncaa-to-stay-out_us_58de6e7ee4b0fa4c09598873

Plummer, K., 2003. *Intimate Citizenship: Private Decisions and Public Dialogues.* Seattle and London: University of Washington Press.

Raymond, J., 1994. *The Transsexual Empire: The Making of the She-Male.* New York, NY: Teacher's College Press.

Richardson, D., 2000. Constructing Sexual Citizenship: Theorizing Sexual Rights. *Critical Social Policy,* 20 (1), 105–135.

Smith, E., et al., 2014. *From Blues to Rainbows: The Mental Health and Well-being of Gender Diverse and Transgender Young People in Australia.* Melbourne, VIC: Australian Research Centre in Sex Health and Society.

South Australia Department for Education and Child Development, 2017. *Transgender and Intersex Student Support.* Adelaide: South Australia Department for Education and Child Development.

Stone, S., 1991. The Empire Strikes Back: A Posttranssexual Manifesto. In: J. Epstein and K. Straub, eds. *Body Guards: The Cultural Politics of Gender Ambiguity.* New York, NY: Routledge, 280–304.

Tasmanian Department of Education, 2012. *Guidelines for Supporting Sexual and Gender Diversity in Schools and Colleges.* Hobart: Tasmanian Government.

Turner, H., Greenblatt, R., and Dominguez, H., 1963. Syndrome of Gonadal Dysgenesis and Abdominal Testis with an XO/XY Chromosome Mosaicism. *The Journal of Clinical Endocrinology & Metabolism,* 23 (1), 709–716.

Turner, S., 1999. Intersex Identities: Locating New Intersections of Sex and Gender. *Gender and Society,* 13 (4), 457–479.

UNESCO, 2016. *Call for Action by Ministers: Inclusive and Equitable Education for All Learners in an Environment Free from Discrimination and Violence.* Paris: UNESCO.

United Nations, 2012. *Born Free and Equal: Sexual Orientation and Gender Identity in International Human Rights Law.* New York, NY and Geneva: United Nations Human Rights Office of the High Commissioner.

United Nations, 2016. *End Violence and Harmful Medical Practices on Intersex Children and Adults, UN and Regional Experts Urge.* Paris: UNESCO.

Urban, R., 2016. Stereotype of Bullied Gay Youth Queried. *The Australian,* 21 April.

Weininger, O., 1906. *Sex and Character.* London: William Heinemann.

Chapter 8

Sexualities education and sexual citizenship

A materialist approach

Pam Alldred and Nick J. Fox

Introduction

In this chapter, we explore the production and reproduction of sexual citizenship and sexual citizens in sexualities education. We explore the impact of different models of sexualities education (constituted around teachers, school nurses and youth workers) upon the sexual and non-sexual capacities produced in young people. These capacities – for instance, a capacity to assert their rights to express specific sexual desires or a capacity to manage their fertility proactively – may contribute *inter alia* to their (sexual) 'citizen-ing'.[1]

Our objective, however, is not only to document these processes of sexual education and associated citizen-ing, but also to develop a relational and materialist perspective on sexual citizenship.

Citizenship has been conceptualised as the foundation for 'modern claims to liberty, equality, rights, autonomy, self-determination, individualism, and human agency' (Nyers 2004, p. 203); though it has been criticised conceptually as 'the worn out offspring of liberal humanism' (Shildrick 2013, p. 153). 'Sexual citizenship' has assessed societal recognition of sexual diversity (Weeks 1998, p. 35), participation in markets and public life (Evans 1993, p. 8) and access to rights of sexual expression and identity (Monro 2005, pp. 155–162, Richardson 2017, p. 211). It has been applied conceptually to study 'the balance of entitlement, recognition, acceptance and responsibility' (Weeks et al. 2001, p. 196) of different sexualities, in a variety of settings (Ammaturo 2015, Mackie 2017), but also as a rallying cry for sexual activism and resistance (Plummer 2001, Weeks et al. 2001, pp. 197–198).

Of course, creating a concept explains nothing, and may itself be the thing that needs to be explained (Latour 2005, pp. 130–131). To that end, in this chapter we develop a relational analysis of sexualities education, which we use to inform an analysis of sexual citizenship. This move, we contend, offers opportunities to step beyond notions of belonging and exclusion/transgression (Ryan-Flood 2009, p. 2, Taylor 2011, p. 588), and a binary opposition between 'citizens' (so defined by their inherent, acquired or ascribed rights or social identities) and those excluded from this attribution (Sabsay 2012, p. 610). A relational framework would instead explore sexual citizenship as emerging from the material network or assemblage of bodies, things (such as money, property), collectivities (communities, nation states), norms and values, legal and policy frameworks, and ideas (nationality, belonging, democracy).

A relational framework for sexual citizenship would concern itself with the micropolitical flows between these assembled elements (Koster 2015, p. 225): a bottom-up exploration of the continued and 'rhizomic' production and reproduction of 'the sexual citizen'. Concerns with which sexual identities are incorporated within sexual citizenship and which are excluded shifts to an investigation of how the micropolitical processes at the interface between sexualities and the social world produce 'citizenship effects' of inclusion and exclusion, security and insecurity, legitimation and transgression. It opens the door, both theoretically and practically, to a 'nomad citizenship' that can 'serve and foster the enrichment of life internally or locally, rather than thrive on and foster external threats' (Holland 2006, p. 202, see also Shildrick 2013). This replaces concern with belonging with an open-ended becoming (Braidotti 2013, p. 169), and with lines of flight rather than boundaries and closure (Alldred and Fox 2015b, Frieh and Smith 2016).

To explore such a relational analysis of sexualities education and its part in producing 'sexual citizens', we adopt a 'new materialist' approach to interactions between people and other materialities. The logic for this choice rests upon new materialism's ontological replacement of essentialist 'relations of interiority' (DeLanda 2006, pp. 9–11) – which define and differentiate people and bodies in terms of their *inherent* and relatively fixed attributes – with 'relations of exteriority' (Deleuze and Parnet 2007, p. 55). As this latter term implies, what a person or a body (or a thing or an idea) can do is an entirely external consequence of its relations to other bodies or things within a particular *contextual* assemblage. For example, in one context, a body may have 'teaching' capacities; in another context, 'cooking' capacities; and in yet a third context, sexual capacities.

This shift has the effect of de-centring analysis away from essential (sexual) 'citizens' and focussing instead upon the relational assemblage, its micropolitics and the capacities it produces in bodies. With this ontological move, 'citizenship' is de-stabilised, as it becomes clear just how contextual and contingent are the assemblages within which sexual citizens are produced (and hence how contingent are such citizen-bodies). Sexual citizenship is no longer mediated at the level of policy, law, social movements and governance, but via a multiplicity of local, contextual, contested assemblages. It is an indeterminate and unstable social flux of power and resistance produced and reproduced, asserted and contested within sexuality assemblages (Fox and Alldred 2013) that draw sexual bodies into contextual relations with many other non-human materialities.

We first set out a new materialist framework for our analysis, with specific reference to sexualities and sexualities education. We then look at empirical data from two studies of sexualities education conducted by the first author, and analyse these in terms of the sexualities-education assemblages that they reflect. We conclude by assessing the implications of these models for sexual citizenship and the possibilities and pitfalls of sexualities education for a nomadic citizenship of becoming and lines of flight.

Sexualities and the new materialism

In both the humanities and social sciences, the new materialism that has emerged since the millennium shifts focus away from post-structuralist concerns with textuality and social *construction* (Coole and Frost 2010, p. 7, Taylor and Ivinson 2013, p. 666), to assert a central role for matter within processes of social *production* (Barad 2003, DeLanda 2006). Drawing on a very wide range of disparate philosophical, feminist and social theory perspectives (Coole and Frost 2010, p. 5, Lemke 2015), these new materialisms recognise materiality as plural and complex, uneven and contingent, relational and emergent (Coole and Frost 2010, p. 29).

These new materialisms do not simply recapitulate historical materialism, and the material factors implicated in producing the world and human history extend far beyond the structural forces regarded as the drivers of social change in the classical Marxist materialism (Edwards 2010, p. 288). The world and history are produced by a range of material forces that extend from the physical and the biological to the psychological, social and cultural (Barad 1996, p. 181, Braidotti 2013, p. 3). Elements as disparate as organic bodies (a tiger, a human), things (a mountain, the wind) and immaterial things (a thought, desire or feeling, 'discourse' or ideology) may be regarded as constituent parts of a relational material universe that interacts, assembles and disassembles continually to produce the flow of events that comprises the world, history and lives – including human sexualities. The new materialisms thus cut across distinctions between mind/body (Braidotti 2011, p. 311), between appearance/essence (Widder 2012, p. 23) and thus also between 'reality' and 'social construction'.

We shall set out now the principal features of a new materialist approach (henceforth, for conciseness, we refer simply to 'materialism') in relation to sexualities. Our efforts to develop a materialist approach to empirical social study of sexuality and sexualities education have used the powerful toolbox of concepts deriving from Gilles Deleuze's (1988) reading of Spinoza, as developed and applied in the work of Deleuze and Guattari (1984, 1988), by social and feminist scholars such as Braidotti (2006), DeLanda (2006), Grosz (1994) and Thrift (2004), and by social researchers such as Fox and Alldred (2013, 2014), Renold and Ringrose (2011) and Youdell and Armstrong (2011). We draw also upon insights from Braidotti's (2011, 2013) development of a post-human philosophy and ethics of engagement that steps beyond the dualisms of nature/culture, man/woman, human/non-human to open up all kinds of possibilities for 'becoming-other' (Braidotti 2013, p. 190), including possibilities for sexualities.

Sexuality has often been treated by biological and medical scientists, as well as many social scientists, as quintessentially an attribute of an organism, be it plant, animal or human. This perspective provides an essentialist and anthropocentric model of sexualities, an outcome of which has been to define quite narrowly what counts as sexuality and sexual identity, for instance in a simplistic classification of sexualities in terms of gendered objects of desire (Lambevski 2004, p. 306). Consequently, practitioners of non-normative (heterosexual, monogamous) sexualities have been labelled as bad, mad or ill and punished/analysed/treated according to essentialist perspectives by the law, medicine, psychotherapy and other social agents (Alldred and Fox 2015a).

By contrast, materialist authors have offered an alternative 'post-anthropocentric' and 'posthuman' conceptualisation of sexuality (Probyn 1995, Lambevski 2004, Braidotti 2006, Holmes *et al.* 2010, Beckman 2011, Renold and Ringrose 2011, Ringrose, 2011). Braidotti (2011, p. 148) describes sexuality as a 'complex, multi-layered force that produces encounters, resonances and relations of all sorts', while Deleuze and Guattari (1984, p. 293) state quite bluntly that 'sexuality is everywhere': in a wide range of interactions between bodies and what affects them physically, cognitively or emotionally, from dancing or shopping to state violence or authority. Inspired by these arguments, we have used the materialist perspective that underpins them to develop an approach (and an ontology) that situates sexuality not as an attribute of a body (albeit one that is consistently trammelled by social forces) but within a new materialist understanding of the 'sexuality-assemblage' (Fox and Alldred 2013, Alldred and Fox, 2015b). Sexuality-assemblages comprise not just human bodies but the whole range of physical, biological, social and cultural, economic, political or abstract forces with which they interact: as such sexuality-assemblages bridge 'micro' and 'macro', private and public, intimacy and polity.

In this ontology, it is not an individual body but the sexuality-assemblage that is productive of all phenomena associated with the physical and social manifestations of sex and sexuality, and that establishes the capacities of individual bodies to do, feel and desire. Sexuality-assemblages shape the eroticism, sexual codes, customs and conduct of a society's members, as well as the categories of sexuality such as 'hetero', 'homo' and so forth (Linstead and Pullen 2006, p. 1299). Sexuality itself may be understood as 'an impersonal affective flow within assemblages of bodies, things, ideas and social institutions, which produces sexual (and other) capacities in bodies' (Fox and Alldred 2013, p. 769). We will now briefly consider the conceptual framework required to establish this materialist perspective of the sexuality-assemblage.

First, the sexuality-assemblage asserts the fundamental *relationality* of all matter: bodies, things and social formations gain their appearance as things in their own right only when in relation to one another. Rather than taking the body or thing or the social organisation as a pre-existing unit of analysis, we look instead at the fluctuating assemblages that coalesce to produce both events and the apparent reality of the relations that they comprise. For example, a sexuality-assemblage accrues around an event such as an erotic kiss, which comprises not just two pairs of lips but also physiological processes, personal and cultural contexts, aspects of the setting, memories and experiences, sexual codes and norms of conduct, and potentially many other relations particular to that event (Fox and Alldred

2013, p. 775). As noted in the introduction, bodies and things do not possess fixed attributes (relations of interiority) but instead gain capacities as they assemble with other materialities (relations of exteriority).

Second, a sexuality-assemblage must be analysed not in terms of human or other agency, but by considering the assembled relations' ability to *affect* or *be affected* (Deleuze 1988, p. 101). Within a sexuality-assemblage, human and non-human relations affect (and are affected by) each other to produce material effects, including sexual capacities and desires, sexual identities and the many 'discourses' concerning sexualities; these affects are qualitatively equivalent regardless of whether a relation is human or non-human. Importantly for the study of sexuality, desire is itself an affect (rather than some essential quality of a body, no matter how culturally shaped), to the extent that it produces specific capacities to act or feel in a body or bodies, be it arousal, attraction, sexual activity, rejection or whatever. An assemblage's 'affect economy' (Clough 2004, p. 15) can be understood as the forces shifting bodies and other relations 'from one mode to another, in terms of attention, arousal, interest, receptivity, stimulation, attentiveness, action, reaction, and inaction'.

Third, this emphasis on affect economies and the changes they produce in relations and assemblages provides a dynamic focus for the micropolitical study of sexuality assemblages. We may ask what a body can do within its relational assemblage, what it cannot do and what it can become. What sexual capacities might be produced in bodies by a particular assemblage of things, ideas, norms, policies and other bodies? Assemblage micropolitics, we suggest (Fox and Alldred 2017, p. 32) can be explored in terms of two affective processes: 'specification' and 'aggregation'.

Specification – founded upon the equivalent DeleuzoGuattarian terminology of 'territorialisation/de-territorialisation' (Deleuze and Guattari 1988, pp. 88–89) – may be understood as an affective process within a (sexuality) assemblage that produces specific capacities in a body or thing; other affects may *generalise* capacities, opening up new possibilities and limits for what a body can do. Sexual arousal, attraction, preferences and conduct can be understood as particular specifications produced by affects and desires within a sexuality-assemblage. So a kiss may specify a body into sexual arousal. Yet that same kiss – say from a new lover, might generalise a body into new possibilities such as polyamory or a new life begun elsewhere, what Deleuze and Guattari (1988, p. 277) called 'a line of flight'.

Aggregation, meanwhile, reflects those affects in assemblages that act similarly on multiple bodies, organising or categorising them to create converging identities or capacities.[2] In the field of sexuality, ideas and concepts such as love, monogamy, chastity or sexual liberation; prejudices and biases; and conceptual categories such as 'women', 'heterosexual' or 'perverted' all aggregate bodies. By contrast, other affects (for instance, a gift from a lover or a smile from a stranger) produce a *singular* outcome or capacity in just one body, with no significance beyond itself, and without aggregating consequences. Singular affects may be micropolitical drivers of generalisation, enabling bodies to resist aggregating or constraining forces, and opening up new capacities to act, feel or desire.

Exploring the micropolitics of sexuality, sexualities education and sexual citizenship in terms of affective movements in assemblages radically shifts the focus of attention. From a materialist perspective, sexuality needs to be seen not as an attribute of an individual human body, but as an impersonal web of intensities and flows of matter, powers and desires within and between bodies, things, ideas and social institutions, producing sexual (and other) capacities in these different materialities. How sexuality manifests has little to do with personal preferences or dispositions, and everything to do with how bodies, things, ideas and social institutions assemble. Specifying forces produce body comportments, identities and subjectivities, 'masculinity' and 'femininity'; and shape sexual desires, attractions, preferences and proclivities according to the particular mix of relations and affects within an assemblage. Sexual codes are culture-specific aggregating affects that establish the limits of what individual bodies can do, feel and desire in specific sociocultural settings. They shape the eroticism, sexual codes, customs and conduct of a society's members, as well as the categories of sexual identity such as 'hetero', 'homo', polyamorous, queer and so forth (Barker 2005, Linstead and Pullen 2006, p. 1299).

These specifications and aggregations mean that while sexuality is a generalising, multiplying, branching flow of affect between and around bodies and other relations, that has the potential to produce any and all capacities in bodies, and indeed 'subversive and unforeseeable expressions of sexuality' (Beckman 2011, p. 11), the flow of affect in the sexuality-assemblage is continuously subject to restrictions and blockages (Deleuze and Guattari 1984, p. 293). Thus specified, sexuality loses its potential, channelling desire into a relatively narrow range of sexual capacities linked to conventional desires. This, sadly, is typical within a contemporary society trammelled by codes, norms and expectations into sexual specification and aggregation, though always still with the possibility of subsequent generalisation or line of flight.

Three approaches to sexualities education

We turn now to address how sexualities education among young people contributes to the social production of sexual citizenship. The data that we subject to materialist analysis is taken from two studies conducted by the first author. The first was the two-year Sex and Relationship Education Policy Action Research (SREPAR) study, funded by the UK Department of Education and Employment as part of its strategy to reduce teenage pregnancy (Alldred and David 2007). Interviews were conducted with 17 teachers with responsibility for sex and relationship education (SRE) and 15 school nurses serving 17 secondary schools and their feeder primary schools. The second study was the 'Sites of Good Practice' study conducted in 2009, during which the first author interviewed 12 youth workers engaged in sexual health work with young people. Data from these studies have been reported elsewhere (Alldred and David 2007, Alldred 2017).

In this section we reanalyse findings from these two studies in terms of the differing material assemblages associated with the practices of teachers, school nurses and youth workers and the capacities these produce in young people. Our method of analysis differs markedly from a traditional qualitative approach.[3] For each group we paint a brief pen-picture of their material practices, before analysing the data to identify the differing sexualities-education assemblages that they reveal. Applying the new materialist conceptual framework described earlier, the first step in this process is to identify – by close reading of the data – the range of relations that assemble around events such as a sexualities education class. This also enables insight into the affective movements that draw these particular relations into assemblage (for example, a teaching affect that transmits factual information to school students). These movements (including the specifications and aggregations described in the previous section) constitute the affect economies (Clough 2004, p. 15) that surround bodies in sexualities-education assemblages. Particular affect economies produce different micropolitical effects in young people's bodies, so from this analysis we can gain an understanding of the consequences of different assemblages for the capacities produced – what these bodies can do (for instance, engage in safer sex or act sexually within a normative moral framework). These include the capacities for sexual citizenship that each assemblage produces in the bodies of young people.

At the time of the SREPAR study, Government guidance to English state schools (DfEE, 2000) located SRE within a 'values framework': to help school students deal with 'difficult moral and social questions', to 'support young people through their physical, emotional and moral development' and to learn the 'importance of values and individual conscience and moral considerations'.[4] For the teachers interviewed, SRE took place within the context of the wider educational environment of the school, and a national educational context of a defined curriculum of academic subjects. The latter underpinned an 'achievement agenda' that aimed to improve educational aspirations and engagement as a means to reduce social exclusion. This context, the study found, had severe knock-on effects upon the delivery of SRE. As a non-examined subject – and one that (like physical education [PE] and manual crafts) was a non-academic topic – it was of low status, and had to compete with academic subjects for timetable space. This was most marked in schools with high levels of academic achievement.

Low status meant less staff training and material resources for SRE, which impacted staff confidence. Teachers in the study resisted involvement in SRE, which for many was an unwelcome add-on to their subject specialism, and one where they considered they lacked educational expertise, adding to their anxieties about teaching SRE classes. One said,

(Teachers) feel underprepared for it. Being under-prepared for it is horrible: I think the biggest fear as a teacher in a situation like that is being asked a question that you just don't know how to answer.

These data enable us to locate teachers' engagement with SRE within a sexualities-education assemblage comprising at least the following relations (in no particular order).

teacher – school students – parents – information – minds – bodies – curriculum – workload – colleagues – 'achievement agenda' – classroom – tabloid newspapers – public outrage – resources – models of education and development – teachers' attitudes/sexualities

These relations assemble as a consequence of a powerful 'educational' affect, by which information/knowledge/values are passed from SRE curriculum to teacher to school student. However, the research interviews revealed a broader affect economy, constituted from the contexts noted earlier concerning schools' and the Government's orientation toward educational achievement, the limited staff, resources and time allocated to SRE as a non-academic subject, and the societal moral attitudes towards sex and sexualities. Many teachers interviewed during the SREPAR study saw SRE as a dubious response to a societal moral panic about sexualisation, and were uncomfortable about being drawn into a moral agenda. They regarded discussions of sexuality with children and young people as a parental responsibility, and only reluctantly accepted their own contribution to SRE. Even those who supported the SRE agenda resented having to take time to prepare a class in which the materials were potentially controversial, particularly as parents in England had the right to withdraw school students from SRE classes. Some (particularly older and male teachers) considered that teaching about intimate and personal matters around sexualities could negatively impact their day-to-day relationships with school students and parents. According to another teacher in the study 'You're a form teacher and you don't just want to go in and suddenly talk about sex'.

These doubts by teachers over an educational framing of SRE all reflect how this broader affect-economy constrained their capacities to deliver effective SRE in schools, in turn, detracting from their effectiveness in delivering on the SRE policy objectives concerning improved sexual health and pregnancy reduction. However, our main concern here is not with the impact upon the professionals delivering SRE, but the effects that different approaches to SRE have upon their recipients – school students and young people. For school students caught up in this teacher-led sexualities-education assemblage, the affect economy produced both a *specification* of capacities, in terms of the perspective on sex and sexualities delivered by this teacher-led educational affect-economy, and an *aggregation* of capacities that locates sexuality and sexual practices within the cultural and moral framing promoted by the SRE curriculum. We shall discuss in greater detail the implications of this specification and aggregation for students' sexual citizenship in the following section of this chapter, along with those deriving from the other assemblages we now assess.

Turning to the school nurses, the SREPAR study found that many regarded themselves as sexual health experts, with a major part to play in the campaign to reduce teenage pregnancy rates. They considered that their role was supplying up-to-date, accessible medical information that empowered school students to make informed decisions, without moral judgement. Most had responsibility for a secondary school and four primary schools, typically teaching classes for school students between 11 and 14 years, and offering drop-in sessions for individual consultations. Unlike teachers, they felt confident about their skills, communication and use of teaching aids and reported positive school student responses to a 'no-nonsense' teaching style (for instance, a competitive 'condom test' to engage boys in learning about safe sex). However, school nurses were rarely involved in curriculum design and were often underused. One nurse described being 'allowed' to sit in a 'cupboard' to run her drop-in, while another said school students 'had to brave a corridor of power' to knock on her door.

The sexualities-education assemblage involving school nurses may be summarised as

school nurse – school students – diseases – bodies – other health professionals – biomedical model of sexual health – medical information – teenage pregnancy reduction agenda – sexually transmitted infections (STIs) – condoms – teaching staff – school spaces – school rules

These relations assemble as a result of a 'health promotion' affect that educates young people's minds and bodies into safe, healthy practices. Nurses generally embraced the UK Teenage Pregnancy Strategy as a framework within which to teach about safer sex. However, study findings reveal a second powerful affective movement in this assemblage. Whether nurses conducted whole class sessions or individual consultations, they described young people as their clients, and their provision as young person-, rather than school-centred. This client-focus ascribed agency and decision-making capabilities to young people treated as possessing legitimate needs for health and sexual health information. Granting young people both sexual and moral agency recognised their potential to be moral and sexual decision makers, and to see the role of sex education as enabling them to make informed life choices. This contrasted with teachers' accounts, in which school students were considered as passive in the face of external pressures to be sexual, and devoid of agency or sexual desire themselves.

Once again, the affects in this latter assemblage produce a *specification* of school students' capacities, by placing sex and sexualities within a health approach, and an *aggregation* of sexualities and sexual practices in terms of health promotion principles that advocate practicing sex rationally, safely and healthily. Concurrent with this, however, the professional/client relationship that the nurse adopted was a *singular* non-aggregating affect that acknowledged students as sexual decision makers in their own right. The significance of these affects for young people's sexual citizenship will be discussed in the next section.

The youth workers in the Sites of Good Practice study provided sexual health and relationships work in youth groups and schools, and one-to-one work with young people. Both practices were framed as supporting young people's well-being, and reflected the general youth work principle of 'giving people the choice and the chance to make informed choices'. Youth workers were increasingly being invited into schools to contribute to SRE, recognising their expertise in engaging with young people on a range of topics. One youth worker described his aim as 'to get young people talking about sex and relationships... to get young men to take responsibility towards young women they see in relation to relationships, consent and sexual health'. Another explained his role as

> raising young people's awareness of the range of decisions and choices open to them around sex and offering opportunities for discussion and debate on the implications of particular choices; offering learning opportunities for young people to develop their capacities and confidence in making decisions ... respecting young people's choices and views, unless the welfare or legitimate interests of themselves or other people are seriously threatened.

The relations in this third sexualities-education assemblage may be represented as follows:

youth worker – young people – youth work principles (voluntarism, participation, equality, social justice) – information – services and resources – autonomy and agency – learning opportunities – responsibility – sexual subjects – schools and teachers

Unlike the assemblages around teachers' and nurses' SRE work, here the principal affect is not around information transmission, but instead supports and resources young people to make active decisions about sex and sexualities. Youth workers in the study engaged with young people as sexual subjects who were potentially sexually active, with desires, fantasies and experiences. Sexuality was a legitimate subject for discussion, not to minimise risks such as STIs or pregnancy, but as a means to enhance positive experiences and relationships, in both present and future selves.

Consequently, the affect economy in these youth work assemblages was both *generalising* and *singular* (non-aggregating) and produced a different and potentially wider range of capacities in young people than those discussed previously, including sexual autonomy, sexual responsibility and a respect for sexual diversity. Young people become sexually affective within these sexuality assemblages, opening up possibilities for their current and future sexual expression. We shall now turn to consider the implications for sexual citizenship of this assemblage, along with the two others discussed earlier.

From sexualities education to sexual citizenship

Sexual citizenship has conventionally been located as a concept that bridges public and private domains (Evans 1993, p. 64, Weeks 1998, p. 36, Plummer 2001, p. 238, Weeks et al. 2001, p. 197, Richardson 2017, p. 212), linking the world of experience, embodiment and identity with the social, economic and political forces of markets, the law and governance. The new materialist approach we have developed in this chapter approaches this connection *micropolitically*, addressing the relationality that produces capacities in bodies, things and abstract notions. Specifically, we have examined the material micropolitics of sexualities education, drawing out the different assemblages and affect economies that emerge in three differing professional approaches to sex and relationship education, and the capacities that these produce in bodies. We wish now to address how the micropolitics of assemblages and capacities contribute to sexual 'citizen-ing', to the emergence of young people with material capacities that mediate their engagement with the social world.

Thus far we have shown how the different material settings of sexualities education (including the inputs of different professionals) can have profound impacts on the sexual capacities produced in school students. As has been noted, each of the three assemblages analysed produced capacities in young people in relation to sex and sexualities. The first assemblage that we explored – the 'teaching assemblage' – revealed an uncomfortable encounter between a profession tasked with educating young minds and a top-down agenda to control their fertility; delivered by often unwilling and anxious staff within strict time constraints. The capacities of students that emerged from this conflicted affect economy were specified and aggregated into a social and moral context for sexual behaviour and reproduction.

The 'health-assemblage' that we analysed next reflected a very different professional focus upon sexual health, in this case delivered by enthusiastic professionals who saw an opportunity to use their expertise to engage students-as-clients to promote safe sex and the Government pregnancy reduction strategy. Once again capacities were specified and aggregated – but this time into a biomedical understanding of sex and reproduction, and the knowledge and skills for healthy, safe and – if possible – non-procreative sex. However, the professional/client model adopted by nurses was singular and non-aggregating, emphasising young people's capacities to make decisions. Finally the 'youth work-assemblage' was shaped by a professional ethos based upon a commitment to young people as partners in learning and decision-making, and to helping young people develop their own values (National Youth Agency 2004). Young people were treated as autonomous and potentially sexually-active, and this affect was generalising and singular, encouraging capacities of sexual autonomy, responsibility and sexual diversity, and hence a potential 'line of flight' from the kinds of specification that the other SRE assemblages produced.

These three material assemblages thus had profoundly different effects on students' capacities. Some capacities were constraining, locating sex and sexuality within narrow framings; others were expansive, opening up potential for sexual exploration and becoming. However, it would be facile simply to celebrate the latter and condemn the former. After all, knowledge of sexual health, contraception and the cultural and moral codes surrounding sexuality are valuable capacities that can limit negative consequences such as unwanted pregnancy or a criminal record; neither of which is likely to be an unmitigated line of flight. On the other hand, sex and sexuality have been the subjects of specification and aggregation for millennia (Foucault 1981) and we need to be vigilant to counter those assemblages that unintentionally impose specifications and aggregations upon sexualities.

This micropolitical analysis of assemblages supplies an innovative insight into sexual citizenship. Earlier we noted that, according to (new) materialist ontology, social production is an emergent outcome of the affective assembling of relations and the capacities these produce – there is no 'other level' of structures or mechanisms at work within this ontology (DeLanda 2013, p. 51, Fox and Alldred 2017, p. 62). Consequently, 'sexual citizenship' (and citizenship more generally) may be reconceptualised as part of the material flux of affects between humans, things, social collectivities and ideas. This flux linking human to non-human produces capacities in all these elements: in what a (sexual) body can do, feel, think and desire but also in non-human things, such as condoms and contraceptive devices or dating apps; in organisations, such as schools and health services; in social institutions, such as the law, marriage and the family; and in abstractions and social constructs, such as monogamy, nationality, democracy or indeed 'citizenship'. These capacities are, of course, themselves affective – that is, they are the means by which human and non-human relations affect and are affected.

This supplies the connection between sexualities education and the phenomenon described by scholars as sexual citizenship. By examining the material relations within SRE, we can discern capacities engendered in young people (such as safe sex, responsibility in sexual relationships or acknowledgement of sexual diversity) that permeate beyond the immediate contexts of a classroom activity or a group discussion, to produce impacts on the capacities of young people as participants in a society and a culture. The sexualities education assemblages we have described – and the knowledge, skills, subjectivities and identities these variously produce – contribute not only to young people's capacities to participate or not participate in sexual encounters, but also to the wider social context within which human sexualities are located.[5]

Of course, young people's capacities are not simply an outcome of the assemblages we have analysed here: what a young body (or young 'citizen') can do sexually will be a consequence of all the events, actions and interactions that together constitute a life, from sexual encounters, interactions with peers (Alldred and Fox 2015b), engagements with sexualised media and pornography (Fox and Bale 2018), interactions not normally considered sexual (Austin 2016) and so on. There will be a myriad of specifications, aggregations, generalisations and dis-aggregations of capacities that together produce 'the sexual' and the phenomena that comprise 'sexual citizenship'. This suggests a research agenda to explore the wider micropolitical production of sexual citizenship in events both sexual and non-sexual.

However, the value of a micropolitical analysis extends beyond mere scholarly interest or a conceptual rethinking of sexual citizenship to suggest practical applications. If we can 'reverse engineer' assemblages such as the educational support and development of young people we looked at in this chapter to understand their micropolitics and the capacities they variously produce, the same ontology may be used to 'forward engineer' or re-design these and other assemblages to foster positive sexual and other capacities in participants. In terms of sexualities education, this opens the way to design pro-actively educational and participation engagements around sexualities that address the needs of students from the earliest days of school through to adulthood, opening up opportunities both for sexual lines of flight and for safe, healthy, diverse, responsible and pleasurable participation in the sexual and sociological world; in other words, of sexual citizen-ing.

By exploring the affective flows and the capacities produced in different sexualities education assemblages we have developed a micropolitical analysis. This not only reveals the specifications and aggregation of young people's capacities, generalisations and lines of flight that sexualities education and development can produce but also makes connections back to the concerns of sexual citizenship scholars with sexual diversity, sexual rights and participation. We have argued that a materialist approach not only offers a means to make sense of different approaches to sexualities education but also to explore how education can be used to support young people's sexual and social engagement (Aggleton and Campbell 2000). It has not escaped our attention that this conclusion may be applied beyond the confines of primary and secondary education, to all those within a society or culture.

In the process, we have unsettled the concept of sexual citizenship. We have stepped away from essentialist and anthropocentric notions founded within the binary of belonging/exclusion to address citizenship instead as an emergent property of a material and more-than-human network or an assemblage of bodies, things, collectivities, ideas and social constructs: a flux that draws human and non-human into an affective engagement that is a part of the wider process of social production. From such a perspective, citizenship can never be a simple process whereby bodies are either assimilated into a cultural milieu or cast out as transgressive, to plough their own counter-cultural furrow (see also Ryan-Flood 2009, p. 186, Taylor 2011, p. 588). Social life is substantially more complex than the notion of citizenship implies, and sexual citizenship is not a state but a continual, becoming, 'citizen-ing' that connects human bodies to a more-than-human assemblage of sexualities and the social and natural world.

Notes

1 We coin this neologism to emphasise the processual character of becoming-citizen that we describe in this paper.
2 This aggregative/singular distinction replaces the equivalent terms 'molar' and 'molecular' in Deleuze and Guattari's (1984, pp. 286–288) conceptual toolkit.
3 For a fuller account of this methodology, see Fox and Alldred (2015).
4 As we write, the Government in England is introducing new frameworks for relationships and sexuality education in primary and secondary schools (Long 2017).
5 Though in the studies we have reported here we have focussed on the production and reproduction of embodied human capacities in sexualities education classes, elsewhere we have explored in greater detail the broader affectivity of sexualities education (Alldred and Fox, 2015b, Alldred *et al.* 2016) and indeed the post-human production of sexualities more generally (Fox and Alldred 2013).

References

Aggleton, P. and Campbell, C., 2000. Working with Young People – Towards an Agenda for Sexual Health. *Sexual and Relationship Therapy*, 15 (3), 283–296.

Alldred, P., 2017. Sites of Good Practice: How Do Education, Health and Youth Work Spaces Shape Sex Education? In: F. Sanjakdar and A. Yip, eds. *Critical Pedagogy, Sexuality Education, and Young People*. New York, NY: Peter Lang.

Alldred, P. and David, M., 2007. *Get Real about Sex. The Politics and Practice of Sex Education*. Maidenhead: Open University Press.

Alldred, P. and Fox, N. J., 2015a. From 'Lesbian and Gay Psychology' to a Critical Psychology of Sexualities. In: I. Parker, ed. *Handbook of Critical Psychology*. London: Routledge, 200–209.

Alldred, P. and Fox, N. J., 2015b. The Sexuality Assemblages of Young Men: A New Materialist Analysis. *Sexualities*, 18 (8), 905–920.

Alldred, P., Fox, N., and Kulpa, R., 2016. Engaging Parents with Sex and Relationship Education: A UK Primary School Case Study. *Health Education Journal*. E-Pub ahead of print: http://hej.sagepub.com/content/early/2016/03/11/0017896916634114

Ammaturo, F. R., 2015. The 'Pink Agenda': Questioning and Challenging European Homonationalist Sexual Citizenship. *Sociology*, 49 (6), 1151–1166.

Austin, J. I., 2016. Dancing Sexual Pleasures: Exploring Teenage Women's Experiences of Sexuality and Pleasure Beyond 'Sex'. *Sex Education*, 16 (3), 279–293.

Barad, K., 1996. Meeting the Universe Halfway: Realism and Social Constructivism without Contradiction. In: L. H. Nelson and J. Nelson, eds. *Feminism, Science and the Philosophy of Science*. Dordrecht: Kluwer, 161–194.

Barad, K., 2003. *Posthumanist* Performativity: Toward an Understanding of How Matter Comes to Matter. *Signs*, 28 (3), 801–831.

Barker, M., 2005. 'This is My Partner, and This is My … Partner's Partner': Constructing a Polyamorous Identity in a Monogamous World'. *Journal of Constructivist Psychology*, 18 (1), 75–88.

Beckman, F., 2011. Introduction: What Is Sex? An Introduction to the Sexual Philosophy of Gilles Deleuze. In: F. Beckman, ed. *Deleuze and Sex*. Edinburgh: Edinburgh University Press, 1–29.

Braidotti, R., 2006. *Transpositions*. Cambridge: Polity.

Braidotti, R., 2011. *Nomadic Theory*. New York, NY: Columbia University Press.

Braidotti, R., 2013. *The Posthuman*. Cambridge: Polity.

Clough, P. T., 2004. Future Matters: Technoscience, Global Politics, and Cultural Criticism. *Social Text*, 22 (3), 1–23.

Coole, D. H. and Frost, S., 2010. Introducing the New Materialisms. In: D. H. Coole and S. Frost, eds. *New Materialisms. Ontology, Agency, and Politics*. London: Duke University Press, 1–43.

DeLanda, M., 2006. *A New Philosophy of Society*. London: Continuum.

DeLanda, M., 2013. *Intensive Science and Virtual Philosophy*. London: Bloomsbury Academic.

Deleuze, G., 1988. *Spinoza: Practical Philosophy*. San Francisco, CA: City Lights.

Deleuze, G. and Guattari, F., 1984. *Anti-Oedipus: Capitalism and Schizophrenia*. London: Athlone.

Deleuze, G. and Guattari, F., 1988. *A Thousand Plateaus*. London: Athlone.

Deleuze, G. and Parnet, C., 2007. *Dialogues II*. New York, NY: Columbia University Press.

Department for Education and Employment (DfEE), 2000. *Sex and Relationship Education Guidance* (Circular 0116/2000). London: DfEE.

Edwards, J., 2010. The Materialism of Historical Materialism. In: D. H. Coole and S. Frost, eds. *New Materialisms. Ontology, Agency, and Politics*. London: Duke University Press, 281–298.

Evans, D., 1993. *Sexual Citizenship: The Material Construction of Sexualities*. London: Routledge.

Foucault, M., 1981. *The History of Sexuality Vol.1: The Will to Knowledge*. Harmondsworth: Pelican.

Fox, N. J. and Alldred, P., 2013. The Sexuality-Assemblage: Desire, Affect, Anti-humanism. *Sociological Review*, 61 (6), 769–789.

Fox, N. J. and Alldred, P., 2014. New Materialist Social Inquiry: Designs, Methods and the Research-Assemblage. *International Journal of Social Research Methodology*, 18 (4), 399–414.

Fox, N. J. and Alldred, P., 2015. Inside the Research-Assemblage: New Materialism and the Micropolitics of Social Inquiry. *Sociological Research Online*, 20 (2), 6. www.socres online.org.uk/20/2/6.html

Fox, N. J. and Alldred, P., 2017. *Sociology and the New Materialism*. London: Sage.

Fox, N. J. and Bale, C., 2018. Bodies, Pornography and the Circumscription of Sexuality: A New Materialist Study of Young People's Sexual Practices. *Sexualities*, 21 (3), 393–409.

Frieh, E. C. and Smith, S. H., 2016. Lines of Flight in Sex Education: Adolescents' Strategies of Resistance to Adult Stereotypes of Teen Sexuality. *Sexualities, 21 (3), 393–409*.

Grosz, E., 1994. *Volatile Bodies*. Bloomington: Indiana University Press.

Holland, E., 2006. Nomad Citizenship and Global Democracy. In: M. Fuglsang and B. M. Sørensen, eds. *Deleuze and the Social*. Edinburgh: Edinburgh University Press, 191–206.

Holmes, D., O'Byrne, P., and Murray, S. J., 2010. Faceless Sex: Glory Holes and Sexual Assemblages. *Nursing Philosophy*, 11 (4), 250–259.

Koster, M., 2015. Citizenship Agendas, Urban Governance and Social Housing in the Netherlands: An Assemblage Approach. *Citizenship Studies*, 19 (2), 214–228.

Lambevski, S. A., 2004. Movement and Desire: On the Need to Fluidify Academic Discourse on Sexuality. *GLQ: A Journal of Lesbian and Gay Studies*, 10 (2), 304–308.

Latour, B., 2005. *Reassembling the Social. An Introduction to Actor Network Theory*. Oxford: Oxford University Press.

Lemke, T., 2015. New Materialisms: Foucault and the 'Government of Things'. *Theory, Culture & Society*, 32 (4), 3–25.

Linstead, S. and Pullen, A., 2006. Gender as Multiplicity: Desire, Displacement, Difference and Dispersion. *Human Relations*, 59 (9), 1287–1310.

Long, R., 2017. *Sex and Relationships Education in Schools (England)*. House of Commons Library briefing paper 06103, 9 June 2017. London: House of Commons.

Mackie, V., 2017. Rethinking Sexual Citizenship: Asia-Pacific Perspectives. *Sexualities*, 20 (1–2), 143–158.

Monro, S., 2005. *Gender Politics*. London: Pluto Press.

National Youth Agency (NYA), 2004. *Ethical Conduct in Youth Work: A Statement of Values and Principles from the National Youth Agency*. Leicester: National Youth Agency.

Nyers, P., 2004. Introduction: What's Left of Citizenship? *Citizenship Studies*, 8 (3), 203–215.

Plummer, P., 2001. The Square of Intimate Citizenship: Some Preliminary Proposals. *Citizenship Studies*, 5 (3), 237–253.

Probyn, E., 1995. Queer Belongings: The Politics of Departure. In: E. Grosz and E. Probyn, eds. *Sexy Bodies*. London: Routledge, 1–18.

Renold, E. and Ringrose, J., 2011. Schizoid Subjectivities? Re-theorizing Teen Girls' Sexual Cultures in an Era of 'Sexualization'. *Journal of Sociology*, 47 (4), 389–409.

Richardson, D., 2017. Rethinking Sexual Citizenship. *Sociology*, 51 (2), 208–224.

Ringrose, J., 2011. Beyond Discourse? Using Deleuze and Guattari's Schizoanalysis to Explore Affective Assemblages, Heterosexually Striated Space, and Lines of Flight Online and at School. *Educational Philosophy and Theory*, 43 (6), 598–618.

Ryan-Flood, R., 2009. *Lesbian Motherhood. Gender, Families and Sexual Citizenship*. Basingstoke: Palgrave Macmillan.

Sabsay, L., 2012. The Emergence of the Other Sexual Citizen: Orientalism and the Modernisation of Sexuality. *Citizenship Studies*, 16 (5–6), 605–623.

Shildrick, M., 2013. Sexual Citizenship, Governance and Disability: From Foucault to Deleuze. In: S. Roseneil, ed. *Beyond Citizenship?* Basingstoke: Palgrave Macmillan, 138–159.

Taylor, C. A. and Ivinson, G., 2013. Material Feminisms: New Directions for Education. *Gender and Education*, 25 (6), 665–670.

Taylor, Y., 2011. Lesbian and Gay Parents' Sexual Citizenship: Costs of Civic Acceptance in the United Kingdom. *Gender, Place & Culture*, 18 (5), 583–601.

Thrift, N., 2004. Intensities of Feeling: Towards a Spatial Politics of Affect. *Geografiska Annaler Series B Human Geography*, 86 (1), 57–78.

Weeks, J., 1998. The Sexual Citizen. *Theory, Culture & Society*, 15 (3), 35–52.

Weeks, J., Heaphy, B., and Donovan, C., 2001. *Same Sex Intimacies: Families of Choice and Other Life Experiments*. London: Routledge.

Widder, N., 2012. *Political Theory after Deleuze*. London: Continuum.

Youdell, D. and Armstrong, F., 2011. A Politics beyond Subjects: The Affective Choreographies and Smooth Spaces of Schooling. *Emotion, Space and Society*, 4 (3), 144–150.

Chapter 9

Constraints and alliances

LGBTQ sexuality and the neo-liberal school

Jessica Fields, Jen Gilbert, Laura Mamo and Nancy Lesko

In the USA, sexuality education has long been a means of not only promoting health and well-being but also constraining models of sexual citizenship. Whether school- or community-based, whether offered explicitly in the classroom or implicitly in the hallway, instruction about sexual decision-making, relationships and puberty deploys 'the discourses and practices of inclusion and exclusion, of belonging and otherness, and the many shades in between' (Cossman 2007, p. 5). As they affirm norms of membership and belonging, school-based lessons about sexuality teach students 'not only how to take care of themselves and others but also how they and others fit (or do not fit) in the world' (Fields and Hirschman 2007). Curricula and instruction regularly associate 'fitness' with normative expectations – pursuing heterosexual partnerships and monogamous coupling, delaying parenting and becoming self-governing autonomous subjects (Fields et al. 2015, Garcia and Fields 2017, Quinlivan 2017).

As teachers educate students in the terms of sexual citizenship, they also participate in creating and reproducing social inequalities (Elliott 2014, see also Connell and Elliott 2009, McAvoy 2013, Bay-Cheng 2017). These inequalities are particularly pronounced for young people of colour, lesbian, gay, bisexual, transgender and queer (LGBTQ) youth and young people living in poverty – all of whom learn about their claims to sexual citizenship within a context of systemic oppression and marginalisation (Santelli et al. 2006, Fields 2008, Quinlivan et al. 2014). Across neo-liberal policies, curricula and pedagogy, students hear that their well-being rests on making good decisions – that is, their health and well-being depend on their becoming what Sinikka Elliott has described as 'responsible sexual agents' who are 'self-managing, self-responsible, and desiring self-advancement' and who 'conform to, rather than challenge, existing institutional arrangements' (2014, p. 212). Responsible sexual agents 'make healthy choices' and do not invite risk into their lives; and they do not adopt sexual behaviours that lead to infection, disease, unwanted pregnancies, or violence. Instead, they pursue relationships, identities, and knowledge that position them to thrive in institutions and communities marked by purportedly meritocratic competition. Systemic disadvantage and the influence of entrenched racism, misogyny, poverty and ableism on people's intimate lives are obscured. So too are the ways students and educators are 'intimately linked with others' through pleasure and violence in relationships that are pursued, chosen, overt, sustained and not (Elliott 2014, p. 222).[1] Mutuality, interdependence, empathy and alliance are muted in favour of lessons about individual responsibility and accountability.

LGBTQ sexualities and lives assume a particular form within these individualising neo-liberal logics. Contemporary debates about schooling, well-being and citizenship increasingly highlight the vulnerability of LGBTQ youth across racial and socio-economic categories to pervasive harassment and discrimination, affecting everything from academic achievement to self-confidence and mental well-being (Kosciw et al. 2013, Watson and Russell 2016). Bullying, harassment, mental health or academic underachievement become the terms through which LGBTQ youth are routinely identified and hailed, even by their advocates. Waidzunas (2011) describes 'the looping effects' of this conflation: the ubiquity of accounts of gay suicide and the reliance on statistics linking LGBTQ youth to suicide creates subjects who understand their sexual identities as linked to self-harm and their struggles for recognition and legitimacy as the product of poor individual choices – not systemic disadvantage. In addition, this individualism 'places responsibility on the sufferer to relieve one's suffering through complacency with oppression and assimilation into heteronormative social structures' (Grzanka and Mann 2014, p. 387). This narrow focus on victimisation affirms the neo-liberal assumption that sexual health and justice for LGBTQ youth rests on individual well-being and young people's capacity to manage, regulate and advance themselves. Even as anti-bullying instruction and programmes address bullying, harassment and other violence as social problems, they may also advance LGBTQ health and citizenship without addressing structural or institutional constraints (Payne and Smith 2013).

In this chapter, we begin by exploring anti-bullying efforts as part of broader neo-liberal, school-based sexuality education efforts. Next, we describe *The Beyond Bullying Project*, a school-based storytelling and research project that aimed to push beyond the thinking that guides many contemporary anti-bullying efforts. The project began with a commitment to examine LGBTQ sexuality as it intersects with other categories of difference and to redefine the bounds of belonging and membership. Once inside high schools, however, we found that racialised expectations of assimilation and accountability shaped not only LGBTQ sexuality but also educators' and administrators' responses to the project's effort to consider LGBTQ sexuality beyond conventional school-based framings of health and citizenship. Through a focussed ethnographic examination of one school, we explore the entanglements of well-being, citizenship and intervention in neo-liberal schooling. We find that neo-liberal forces locate not only schools but also LGBTQ sexualities and gender inside racialised educational markets that require students to become self-regulating actors. And yet, in the midst of these constraining conditions, possibilities for unlikely alliances that interrupt this persistent neo-liberal script emerged, however fleetingly. In conclusion, we consider possibilities for fostering and asserting alternative models of citizenship, membership and belonging.

Anti-gay bullying and neo-liberal interventions

Neoliberalism has done 'profound damage to democratic practices' (Shenk 2015, see also Brown 2015). Principles of participation, access and protection are compromised as concerns with systemic obstacles and institutionalised violence are muted, even as long-standing racialised, gendered, sexual and classed hierarchies continue to shape people's access to social inclusion, mobility and prosperity. On the one hand, neoliberalism promises that self-regulating and -disciplined actors can succeed as citizens in a just society. On the other hand, it masks the social inequalities that advantage some (usually white, affluent, straight, able-bodied, cisgender, men) at the expense of others (for example, people of colour, LGBTQ people, poor people, people with disabilities, women).

In the peer relationships that fill young people's days at school, students meet this tension between the possibilities and limits to the support and resources they expect from others. Despite an increasing awareness and official intolerance of anti-gay sentiment, 'gay' remains a slur among young people (Pascoe 2011) and students and staff routinely ignore anti-gay bullying (Russell et al. 2016). Routinely, the educational institutions preparing young people for adulthood and citizenship – the institutions in which most young people spend most of their days – offer limited guidance, or worse, lessons that compromise LGBTQ young people's well-being (Biegel 2010, Robinson and Espelage 2011, Gilbert 2014).

The problem is not always inadequate or misplaced attention. A sense of crisis surrounding LGBTQ young people's well-being has sparked legal, policy and curricular reform focussed on protecting LGBTQ youth from bullying; minimising risks of depression and suicide for LGBTQ youth; and reforming or, if all else fails, punishing those who violate expectations of tolerance. Education researchers and community workers have advocated and studied a range of anti-bullying programmes and policies from educational curricula (Greytak et al. 2013, C. Mayo 2013, Meyer, 2015, 2016) to Gay-Straight Alliance (GSAs) (Walls et al. 2010, J. B. Mayo 2013, Fetner and Elafros 2015) to 'safe space' policies (Loutzenheiser and Moore 2009) to zero-tolerance policies (Snapp et al. 2015).

An emphasis on self-regulation and a denial of systemic inequalities shapes many of these contemporary efforts. The commitment to confront sexual injustice and inequality and to stem the anti-gay sentiment that threads through most school days cannot be separated from neo-liberal institutions and cultural logics. Inevitably, the care that contemporary anti-bullying efforts offer LGBTQ people is entangled with individualising narratives of success and well-being (Meyer 2016). Anti-bullying sexuality education may imagine a kinder, gentler school in which LGBTQ sexuality is valued and homophobic bullies are reformed. However, the path to that school 'has allowed for expanding mechanisms

of control' (Meyer 2016, p. 357). Too often, neo-liberal anti-gay bullying education locates the violence in the poor choices an individual student or teacher
makes, not in the cultural or structural conditions of schooling. Individual
pathologies – not social forces – are cast as the source of homophobic violence
and thus the preferred site of intervention. A 'gentle neoliberalism' emerges, a
discourse that presents itself as addressing a social problem – bullying in this
case – in a purportedly humane way while simultaneously encouraging more
surveillance (Meyer 2016). Like other neo-liberal projects, this focus on individual risks obscuring inequalities systemic to heterosexist and patriarchal social
conditions (Talburt 2004, Garcia 2012, Payne and Smith 2012).

Rethinking health, citizenship and sexuality: an attempt to think 'beyond'

The Beyond Bullying Project, a storytelling and research project located in US high
schools and funded by the Ford Foundation, sought to interrupt this obfuscation
by moving away from understanding LGBTQ health and well-being through
discourses of bullying and vulnerability towards recognising the ordinary and
conflicted renderings of membership, belonging, and LGBTQ sexuality and gender that circulate in schools (Fields et al. 2014). The project team used storytelling
as a means to recognise the 'complex personhood' (Gordon 2008) of LGBTQ
students and teachers, and the diverse relationships that *all* members of school
communities have with LGBTQ sexuality and gender. The project invited, archived and analysed student and educator stories of LGBTQ sexuality and gender, asking how school communities might welcome 'complicated conversations'
(Pinar 2012) that push beyond bullying and that cast health and citizenship as
capaciously as possible. Central to our approach was an insistence that LGBTQ
sexuality is not simply an attribute of the self, cordoned off in the body of gay
teenagers, but rather a relation or network of relations, moving through the
school corridors, pulling some people together and holding others apart.

The authors of this chapter, all lead *Beyond Bullying Project* researchers, hired
and trained graduate student research assistants, secured institutional review
board (IRB) approval, and established a local school partnership in three cities –
Minneapolis, New York and San Francisco. The team worked with the Bay Area
Video Coalition to install a storytelling booth, an 8' × 5' × 7.5' wooden box, in
each school for two weeks. On the first Monday, graduate students and faculty
researchers began inviting students, teachers and staff to enter the booth and tell
a story about LGBTQ sexualities. The pitch invited ambivalence and ambiguity:
stories could be about storytellers, their families, their friends, or a cultural or
political event; stories did not need to be true. Student ambassadors made the
booths part of the school: they decorated the boxes with construction paper, ban-
ners and rainbow boas; made announcements about the project in classrooms
and assemblies; and gathered outside the booth during lunches, between classes
and when they could get out of class.

Before entering the booth, storytellers completed a brief demographic survey and provided their informed consent or assent to record and/or share their stories. Once inside the booth, storytellers encountered a high-quality digital camera on a tripod. A small carpet covered the floor, and foam covered the walls; storytellers might be able to hear murmurings beyond the booth, especially during lunch periods and between classes, but no one outside could hear what they said inside. Once storytellers were seated, a member of the research team clipped a microphone to their shirt and adjusted the camera angle. During this preparatory work, storytellers wrote their names on a clapperboard. Then the researcher left the booth and shut the door. Storytellers held the slate in front of them, called out 'Action!' and began telling a story. When they had finished, they unclipped the mic, knocked on the door and waited briefly for a researcher to let them out. Across three schools, we recorded 367 visits to the booths by 306 unique storytellers. Some recordings included several storytellers with multiple, competing stories, yielding a total of over 450 stories told. Stories run from a few seconds to over 30 minutes long. They include goofing around, pleas for justice, memories of middle school, tales of friends and family, commentary on political and cultural issues, and personal narratives of desire and its obstacles. The stories documented the landscapes of LGBTQ sexualities in education, rhythms of the school day and new relational modes that complicate the narrative about LGBTQ sexualities in schools (Gilbert et al. forthcoming).

We also conducted what the team calls 'flash ethnography', an intensive, immersive participant observation effort that explored the implications of the project for schools. Throughout the day, researchers jotted notes and then wrote extensive field notes in which they recorded student, teacher and staff interaction with the booth and the project. The team also interviewed approximately 25 students, teachers and staff members in each school to learn more about the school climate, the conversations underway about LGBTQ sexualities and the impact of *The Beyond Bullying Project* on those conversations (see Gilbert et al. 2018 for an overview). This data helped us understand the booth and larger project as objects that students, teachers and staff encountered. The flash ethnography afforded a picture of the specific ways the discourse of bullying and neo-liberal anti-bullying interventions filled students' and teachers' imaginations. The participant observation and interviews also illuminated how efforts to move 'beyond bullying' interrupted or failed to interrupt that discourse and its neo-liberal determinants (Lesko et al. 2018).

Our team began the study with a series of questions about schools as sites of citizenship and health education: what would be required of school that decided to welcome stories of LGBTQ sexuality that reached beyond bullying discourse and interventions? How might a school have to reimagine sexual citizenship? How might our framing of LGBTQ sexuality contest or support school-based renderings of health and well-being as matters of self-regulation and responsibility? In each school, neo-liberal ideologies and practices impacted our efforts to address these questions. For example, in San Francisco, anti-bullying tenets of tolerance, intervention and vulnerability influenced educators' welcome of the project. In New York, *The Beyond Bullying Project* helped the school principal satisfy requirements that the school affirm LGBTQ belonging; superficial engagement with the project averted a more substantial rethinking of sexual citizenship. Although neo-liberal conditions were present in each of the three schools, we focus in this chapter on a single school in order to provide a detailed discussion of constraints and alliances present. Central High School,[2] a comprehensive public school in Minneapolis, embraced the project with particular enthusiasm, reflecting the school's vulnerability in a racialised neo-liberal educational market and the power of LGBTQ-affirming instruction in that market.

Beyond Bullying goes to school: the neo-liberal conditions of Central High School

After an initial introduction by Professor J. B. Mayo, a colleague from the University of Minnesota and a *Beyond Bullying Project* collaborator, Central High School's principal James Nivens welcomed us to the school. Nivens was a white man with a graduate degree from an elite West Coast US university, which had a long-standing reputation for social justice education. He appreciated the team's critique of conventional anti-bullying policies and our interest in stories of LGBTQ sexuality and well-being that are muted by concerns with victimisation. He also understood the project to be a source of additional resources – including increased status, reputation and an opportunity to demonstrate that Central High School was a diverse and progressive community. The team learned on our first day of fieldwork that the school would host a meeting for the families of incoming ninth graders the following week; Nivens planned to boast about the project to them. A few days before that meeting, Nivens wrote about *The Beyond Bullying Project* on his school blog. He explained to blog readers that the project was pivotal to his aim of 'empowering' young people to share their stories about LGBTQ issues. He also welcomed the opportunity to think about LGBTQ sexuality, health and community beyond concerns about violence and harassment.

As Nivens discussed on his blog, an invitation to stories of LGBTQ sexuality was integral to his goal of creating an inclusive learning community in which all students are supported in their pursuit of success; the project also enhanced his commitment to creating a school characterised by clear expectations and rewards for positive student behaviour. For Nivens, such a community was a goal always in sight and strived for, even if never fully reached. He understood inclusion and welcome to be processes, not endpoints, and he was willing to think within that ambiguity. And yet Nivens could not be endlessly patient; his enthusiasm for *The Beyond Bullying Project* reflected pressing ambitions for Central. In 2011, Minneapolis Public Schools had charged Nivens with rebuilding Central High School's reputation, intellectual standing and disciplinary culture, and, according to many measures, he had been successful. He closed the campus at lunch, allowing only junior and senior students with perfect attendance records to leave the building. He and his staff also instituted regular 'hall sweeps' to encourage students to become the self-regulating students Nivens believed Central needed: in class and ready to work when the bell rang.

These disciplinary efforts were beginning to pay off when *The Beyond Bullying Project* arrived. While *no* families had listed Central High as their first choice in the city's school lottery in 2012, Central was the first choice of over 250 students in 2014. Student participation in extracurricular activities was up, and the school had raised funds to support a public art installation. Nivens established a partnership with the University of Minnesota to recruit a racially diverse pool of student teachers who would partner with established teachers. The aim was twofold: to help novice teachers learn from mentors with long-term classroom experience; and to help experienced teachers gain access to innovative ideas in pedagogy and curriculum. Nivens planned to recruit the mentored novice teachers to join Central's full-time teaching staff. Morale was improving at Central.

Through these efforts, Nivens hoped to secure Central's long-term survival in a neo-liberal educational market marked by competition and calls for self-regulating citizens. However, he also wanted to respond to the public health problems of racialised divestment in poor neighbourhoods and schools and the racist policing and criminalisation of disadvantaged areas (Cohen 2015). In the year *The Beyond Bullying Project* visited, Central had the highest proportion of students of colour and more students living in poverty than any other city high school. Its teachers were predominantly white (80%), while the student population was predominantly Black/African American and Latina/o/x (75% combined). Almost nine out of 10 students received a free or reduced-price lunch. One-third of Central's students were English language learners. Somali- and Oromo-American Muslim students constituted a visible minority. Some girls wore hijab, and 20 to 30 Muslim students gathered three times a day to pray in the school auditorium. Few of the families in the white working- and lower-middle-class neighbourhood that houses Central sent their children there.

The racialised project of recovery

Nivens understood that Central's precarity in the city-wide school system reflected the sustained attack on social support in the USA. As Cathy Cohen has argued,

> [T]here [has] had to be a process of misrepresenting those who benefitted from the social safety net. The trope of urban Black and Brown boys [and girls] who are remorseless 'super-predators' has helped create and solidify an 'other' that whites and middle-class people of color could rally against.
>
> (2015, p. 282)

These predators stand in sharp contrast to the responsible citizens who do not cause trouble, either through needing state assistance or by posing a physical threat. The predominantly low-income, students of colour at Central High School have long been marginalised and maligned in the Minneapolis school system; and when *The Beyond Bullying Project* arrived at the school, this othering had recently re-asserted itself. Earlier in the school year, local news stations reported a sexual assault at Central. Central teachers, staff and students were indignant about another recent news story reporting an assault that had taken place in the neighbourhood. At the end of the school day, three girls had attacked another girl, beating her on the sidewalk and stealing her smartphone. With no evidence beyond its timing, television, newspaper and online reporting linked the fight to Central High. Brianna, a white, 15-year-old ninth grader,[3] explained in an interview, 'On the news, they try to make Central look horrible. So, if there's a fight at [a nearby high school], they'll be say "six miles from Central"'. News stories about student violence affirmed stereotypes that Central was, as Brianna described, 'that school where all the ghetto kids go'.

Such stories and stereotypes undermined Nivens' efforts to boost the reputational and health status of the school. Its students and school staff alternated between feelings of outrage, despair and defeat as they recounted the predicament to *The Beyond Bullying Project* team. In hallway conversations and formal interviews, teachers described being unsure how to defend their students and school against such vilification. During a lunch which the project hosted for teachers and staff, 'people complained about the perception of Central as a bad school, a place with bad students'. But even amidst these complaints, teachers and administrators themselves considered fighting a concern at Central and relied on policing mechanisms when Central students failed to meet neo-liberal expectations of self-regulation. Teachers described ongoing tensions between African American students and recent East African immigrant students that occasionally erupted in violence. One day, as we walked with a teacher to conduct an interview, the teacher explained it had been 'a weird day' marked by rumours of a fight. Once the teachers know about fights, though, she said, they would call in the school 'peace officer' to clear things up. Stationed across the hallway from the counselling office and near the front entrance to the school, our team often witnessed disciplinary responses to student misbehaviour and fighting. In field notes, researchers noted 'very intense' exchanges between disciplinary deans and students: '"Don't come back without a parent," said one dean sternly as he essentially pushed a student out the door'.

In the midst of this turbulence, Nivens and his staff had to convince Minneapolis families that their school was a safe and appealing place to send their children. Producing self-regulating students through rules and hall sweeps would not be enough. The school also held open houses, touted accomplishments on social media and sought positive news coverage that would alert the city's residents to their efforts. A health fair in the school gymnasium featured community-based organisations and district offices that addressed nutrition, bullying and harassment, sexual health and self-defence. Nivens and an out lesbian teacher promoted the school's GSA as a place for students to work together towards sexual justice. The school's community liaison office hired a local Latina artist to paint a mural in the school's entrance; student artists contributed to the mural after school. The school was celebrating a successful 'arts walk' – an evening event that featured student improvisation troupes, concert and dance performances, drawing and fashion design. *The Beyond Bullying Project* – being university affiliated, staffed by a racially and sexually diverse team led by white lesbian researchers, funded by the Ford Foundation and committed to challenging homophobia – fit right in. Such academic, artistic and social exceptionalism promised to reassure white, lower-middle- and middle-class families suspicious about the safety and progressivism of a school with a majority of Black/African American, Latina/o/x and immigrant students assaulting one another in the streets and in the hallways.

But securing Central's place in Minneapolis's educational market also risked denigrating the students the school had long served. Central High's reputation as a school for struggling students of colour was a source of pride for many of its teachers – a reflection of their commitment to serving students who were not otherwise cared for. In an interview, Kenneth Taylor, Central's African American assistant principal, described with pride what he considered to be the school's long-standing strength:

> [S]tudents would get kicked out of other schools… They would come to Central and they would find a home. We would put our arms around them and make sure that they were successful. Students hated to leave Central. They didn't like it coming in because they had all the negative stigmas about what Central was. But once they came into our doors and saw how we treated them, saw how we responded to them, saw how we supported them, they were like "Dang, I really like Central. This is a place that is for me." Families felt the same way.

As Taylor noted, any talk of 'school improvement' risked casting the students of colour who had long made Central their home, as problems to be solved or deficits to be overcome.

> I'm careful about saying Central is getting better because—it scares me to say that because there's always underlying messages and tones and statements…. When you hear it's getting better, [the number of white students] is the only demographic that's changing. So, are we saying we're getting better because we're more white?

Taylor had good reason to be sceptical. Brianna was aware that, in a school stereotyped as for 'ghetto kids', she enjoyed special treatment from many teachers: among her peers, 'I'm not very liked here'. However, 'because I'm white, I'm a teacher's pet'. She continued,

Every teacher loves me. So, "Why are you in the hall?" "I have——, just going to the bathroom. I don't have a pass." "OK. I believe you." And they do that because I'm white. But if someone, other colour probably said it they'd probably act, make them go back to class. You see it a lot.

Brianna *was* special in a school whose survival depended on filling empty classrooms with white students who had chosen to come to Central. Nivens' embrace of LGBTQ acceptance and the arts was a subtle suggestion to white families in the surrounding community that the school's values and future lay with white, progressive families and not with serving the Black and Somali-American families who historically had sent their children there for English language instruction or for support after having been pushed out of other local high schools. As sexuality scholars have noted, support for LGBTQ rights – especially when those rights are tied to neo-liberal values like marriage equality – is often insidiously coded 'white' (Ferguson 2004, Puar 2007).

Neglect, repair, renewal: Central High School's auditorium

And yet, despite the power and ubiquity of these discourses of neoliberalism, students' everyday lives in school pushed back against apparently totalising logics of neoliberalism. If neoliberalism's tactics can be gentle, they can also have only limited reach. Against the mantra of 'personal responsibility', Elliott (2014) describes 'intimate relations' as constituting the hidden curriculum of sexuality education: what a neo-liberal sexuality education cannot admit is that we are vulnerable and dependent on others for support and recognition. Across our two weeks at Central, we witnessed unlikely alliances. Students from families that rejected same-sex marriage joined Central's GSA; boys who went into the booth to tease one another about being gay later entered alone to tell stories about having been targets of anti-gay bullying; girls who identified as straight wondered aloud how to support best friends who had recently come out as lesbian, even as their friends' revelations left them unsettled.

These alliances abutted the individualism of neoliberalism. Sitting at our recruitment table, we watched students pull out their ID as they entered the school, visited the disciplinary deans' offices, or met with guidance counsellors. Behind us, a set of wooden double doors opened into the high school auditorium where, with help from Central's woodworking and carpentry class, the team installed the project's storytelling booth. The auditorium was a large and crowded space. One of many sites of quiet disrepair in the high school building, it featured a piano, a curtained stage, and rows of orchestra and balcony seating. Many of the wooden seats were broken, the sound system was weak and the carpeted floors were littered. Scraps of paper, abandoned pens and pencils, handouts left behind after an open house, food wrappers and drink bottles felt like the ordinary detritus of a high school day. Where was the funding to support a staff that would keep the space clean? A sense of disregard extended across the school. For example, during the initial tour of the school, months before beginning story collection, researchers walked past multiple dark and empty classrooms stacked with unused chairs and desks. The building felt too big for its students and teachers: Central High School did not have enough people to fill the available rooms.

But the school's occupied classrooms were filled with books, posters and other declarations of teachers' commitments; hallways were filled with students between classes making their way to the next tasks and lessons; and the auditorium was a mess in part because students and educators put it to use. During our time at Central, the vast room hosted a city-wide choral competition and an open house for prospective students and their families. And, each day, inside the auditorium, dozens of students waited their turn to tell a story in *The Beyond Bullying Project* booth. A regular in that line was Valerie, a 15-year-old Asian/Native American girl who, over the course of two weeks, told six stories about her experiences as the daughter of a lesbian. When asked in an interview how the school might support her and others concerned about LGBTQ sexuality, Valerie imagined the administration could 'just like have like where all the students come into the auditorium and we just talk about [LGBTQ issues] …. I don't know, just somehow to make us all feel comfortable with each other'. For Valerie, the auditorium was a site of promise.

The potential extended beyond what Valerie might have imagined. The storytellers were a diverse bunch. Most were students who might not easily claim membership in Central's community: low-income students, immigrants, girls in hijab and niqab, students with developmental disabilities, students in regular trouble with Central's principal, out LGBTQ students and students with family members and friends who identified as LGBT or Q. As these young people lined up to participate in a school-based effort to affirm LGBTQ sexuality and lives, they shared space with observant Muslim students. Three times a day, a dozen or so Muslim students and staff would arrive at the auditorium to pray. Storytellers also shared the auditorium with students being punished for missing class. After each hall sweep, disciplinary deans and administrators gathered up the students caught without a hall pass and sent them to the auditorium to receive detention slips. *Beyond Bullying* storytellers and researchers regularly waited in the hallway while students, some of whom had previously told stories, now lined up inside the auditorium to pray or to receive their punishment.

The boundaries between the different projects the auditorium housed were permeable, and in that porousness resided hope. The queerness of the booth was a marketing boon *and* a fixture in the dirty auditorium with its stories about LGBTQ sexuality, Muslim prayer and authoritarian punishment. Misbehaving, religious and LGBTQ students constituted overlapping communities, bumping up against each other, stepping around each other and navigating porous boundaries. These students felt like queers, in the broadest sense of the word: those who stand outside the centre, share a history of oppression, and hold the capacity for radical solidarity (Cohen 1997).

Contradictions and conclusions

In the year after our time at Central, Nivens and his staff secured funding from the school district to replace the auditorium's broken seating, soiled carpet, and inadequate lighting and sound systems. The school also established an expanded arts programme that would extend into special education and Spanish language immersion classes. Nivens also suspended the hall sweeps: students were no longer wandering the halls; they were in class. Both changes are major accomplishments in the effort to market Central as a desirable school. During the team's last visit to the school, a year and a half after *The Beyond Bullying Project* first arrived at Central, workers were in the midst of renovating the auditorium. Peering inside the construction site, questions arose: where will the students pray, the stories be told and the queer alliances form? As Central advances, even gently, in a neo-liberal educational market, where will students find room to cultivate the alliances that *The Beyond Bullying Project* supported?

Even as research supports arguments for schools and educators to affirm non-normative sexual expression and advance an expansive understanding of sexual justice and inclusion, neoliberalism's hold on US schools poses a profound challenge for any effort to promote the sexual health and citizenship of all students. *The Beyond Bullying Project* visited schools with the aim of thinking outside the logics of personal responsibility that usually govern sexuality and anti-bullying education. Stories about LGBTQ sexuality and lives pointed to the queerness already circulating in schools and welcomed the mutuality, interdependence, empathy and alliance that queerness signals. However, even as queerness flourished, it also became another market strategy deployed to signal progressive thinking already underway – not to herald a radical rethinking of educational practice or redistribution of scarce resources.

The history of US public schooling is, in part, a history of ongoing efforts to cultivate citizens who will act in the interests of the status quo. School-based instruction about sexuality – in health classes and in anti-bullying programming – has long contributed to this project of promoting norms of membership and belonging. Under neoliberalism, sexuality education, broadly defined, asserts models of sexuality and citizenship that emphasise accountability, self-regulation, conforming to institutional demands at the expense of mutuality. This model circulated throughout Central, as witnessed in the surveillance of students, the marketing of the school, the emphasis on choice as the key to school success. However, despite the pervasiveness of these beliefs, contradiction also travelled across the school. The auditorium was at once a site of neglect and punishment, a space for prayer and contemplation, a hiding spot for queer youth escaping class, and home to our booth and the stories of queerness it invited. And like the heterogeneity of the auditorium, Nivens, Taylor, and the other teachers and students operated within and against the demands of a school system responding to neoliberalism. *The Beyond Bullying Project* offered a welcome critique of neo-liberal anti-bullying programmes. We also, despite our intentions, supported neo-liberal efforts to cast Central as a safe and inclusive environment for white, middle-class families.

These contradictions cannot be resolved; these days, to work in schools as students, educators or researchers is to be incorporated into the whirl of neo-liberal discourses, texts, practices and ideologies. However, noticing the contradictions, charting their contours and mapping out their contingent paths create spaces for intimate links – pleasurable and otherwise – to emerge, even as a school, its teachers and its students struggle to survive in that market. Learning to recognise and foster these possibilities is crucial to asserting and sustaining alternative models of young people's sexual well-being and citizenship.

Notes

1 The impact of neoliberalism on sexuality policy across a range of contexts, including school-based sexuality education, is explored in a special issue of *Sexuality Research and Social Policy* (Grzanka et al. 2016). Articles in that issue trace, in part, the insidious effects of neoliberalism on the conception, design and implementation of sexuality education.
2 School and participant names are pseudonyms.
3 Participants provided demographic characteristics in response to open-ended questions. We retain their language unless doing so would compromise confidentiality.

References

Bay-Cheng, L. Y., 2017. Critically Sex/ed: Asking Critical Questions of Neoliberal Truths in Sexuality Education. In: L. Allen and M. L. Rasmussen, eds. *The Palgrave Handbook of Sexuality Education*. Basingstoke: Palgrave Macmillan, 343–367.

Biegel, S., 2010. *The Right to Be Out: Sexual Orientation and Gender Identity in America's Public Schools*. Minneapolis, MN: University of Minnesota Press.

Brown, W., 2015. *Undoing the Demos: Neoliberalism's Stealth Revolution*. New York, NY: Zone Books.

Cohen, C. J., 1997. Punks, Bulldaggers, and Welfare Queens: The Radical Potential of Queer Politics. *GLQ: A Journal of Lesbian and Gay Studies*, 3 (4), 437–465.

Cohen, C. J., 2015. Afterword: When will Black Lives Matter? In: E. Nielson, ed. *The Hip Hop & Obama Reader*. Oxford: Oxford University Press, 280–289.

Connell, C. and Elliott, S., 2009. Beyond the Birds and the Bees: Learning Inequality through Sexuality Education. *American Journal of Sexuality Education*, 4 (2), 83–102.

Cossman, B., 2007. *Sexual Citizens: The Legal and Cultural Regulation of Sex and Belonging*. Stanford, CA: Stanford University Press.

Elliott, S., 2014. "Who's to Blame?" Constructing the Responsible Sexual Agent in Neoliberal Sex Education. *Sexuality Research and Social Policy*, 11 (3), 211–224.

Ferguson, R. A., 2004. *Aberrations in Black: Toward a Queer of Color Critique*. Minneapolis, MN: University of Minnesota Press.

Fetner, T. and Elafros, A., 2015. The GSA Difference: LGBTQ and Ally Experiences in High Schools with and without Gay-Straight Alliances. *Social Sciences*, 4 (3), 563–581.

Fields, J., 2008. *Risky Lessons: Sex Education and Social Inequality*. New Brunswick, NJ: Rutgers University Press.

Fields, J., Gilbert, J., and Miller, M., 2015. Sexuality and Education: Toward the Promise of Ambiguity. In: J. DeLamater and R. F. Plante, eds. *Handbook of the Sociology of Sexualities*. Cham: Springer, 371–387.

Fields, J. and Hirschman, C., 2007. Citizenship Lessons in Abstinence-Only Sexuality Education. *American Journal of Sexuality Education*, 2 (2), 3–25.

Fields, J., et al., 2014. Beyond Bullying. *Contexts*, 13 (4), 80–83.

Garcia, L., 2012. *Respect Yourself, Protect Yourself: Latina Girls and Sexual Identity*. New York: NYU Press.

Garcia, L. and Fields, J., 2017. Renewed Commitments in a Time of Vigilance: Sexuality Education in the USA. *Sex Education*, 17 (4), 471–481.

Gilbert, J., 2014. *Sexuality in School: The Limits of Education*. Minneapolis, MN: University of Minnesota Press.

Gilbert, J., et al., forthcoming. Tending Toward Friendship: LGBTQ Sexualities in School. *Sexualities*. Online Frst: doi:10.1177/1363460717731931

Gilbert, J., et al., 2018. Intimate Possibilities: The Beyond Bullying Project and LGBTQ Sexuality and Gender in US Schools. *Harvard Educational Review*, 88 (2), 163–183.

Gordon, A. F., 2008. *Ghostly Matters: Haunting and the Sociological Imagination*. Minneapolis, MN: University of Minnesota Press.

Greytak, E. A., Kosciw, J. G., and Boesen, M. J., 2013. Putting the "T" in "Resource": The Benefits of LGBT-Related School Resources for Transgender Youth. *Journal of LGBT Youth*, 10 (1–2), 45–63.

Grzanka, P. R. and Mann, E. S., 2014. Queer Youth Suicide and the Psychopolitics of "It Gets Better." *Sexualities*, 17 (4), 369–393.

Grzanka, P. R., Mann, E. S., and Elliott, S., eds., 2016. Special Issue on Neoliberalism in Sexuality Research and Social Policy. *Sexuality Research & Social Policy*, 13 (4), 297–427.

Kosciw, J. G., et al., 2013. The Effect of Negative School Climate on Academic Outcomes for LGBT Youth and the Role of In-school Supports. *Journal of School Violence*, 12 (1), 45–63.

Lesko, N, et al., 2018. "An Island Just for the Gays": Affective Geographies of a High School in a Historically Gay Neighborhood. In: S. Talburt, ed., *Youth Sexualities: Public Feelings and Contemporary Cultural Politics*. Westport, CT: Praeger, 207–228.

Loutzenheiser, L. W. and Moore, S. D. M., 2009. Safe Schools, Sexualities, and Critical Education. In: M. W. Apple, Au, W., and Gandin, L. A., eds. *The Routledge International Handbook of Critical Education*. New York, NY: Routledge, 150–162.

Mayo, C., 2013. *LGBTQ Youth and Education: Policies and Practices*. New York, NY: Teachers College Press.

Mayo, Jr, J. B., 2013. Critical Pedagogy Enacted in the Gay-Straight Alliance: New Possibilities for a Third Space in Teacher Development. *Educational Researcher*, 42 (5), 266–275.

McAvoy, P., 2013. The Aims of Sex Education: Demoting Autonomy and Promoting Mutuality. *Educational Theory*, 63 (5), 483–496.

Meyer, D., 2016. The Gentle Neoliberalism of Modern Anti-Bullying Texts: Surveillance, Intervention, and Bystanders in Contemporary Bullying Discourse. *Sexuality Research and Social Policy*, 13 (4), 356–370.

Meyer, E. J., 2015. *Gender, Bullying, and Harassment: Strategies to End Sexism and Homophobia in Schools*. New York, NY: Teachers College Press.

Pascoe, C. J., 2011. *Dude, You're a Fag: Masculinity and Sexuality in High School, with a New Preface*. Berkeley, CA: University of California Press.

Payne, E. and Smith, M., 2012. Rethinking Safe Schools Approaches for LGBTQ Students: Changing the Questions We Ask. *Multicultural Perspectives*, 14 (4), 187–193.

Payne, E. and Smith, M., 2013. LGBTQ Kids, School Safety, and Missing the Big Picture: How the Dominant Bullying Discourse Prevents School Professionals from Thinking About Systemic Marginalization or... Why We Need to Rethink LGBTQ Bullying. *QED: A Journal in GLBTQ Worldmaking*, 1, 1–36.

Pinar, W. F., 2012. *What Is Curriculum Theory?* New York, NY: Routledge.

Puar, J. K., 2007. *Terrorist Assemblages: Homonationalism in Queer Times*. Durham, NC: Duke University Press.

Quinlivan, K., 2017. 'Getting It Right'? Producing Race and Gender in the Neoliberal School-based Sexuality Education Assemblage. In: L. Allen and M. L. Rasmussen, eds. *The Palgrave Handbook of Sexuality Education*. Basingstoke: Palgrave Macmillan, 391–413.

Quinlivan, K., et al., 2014. Crafting the Normative Subject: Queerying the Politics of Race in the New Zealand Health Education Classroom. *Discourse: Studies in the Cultural Politics of Education*, 35 (3), 393–404.

Robinson, J. P. and Espelage, D. L., 2011. Inequities in Educational and Psychological Outcomes between LGBTQ and Straight Students in Middle and High School. *Educational Researcher*, 40 (7), 315–330.

Russell, S. T., et al., 2016. Are School Policies Focused on Sexual Orientation and Gender Identity Associated with Less Bullying? Teachers' Perspectives. *Journal of School Psychology*, 54, 29–38.

Santelli, J., et al., 2006. Abstinence and Abstinence-only Education: A Review of US Policies and Programs. *Journal of Adolescent Health*, 38 (1), 72–81.

Shenk, T. 2015. Booked #3: What Exactly Is Neoliberalism? (Interview with Wendy Brown). *DISSENT Magazine*, 2 April.

Snapp, S. D., et al., 2015. Messy, Butch, and Queer: LGBTQ Youth and the School-to-Prison Pipeline. *Journal of Adolescent Research*, 30 (1), 57–82.

Talburt, S., 2004. Constructions of LGBT Youth: Opening Up Subject Positions. *Theory into Practice*, 43 (2), 116–121.

Waidzunas, T., 2011. Young, Gay, and Suicidal: Dynamic Nominalism and the Process of Defining a Social Problem with Statistics. *Science, Technology & Human Values*, 37 (2), 199–225.

Walls, N. E., Kane, S. B., and Wisneski, H., 2010. Gay-Straight Alliances and School Experiences of Sexual Minority Youth. *Youth & Society*, 41 (3), 307–332.

Watson, R. J. and Russell, S. T., 2016. Disengaged or Bookworm: Academics, Mental Health, and Success for Sexual Minority Youth. *Journal of Research on Adolescence*, 26 (1), 159–165.

Section 4

Communication technologies

Chapter 10

Twenty years of 'cyberqueer'

The enduring significance of the Internet for young LGBTIQ+ people

Brady Robards, Brendan Churchill, Son Vivienne, Benjamin Hanckel and Paul Byron

Introduction

Over the past 20 to 30 years, the Internet has come to serve as a key channel for communicating and connecting, but also engaging in civic participation. For lesbian, gay, bisexual, transgender, intersex, and queer or questioning (LGBTIQ+) people, who continue to experience disproportionate health risks and high rates of discrimination (Leonard et al. 2012), the significance of the Internet as a social resource is further magnified (Gray 2009, Hanckel and Morris 2014). While digital social spaces have evolved, many of the motivations for using these platforms remain the same. Different platforms offer different opportunities to connect with queer peers and others, for discussing, documenting and exploring sexuality away from heteronormative spaces (Hillier et al. 2001, 2010, O'Neill 2014). From text-based 'virtual' worlds and discussion boards through to sites and apps such as Facebook, Instagram, Twitter, Snapchat, Tumblr, YouTube, Reddit, Tinder, Grindr and Her, the digital social media landscape is now more complex than ever. What new challenges and opportunities does this evolution present? A better understanding of digital engagement (and disengagement) is useful not only for researchers and platform designers but also for a broad range of social service providers, educators and policymakers who are routinely tasked with both the regulation and the support of young LGBTIQ+ people.

This chapter draws on data from the *Scrolling Beyond Binaries* study, centred on a national survey of 1,304 young LGBTIQ+ Australians. The survey addresses a key gap in our understanding of social media use among LGBTIQ+ people in Australia. We begin by providing a brief background on Internet use among LGBTIQ+ young people over the past 20 years before presenting some key findings from the study in two parts: (a) differences across our four age cohorts (16–20, 21–25, 26–30, 30–35) in terms of their identities (gender and sexuality) and the social media platforms they use; and (b) the argument that the Internet continues to be significant for our respondents for social connection and learning. In doing so, we explore the complex and evolving ways in which young LGBTIQ+ people use and thus (re)produce digital social spaces, returning to Nina Wakeford's (2000 [1997]) consideration of 'cyberqueer spaces'.

Background: the story thus far

> If you have ever stepped off the ferry on to Fire Island or pulled into Provincetown or any other gay and lesbian enclave, you know the feeling. It's as if a desert dweller had walked through a magical wall into lush tropics. The natives seem exotic and utterly normal... a door opening into a world where gays and lesbians are the natural majority.
>
> (Dawson 1996 in Wakeford 2000 [1997], p. 404)

In her influential essay, *Cyberqueer*, Nina Wakeford (2000 [1997]) begins by invoking Dawson's description of entering digital social spaces for gay and lesbian people as akin to arriving in a gay enclave. The affective dimensions of 'arriving' and no longer feeling in the minority in a digital space that Dawson sets out here, and that Wakeford further explores, resonate even today, 20 years later. At the same time, there are significant differences in how we conceptualise the Internet today. Scholarship from the 1990s is replete with metaphors, like Dawson's, that tell tales of 'arriving at' or 'on' or 'in' the Internet. Another example is Julian Dibbell's (1998) pioneering work on the LambdaMOO MUD (a text-based Multi-User Domain), where Dibbell found himself 'tripping now and then down the well-travelled information lane that leads to LambdaMOO, a very large and very busy rustic mansion built entirely of words' (Dibbell 1998, p. 11). Sherry Turkle's work around this time, which acknowledged the ways in which digital media were becoming embedded in the 'routines of everyday life' (1995, p. 9), dealt in descriptions of 'cyberspace' as a place people went to and spent time in, away from their 'real lives'. At the time, these kinds of metaphors and spatial conceptualisations of the Internet made sense as people were interacting through shared 'virtual worlds' like MUDs where imagination – imagining a room, characters, responses – was key.

More recent conceptualisations of the Internet have called for doing away with dualisms that seek to inscribe a distinction between 'real' and 'virtual'. Rather than engage in this 'digital dualist' thinking, Jurgenson (2011), for instance, has argued for seeing the online and offline as overlapping and integrated within individuals' lives. As Hine (2015, p. 192) explains, the Internet can be understood as 'a culturally embedded phenomenon, as online activities acquire meaning and significance in so far as they are interpreted within other online and offline contexts'. In this way, the on/offline converge and their meaning is made through the spaces in which they develop, and are used.

Meanwhile, the digitally mediated social 'spaces' and 'places' people spend time in have also changed. For our survey respondents, many of whom felt 'always connected' to social media, the idea of arriving at and departing from the Internet in Dawson's analogy would seem antiquated. Rather, digital media are embedded in everyday life. Nevertheless, there are many dimensions of these early conceptualisations of 'cyberqueer spaces' that continue to be salient. As Wakeford explains, 'cyberqueer spaces are constantly reconstituted as points of resistance against the dominant assumption of the normality of heterosexuality' (Wakeford 2000 [1997], p. 408). Our research findings suggest that, for young LGBTIQ+ people, digital social spaces are still significant because the 'different heteronormative/homophobic burdens' (Gray 2009, p. 21) that they confront are persistent, albeit with variations to those of 20 years ago.

Digital spaces have been shown to assist LGBTIQ+ young people in coming to terms with a sense of self (Hillier et al. 2010, Hanckel and Morris 2014) and connecting with like-minded others (Russell 2002). These interactions provide young people with important knowledge about LGBTIQ+ identities, the opportunity to refute the negative stereotypes and perceptions of non-heterosexual people (Castañeda 2015) and connection to sexual health information (Mustanski et al. 2011). Taken together, these uses allow for a broad reading of the Internet as a forum for the transfer of (sub)cultural capital, including knowledge about what it is to be queer (Munt et al. 2002). Not only does this circumvent some of the stigma LGBTIQ+ people live with, but it also presents a 'valuable performative and discursive space' (O'Neill 2014), and opportunities to engage in civic life (Hanckel and Morris 2014, Vivienne 2017). Put simply, the Internet provides opportunities for exploring sexuality and gender, and engaging in forms of queer world-making.

In Australia, 79% of Internet users aged 18–29 accessed some form of social media at least once per day, ahead of the national average of 50% of the general Internet-using population (Sensis Social Media Report 2016). While we do not have explicit data on Internet usage rates among the LGBTIQ+ population, given the aforementioned and Dawson's (in Wakeford 2000 [1997]) still resonant description of the comfort and safety of queer digital spaces, we wondered if these perceptions still held. More specifically, given the transformation of the web to the participatory 'web 2.0', we aimed to explore how social media is being used by LGBTIQ+ young people in Australia. As we will discuss, the findings reveal not just the enduring significance of 'cyberqueer spaces' in the lives of young LGBTIQ+ people, but also clear differences in use across age cohorts and in the way our different cohorts conceptualise their own genders and sexualities.

The *Scrolling Beyond Binaries* project

The *Scrolling Beyond Binaries* study began in 2016. First, we surveyed a range of young LGBTIQ+ people in Australia from June to November 2016 on their social media use. These data comprise 1,304 survey responses from young people aged 16 to 35 years (average age: 21.9 years). In the second phase of the study, we undertook in-depth Skype interviews with self-elected survey participants (n = 23). In this chapter we focus on survey data from Phase One of the study.

The project began at a curious point in Australian history, where the inclusion of LGBTIQ+ people remains controversial in popular discourse. On the one hand, LGBTIQ+ people are becoming more represented in the sporting arena and mass media more generally, which is important for responding to the earlier 'symbolic annihilation' (Gross 1991, p. 26) of sexual minorities in the media. For example, the Australian Football League (AFL), a traditionally masculine and heteronormative sporting context, has begun to promote 'pride games' (ABC News 2016). Australian television programmes and films, such as *Please Like Me* (2013–2016), *The Principal* (2015–2016) and *Barracuda* (2016) increasingly have central queer characters and actors. However, whilst such representations are increasing, there is evidence to suggest that there is a persistence of invisibility of diverse LGBTIQ+ narratives in mainstream media. Reports and stories often emphasise heterosexual lives, and assume this to be the norm (see for example McKinnon et al. 2017). Furthermore, 'Safe Schools', the anti-bullying campaign designed to foster more inclusive schools for LGBTIQ+ people, came under attack from conservatives in 2016, who framed the programme as 'a gateway drug for children to experiment with sex' (Rhodes et al. 2016; see also Law 2017). The family-rated and award-winning documentary *Gayby Baby* (2015), which tells the story of children of same-sex parents, was also banned from being screened during school hours by the New South Wales Education Minister (Safi 2015). More broadly, the long marriage equality 'debate' in Australia that culminated in a change to the legislation in 2017, created the space for highly contentious debate, with comments against LGBTIQ+ people circulating throughout popular media. There is evidence this impacted young LGBTIQ+ peoples' lives, with mental health support services reporting a '40 per cent surge in young people accessing help since the same sex marriage postal survey began' (ReachOut 2017).

Internationally, gross human rights violations and news of a 'gay purge' in Chechnya (Andreevskikh 2017), alongside the conservatism behind populist movements in the USA and the UK, continue to make the world seem hostile and threatening for LGBTIQ+ people. Meanwhile, in predominantly digital spaces (where national identity is often less marked) and Tumblr in particular, there is evidence of a proliferation of non-binary gender identities (including gender-queer, enby, agender, two spirit, etc.). This phenomenon is also marked by increased options on dating sites and hook-up apps for self-selecting diverse combinations of gender and sexuality. For example, as early as 2014, OKCupid announced more inclusive options and currently offers 22 choices of gender and 13 sexual 'orientations'. OKCupid further encourages the expansion of categories via online submission: 'Language and words evolve just as the people who use them do. Help us add your perspective and share with the world what terms of identification mean to you' (OKCupid 2017). Transgender author and activist Riki Wilchins, argues that while non-binary and gender-queer people have existed in various forms, cultures and nominalisations across time, recent social changes indicate that 'we are unconsciously and finally treading toward the end of gender. In my opinion, that step is long overdue' (Wilchins 2017).

With this context in mind, how do young LGBTIQ+ people in Australia reconcile these competing discourses? And in what ways might Plummer's (2003) arguments about sexual citizenship be realised through social media? While there is some detailed work on specific digital spaces (Hanckel and Morris 2014) and approaches to inclusion through digital media (Vivienne 2016), there is a gap in wider understandings of the complex ways young people simultaneously juggle a variety of social media platforms with different affordances for privacy and disclosure, among multiple networked publics. These negotiations, good and bad, have consequences for health and well-being. Feelings of connectedness are themselves indicators for engaged citizenship and living a meaningful life. The *Scrolling Beyond Binaries* project sought to address this gap, and we present some preliminary findings here.

Generational differences

In this section, we tease out some useful distinctions between our four cohorts, in terms of differences between gender, sexuality and the platforms they use, before returning to the more substantive issue of the enduring significance of the Internet in the lives of young LGBTIQ+ people. Our largest age cohort was the youngest category. Over half (54%) of respondents were from the 16- to 20-year-old cohort, with progressively smaller cohorts for each group.

Gender

Our two younger cohorts were more likely to identify as non-binary when it comes to gender (Table 10.1). Notably, the number of respondents who identified as men almost doubled from 21% in the youngest cohort (16–20) to 37% in the older cohort (31–35). In addition to male, female and non-binary, we invited respondents to complete an open-ended field to name their own gender identity. Approximately 9% of the respondents made use of this box, with the most common responses being gender-fluid, agender and trans.

The high percentage of non-binary participants, particularly in the younger age groups, reflects a diversification away from binary gender categories, and is consistent with recent findings in this area. For instance, in the third *Writing Themselves In* study, the authors revised the survey to include the identity category

Table 10.1 Gender identity across four age cohorts, %.

%	16–20 (n = 712)	21–25 (n = 251)	26–30 (n = 193)	31–35 (n = 156)
Male	20.79	27.89	38.34	36.54
Female	48.31	40.64	40.93	44.87
Non-binary	20.51	25.5	13.99	9.62
Self-identified	10.39	5.98	6.74	8.97
Gender-fluid	3.5	0.8	1.55	1.28
Agender	1.5	1.19	0.5	1.28
Trans	1.0	1.6	1.0	1.28

of 'genderqueer' (Hillier et al. 2010), with 1.7% of participants (14–21 years) identifying as genderqueer or 'other' (2010, p. 13). In a 2014 Australian survey of gender-diverse, trans and intersex young people (14–25 years), the authors found that more than one-third of participants identified as a non-binary gender (Smith et al. 2014), and in the most recent survey of LGBTIQ young people in Australia, 22.4% of participants (16–25 years) nominated a non-binary gender (Byron et al. 2017, p. 16). While these surveys and our own involved different age groups, used different survey questions and emphasised different aspects of queer life (e.g. well-being, mental health and/or social media use), it is evident both here and elsewhere (Richards et al. 2016) that non-binary gender identities are increasingly used among this cohort. What role might 'cyberqueer spaces' play in these trends?

While 'non-binary' and 'gender-queer' are not wholly new terms, identities or ways of being, tracing their histories is complicated by the very process of measurement, categorisation and nominalisation. When gender-diverse people are offered binary alternatives for self-documentation they can only comply or refuse the service. Sexual and/or gendered citizenship becomes much more than a quest for the right to incorporate sexed/gendered aspects of self, as it is also concerned with the ongoing threat of exclusion. Much as the gender and bathroom/toilet access debate (McAvan 2017), which continues to unfold in public discourse in Australia and globally, symbolically evokes categorisation and exclusion. Survey questions and other processes of measurement, including the national census, represent a fundamental challenge to fluid or multiple or non-compliant identities. As such, tracing the antecedents of non-binary identities across generations in archives or public records is thwarted by the fact that these categories have not previously been available, despite the likelihood that gender-diverse people have long existed. Through categorisation they are inevitably folded in normative forms. In our own survey, we address this issue by offering open fields and, where possible, seeking expansion of non-conforming gender/sexual identities through interviews and qualitative evaluation. What is clear, however, is that 'cyberqueer' spaces (like Tumblr, which we describe later) have become central for the forming of connections and the discovery of a common language, a subcultural knowledge, by which to describe the non-binary, fluid and trans experiences of gender.

Sexuality

Like gender, when it comes to sexuality, our older respondents were more likely to identify with a more 'long-standing' and binary category like lesbian, gay or homosexual: 48.08% for the 31- to 35-year-old cohort compared to 27.35% for the 16- to 20-year-old cohort. In fact, more of our youngest respondents (16–20 years) identified as bisexual than they did as lesbian or gay. As with gender diversity, a movement away from binary sexual identities is reflected in recent Australian studies. Of the young women in their survey, Hillier et al. (2010, p. 27) found that most identified as bisexual (42%) rather than lesbian (39%); 25.4% of Robinson et al.'s

Table 10.2 Sexuality across four age cohorts.

%	16–20 (n=713)	21–25 (n=251)	26–30 (n=192)	31–35 (n=156)
Lesbian or gay	27.35	34.26	44.79	48.08
Straight	3.65	2.39	2.08	6.41
Bisexual	30.43	19.92	19.79	12.82
Queer	13.88	22.71	18.75	26.92
Self-identified	24.68	20.72	14.58	5.77
Pansexual	13.6	11.15	8.85	2.56
Asexual	6.31	5.58	2.08	1.28
Panromantic	3.37	0.8	0	0.64

(2014, p. 45) participants identified as bisexual; and in Byron et al.'s study (2017, p. 17), more young people identified as bisexual (32.3%) than lesbian (21.5%) or gay (18.5%).[1] A large number of participants in Byron et al.'s (2017) study also identified as pansexual (19.1%) and asexual (9.2%). Again, it is worth noting the historical and cultural specificity of these nominalisations, and the different survey tools used. For example, Byron et al. (2017) allowed participants to list multiple sexual identity categories, and 42.6% of participants did so (Table 10.2).

Increased discussion of non-binary genders arguably relates to an increase in plurisexual identities, including bisexual, pansexual and queer (Galupo et al. 2017). Galupo et al.'s study notes that their pansexual participants, in particular, were unlikely to evoke gender binaries when discussing their sexualities. As with gender diversities, young people's awareness of, and identification with, plurisexual identities has been attributed to Tumblr, Instagram and other social media spaces that reflect and contemplate a diversity of gender and sexual identities (Oakley 2016). An increased awareness of asexuality has also been attributed to Tumblr-based counterpublics (Renninger 2015).

Is the queer umbrella getting bigger, and including more people beneath it?

It is important to note the generational differences in labels and categories that our respondents are using. Our younger respondents were more likely to fill in their own descriptions of gender and especially sexuality, both to be more specific but also to provide detail and nuances to their responses. These findings also align with Cover's (2018) arguments around the emergence of new sexual subjectivities, categories and labels amongst young people.

Some respondents positioned these ideas as temporal, with one respondent describing their gender as 'whatever feels right at that time in my life'. Some were also combinations of other labels and categories, with one describing their sexuality as 'bisexual with a 90% female preference - publicly I identify as a lesbian', and another explained their gender as 'queer but usually say female when asked', and for another still, 'trans masculine gender non-conforming femme'. One respondent explained how they were using a term coined by a friend to describe their sexuality: 'predominantly homosexual; I've used "homo-flexible lesbian" and a friend coined "pangynic"'. For us, these examples point to a complex process of re-working language to suit individual experiences that are not confined to singular pre-existing categories. These findings support and ex-tend previous work (e.g. Russell et al. 2009) that found younger youth were more likely to present alternative labels about their sexuality than lesbian, gay and bisexual (LGB).

As suggested earlier, the fact that more personalised descriptions seem to pre-vail among our youngest respondents raises a number of questions. Is there a link here between the role of digital media in exposing young people to more complex language around gender and sexuality? As we have described elsewhere (see Byron and Robards 2017), our respondents single out Tumblr as a site of learning a new language, so it is possible that this plays a role here. Or, is there a wider generational effect at work, where young people are more likely to reject categorisation in general?

Russell et al. (2009, p. 888) suggest that over time, people 'may be more likely to have developed a stable and solidified LGB identity, and/or they may adapt to community norms and use traditional terms as they become integrated into LGB communities'. While we are sceptical of the notion that new terms and emerging identity descriptions are not 'stable', it will be important to trace the longevity of emerging terms to describe gender and sexuality. This language seems to find coherence and amplification on platforms like Tumblr, providing evidence of emerging forms of (sub)cultural capital around gender and sexuality.

Recent research in the UK also indicates there is a generational shift in how young people describe sexuality. Re-applying the 1948 Kinsey Scale (Kinsey et al. 1948), a YouGov UK study found that one in two young people say they are not fully heterosexual, with more young people than ever identifying somewhere along the Kinsey scale (Dahlgreen 2015). While the Kinsey scale has been widely circulated, adapted and modified in various digital spaces, Drucker (2012, p. 259) argues that it 'remains a powerful tool for sexual understanding, self-reckoning, and nurturing compassion for sexual others'.

While some might be critical of the growing LGBTIQ+ 'alphabet soup', it is our contention that this proliferation of terms points to a form of personal citizen-ship. Naming one's experiences – and offering that naming to others with shared experiences – is a productive act in itself, allowing for groups to form and voices to be heard. That language is becoming more complex, distinguishing, for instance, between bisexual and pansexual, naming up intensities of sexuality (with terms like asexual and greysexual), and drawing markers between romantic and sexual attraction. However, while young people are sharing experiences of gender tran-sition on YouTube and theorising asexuality on Tumblr, physical spaces continue to be marked out in rigid ways. As we've noted, debate continues over gendered bathrooms while digital spaces have provided opportunities for response via self-ies and hashtags like #WeJustNeedToPee (Kellaway 2015, Vivienne 2017).

Platforms

The link between 'everyday activism' (Vivienne 2016), digital platforms and social change can no longer be disputed. Greater choice in platforms for debate
has led to more complex discussion and self-expression. There are also clear differences in patterns of social media use in our four age cohorts. Generally, the
use of almost all platforms declines for each subsequent older cohort, with some
exceptions (Figure 10.1).

The main exception to this trend is the use of Twitter, which increases from
40% of 16- to 20-year-olds to almost 70% of our 31- to 35-year-old respondents.
Facebook, Instagram and YouTube are commonly used platforms for all of our
respondents and there is little variation amongst usage across age cohorts in our
study. There were, however, significant differences in other platforms. There was
an age gradient in the use of apps like Snapchat and Tumblr, where usage was
highest amongst younger cohorts. Snapchat, for instance, was used by 80% of
our 16- to 20-year-old cohort but by just 34% of our 31- to 35-year-old cohort.
Reddit use was also higher for the middle cohort (almost one-quarter of 21 to
25-year-olds and 21% of 26- to 30-year-olds) but lower amongst our youngest
and oldest cohorts (13% of 16- to 20-year-olds and 16% of 31- to 35-year-olds).
When mapped proportionately across our age cohorts, the differences are also
clear (Figure 10.2).

Figure 10.2 further highlights the changing patterns of social media use across
our four age cohorts. The 21 to 25-year-old cohort appears to be the most so-
phisticated in terms of platform diversity, although there was clearly a wide
range of platforms in use across each cohort. This diversity in platforms that our

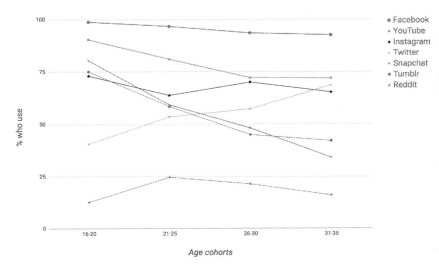

Figure 10.1 Usage of Social Media Platforms, by Age Cohort (Line Graph) (%).

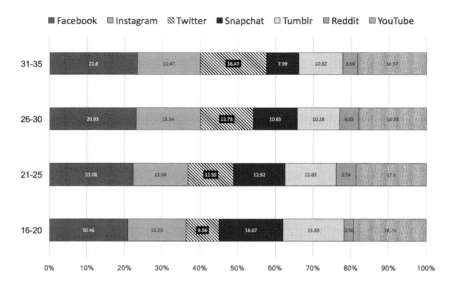

Figure 10.2 Usage of Social Media Platforms, by Age Cohort (Stacked Bar Graph) (%).

respondents are actively using is significant, as 'cyberqueer space' can cut across these platforms in complex and contested ways. We will return to this point in the final section before the conclusion, when reflecting on some of the responses to our open-ended questions on the significance of these platforms.

There are also interesting patterns of use of hook-up and dating apps across our age cohorts. Overall, Tinder was the most popular, with 21% of respondents using it; followed by Grindr (11%); OKCupid (7.5%); Her (6%); Scruff (5%); and to a lesser extent Hornet (3%), Happn (1%) and Bumble (1%). When we combine these apps and instead divide them into categories that allow for multiple sexual orientations or interests (like Tinder or OKCupid) versus apps that are more specific – for gay men or women (like Grindr, Her, Scruff and Hornet) – there is an evident age gradient (Figure 10.3).

The youngest cohorts in this study were more likely to use platforms such as Tinder, Happn and Bumble that allow for users to engage with more than one sex (e.g. Happn allows for users to 'find' men and women). In contrast, the older cohorts were more likely to use targeted hook-up/dating apps like Grindr or Her. This significant difference in usage of these two platform groups may reflect the historical development of hook-up and dating apps, where apps like Grindr and Scruff were amongst the first hook-up/dating apps available and thus older co-horts are more familiar, long-term users. These apps were preceded by dating sites specifically for gay men, like Gaydar (see Light et al. 2008), potentially offering further explanation for this age gradient.

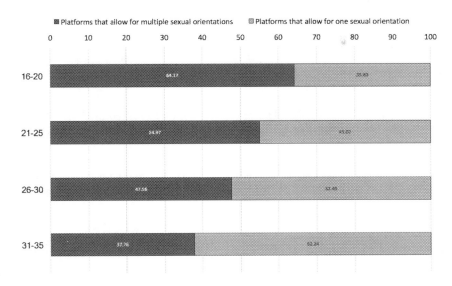

■ Platforms that allow for multiple sexual orientations   ▨ Platforms that allow for one sexual orientation

Figure 10.3 Usage of Dating/Hook-up Apps by Age Group (Stacked Bar Graph) (%).

This difference across age cohorts may also reflect the fluidity in sexuality and sexual preferences of users at younger ages, in which apps that allow for more 'choice' may be preferable. It is also worth noting the many complex distinctions between the affordances of particular platforms – some of which are mobile apps rather than web-based, some that are more appealing to text and/or image-based literacy – and how these distinctions influence take-up and popularity. A growing body of work focussing on these nuances is emerging (Jørgensen 2016, Light et al. 2016). For us, one of the key points in this age gradient points to evidence of the changing patterns in the way young people describe their own gender and sexual identities, and how digital media might map to these changing conceptualisations and the evolution of cyberqueer spaces.

Community and connection: the enduring significance of 'cyberqueer' spaces

In open-ended questions, many respondents explained the various ways in which digital media helped them to learn and feel connected, describing the enduring significance of 'cyberqueer spaces', some 20 years on from Wakeford's (2000 [1997]) essay:

> I used [Grindr] when I began to more actively explore my sexuality.
>
> (25, gay male)

Before Tumblr, I had no idea that lgbt+ people existed (my parents are quite homophobic and very strict…) and by using Tumblr I was able to fully immerse myself within its very lgbt+ culture.

(17, lesbian female)

Reddit was significant in the way it introduced me to a social media platform of pure discussion and expression of other people's opinions. Subreddits specifically for lesbians/bisexuals were very helpful in making me more aware of my sexuality.

(19, queer female)

social media helped me embrace my sexuality and feel like I am not alone.

(18, bisexual female)

Grindr allowed me to meet other guys while I was coming out and didn't really know any gays.

(29, gay male)

Lesking.com.vn was a really significant website that helped me discover my transness and embrace my gender. I got to know different trans, gender diverse and same-sex attracted people who were assigned female at birth and of Vietnamese heritage.

(18, non-binary trans guy)

As these quotes show, the Internet continues to operate as a significant resource for young LGBTIQ+ people, perhaps now more than ever. Since the 1990s when 'cyberqueer spaces' were being interrogated and conceived of as political sites of connection and citizenship, the wider sociopolitical landscape may have changed but the significance of the Internet for LGBTIQ+ people remains. Instead of mailing lists, bulletin boards and text-based 'virtual worlds' (like MUDs), LGBTIQ+ people now connect through dominant mainstream platforms like Facebook and Instagram, but also find more queer spaces on Tumblr (Byron and Robards 2017) and Reddit, or through hook-up apps like Grindr and Her. Although these quotes are just a brief insight into the 653 responses (50% of respondents) to open-ended questions on the significance of social media, they go some way to sketching out the enduring significance of the Internet in the lives of LGBTIQ+ people – from exploring sexuality and gender, gaining important 'subcultural knowledge', to finding friends and feeling 'not alone'.

Being part of a community of like-minded people is core to feelings of connection. Similarly, understanding that one plays a significant role in the community is core to understandings of citizenship. In 2003, Plummer argued that 'intimate citizenship' was becoming increasingly important and related to the decisions people have to make over *the control (or not) over* one's bodies, feelings, relationships; *access (or not) to* representations, relationships, public spaces etc.; and *socially grounded choices (or not) about* identities, gender experiences, erotic experiences.

(emphasis added, Plummer 2003, p. 14)

While not reserved to LGBTIQ+ people, it is easy to see how identifying as 'non-normative' in body and law mandates a particular kind of everyday activism (Vivienne 2016), without which one can scarcely claim to be a citizen or a part of the whole.

As the quotes from our participants demonstrate, an important part of the significance of digital media is the role it plays in facilitating expression of both united and disparate voices of difference. 'Digital Citizenship' in turn has been explored both as an always-ongoing way of being and as an interface via which people utilise technology to negotiate and contest control, sometimes through cultural expression. McCosker et al. (2016) understand digital citizenship as both formal processes of governance, social policy and education, and a suite of informal practices, inclusive of workarounds that elude categorisation and measurement. Building upon this work we understand sexual citizenship as an ever-changing collection of practices that challenge and redefine ways of being in the world, among other people and alone, simultaneously in one's body and in digital spaces. Simply being visible in digital and physical spaces is an act of citizenship and activism for many LGBTIQ+ people, and this has been the case for more than two decades now.

Conclusion

In the 1990s, Wakeford argued that 'cyberqueer spaces are necessarily embedded within both institutional and cultural practices, and are a means by which the lesbian/gay/transgendered/queer self can be read into the politics of representation and activism confronting homophobia' (2000 [1997], p. 408). While there might be cause for optimism 20 years later, amidst 'it gets better' narratives (Gal et al. 2016), LGBTIQ+ people continue to experience significant challenges. Within this context, it is important to explore how young people are engaging with a diverse number of media platforms to explore sexuality and gender identity, and find other people like themselves. Often these assist them and contribute to important queer (sub)cultural capital (Munt et al. 2002) that works to mitigate against the effects of homophobia, transphobia and isolation.

Assemblages of social media platforms are used according to particular needs and affordances. Respondents in our study describe the importance of social connection and belonging, but also indicate that these spaces can become problematic and even toxic. Forty per cent of respondents reported experiencing some form of isolation, exclusion or harassment through social media. These findings challenge the narrative that these spaces only provide experiences of connection, learning and community; the 'productive' dimensions of cyberqueer spaces and digital citizenship. Evidently, digital social spaces are like all social spaces, in that they can be both good and challenging, and embedded within the contexts of their use. While young LGBTIQ+ people may experience harassment and bullying on 'mainstream' sites like Facebook and Tinder, there are also experiences of disconnection, harassment, isolation and exclusion *within* contemporary 'cyberqueer' spaces, such as racism on Grindr and the exclusion of trans women in some feminist subreddits and threads on Tumblr. This is notable for future analysis and discussion.

For participants in this study, it is this assemblage of platforms, and their movement between them, that is crucial to participation in everyday life, regardless of whether they conceive of themselves as sexual/digital/intimate citizens or disconnected from an amorphous community. For researchers, and by extension the stakeholders we aim to engage with – educators, social service/health providers and policymakers – understanding how young people, as 'digitally augmented subjects', adapt to and modify online spaces and tools to suit their needs is imperative.

Acknowledgements

We acknowledge the participants in the *Scrolling Beyond Binaries* project (scrollingbeyondbinaries.com). We also thank our advisory group for input on the design and dissemination of our survey: Angela Dwyer, Kirsten McLean, Kim McLeod, Bob Buttigieg, Natalie Hendry, Andrew Badcock, Ruby Grant and Stefanie Duguay.

Note

1 This may also be the case for our study and Robinson et al.'s study (2014), in which 'lesbian, gay & homosexual' identities were grouped together.

References

ABC News, 2016. Rainbow Flags to Feature at AFL's Pride Game between Sydney Swans and St Kilda. *ABC News*, 9 August. Available from: www.abc.net.au/news/2016-08-09/afl-launches-first-pride-game-between-sydney-swans-and-st-kilda/7703642 [Accessed 29 May 2017].

Andreevskikh, O., 2017. Report Reveals the Full Brutality of Anti-gay Purges in Chechnya. *The Conversation*, 30 May. Available from: https://theconversation.com/report-reveals-the-full-brutality-of-anti-gay-purges-in-chechnya-78373 [Accessed 16 June 2017].

Byron, P. and Robards, B., 2017. 'There's Something Queer About Tumblr', *The Conversation*, 29 May. Available from: https://theconversation.com/theres-something-queer-about-tumblr-73520 [Accessed 12 June 2017].

Byron, P., et al., 2017. *'You Learn from Each Other': LGBTIQ Young People's Mental Health Help-Seeking and the RAD Australia Online Directory.* Sydney, NSW: Western Sydney University & Young and Well Cooperative Research Centre. Available at: http://researchdirect.westernsydney.edu.au/islandora/object/uws:38815

Castañeda, J. G. M., 2015. Grindring the Self: Young Filipino Gay Men's Exploration of Sexual Identity Through a Geo-Social Networking Application. *Philippine Journal of Psychology*, 48 (1), 29–58.

Cover, R., 2018. Micro-Minorities: The Emergence of New Sexual Subjectivities, Categories and Labels Among Sexually-Diverse Youth Online. In: S. Talburt, ed. *Youth Sexualities: Public Feelings and Contemporary Cultural Politics.* New York, NY: Praeger.

Dahlgreen, W., 2015. 1 in 2 Young People Say They Are Not 100% Heterosexual. *YouGov.co.uk Website.* Available from: https://yougov.co.uk/news/2015/08/16/half-young-not-heterosexual/ [Accessed 12 June 2017].

Dibbell, J., 1998. *My Tiny Life: Crime and Passion in a Virtual World.* New York, NY: Holt.

Drucker, D. J., 2012. Marking Sexuality from 0–6: The Kinsey Scale in Online Culture. *Sexuality & Culture*, 16 (3), 241–262. doi:10.1007/s12119-011-9122-1

Gal, N., Shifman, L., and Kampf, Z., 2016. "It Gets Better": Internet Memes and the Construction of Collective Identity. *New Media & Society*, 18 (8), 1698–1714.

Galupo, M. P., Ramirez, J. L., and Pulice-Farrow, L., 2017. "Regardless of Their Gender": Descriptions of Sexual Identity among Bisexual, Pansexual, and Queer Identified Individuals. *Journal of Bisexuality*, 17 (1), 108–124.

Gray, M. L., 2009. *Out in the Country: Youth, Media and Queer Visibility in Rural America.* New York: University Press.

Gross, L., 1991. Out of the Mainstream: Sexual Minorities and the Mass Media. *Journal of Homosexuality*, 21 (1–2), 19–46.

Hanckel, B. and Morris, A., 2014. Finding Community and Contesting Heteronormativity: Queer Young People's Engagement in an Australian Online Community. *Journal of Youth Studies*, 17 (7), 872–886.

Hillier, L., Kurdas, C., and Horsley, P. A., 2001. *It's Just Easier: The Internet as a Safety-Net for Same Sex Attracted Young People.* Melbourne, VIC: Australian Research Centre in Sex, Health and Society, La Trobe University.

Hillier, L., et al., 2010. *Writing Themselves in 3: The Third National Study on the Sexual Health and Wellbeing of Same Sex Attracted and Gender Questioning Young People.* Melbourne, VIC: Australian Research Centre in Sex, Health and Society, La Trobe University.

Hine, C., 2015. *Ethnography for the Internet: Embedded, Embodied and Everyday.* New York, NY: Bloomsbury.

Jørgensen, K. M., 2016. The Media Go-Along: Researching Mobilities with Media at Hand. *MedieKultur: Journal of Media and Communication Research*, 32 (60), 32–49.

Jurgenson, N., 2011. Digital Dualism and the Fallacy of Web Objectivity. *Cyborgology*, 13 September. Available from: https://thesocietypages.org/cyborgology/2011/09/13/digital-dualism-and-the-fallacy-of-web-objectivity/ [Accessed 7 June 2017].

Kinsey, A. C., Pomeroy, B. P., and Martin, C. E., 1948. *Sexual Behavior in the Human Male.* Philadelphia, PN: W.B. Saunders.

Kellaway, M., 2015. Trans Folks Respond to 'Bathroom Bills' with #WeJustNeedtoPee Selfies [GLBTQIS News & Commentary], *The Advocate*, 14 March. Available from: www.advocate.com/politics/transgender/2015/03/14/trans-folks-respond-bathroom-bills-wejustneedtopee-selfies [Accessed 3 July 2016].

Law, B., 2017. 'Moral Panic 101: Equality, Acceptance, and the Safe Schools Scandal'. *Quarterly Essay*, 67, 1–81.

Leonard, W., et al., 2012. Report. In: *Private Lives 2: The Second National Survey of the Health and Wellbeing of GLBT Australians*, Australian Research Centre in Sex, Health & Society, LaTrobe University, 1–75. Available from: www.glhv.org.au/sites/default/files/PrivateLives2Report.pdf

Light, B., Burgess, J., and Duguay, S., 2016. The Walkthrough Method: An Approach to the Study of Apps. *New Media & Society*, 20 (3), 881–900.

Light, B., Fletcher, G., and Adam, A., 2008. Gay Men, Gaydar and the Commodification of Difference. *Information Technology & People*, 21 (3), 300–314.

McAvan, E., 2017. 'The Politics of Transgender Bathroom Access in Australia'. *SBS In Focus*, 16 January. Available from: www.sbs.com.au/topics/sexuality/agenda/article/2017/01/16/politics-transgender-bathroom-access-australia [Accessed 28 August 2017].

McCosker, A., Vivienne, S., and Johns, A., eds., 2016. *Negotiating Digital Citizenship: Control, Contest, Culture*. Lanham, MD: Rowman and Littlefield.

McKinnon, S., Gorman-Murray, A., and Dominey-Howes, D., 2017. Disasters, Queer Narratives, and the News: How Are LGBTI Disaster Experiences Reported by the Mainstream and LGBTI Media? *Journal of Homosexuality*, 64 (1), 122–144.

Munt, S. R., Bassett, E. H., and O'Riordan, K., 2002. Virtually Belonging: Risk, Connectivity, and Coming Out On-Line. *International Journal of Sexuality and Gender Studies*, 7, 125–137.

Mustanski, B., Lyons, T., and Garcia, S. C., 2011. Internet Use and Sexual Health of Young Men Who Have Sex with Men: A Mixed-Methods Study. *Archives of Sexual Behavior*, 40 (2), 289–300.

O'Neill, M., 2014. Transgender Youth and YouTube Videos: Self-Representation and Five Identifiable Trans Youth Narratives. In: C. Pullen, ed. *Queer Youth and Media Cultures*. New York, NY: Palgrave Macmillan, 34–45.

Oakley, A., 2016. Disturbing Hegemonic Discourse: Nonbinary Gender and Sexual Orientation Labeling on Tumblr. *Social Media + Society*, 2 (3), 1–12.

OKCupid, 2017. Identity Spectrum | Orientation and Gender Expression as Told by Real, Actual Humans. Available from: www.okcupid.com/identity [Accessed 14 June 2017].

Plummer, K., 2003. *Intimate Citizenship: Private Decisions and Public Dialogues*. Washington, DC: University of Washington Press.

ReachOut, 2017. Postal Survey Distress "Indisputable", Calls for Calm [Press release]. Available from: https://about.au.reachout.com/postal-survey-distress-indisputable-calls-for-calm-2017/ [Accessed 11 January 2018].

Renninger, B. J., 2015. "Where I Can be Myself… Where I can Speak My Mind": Networked Counterpublics in a Polymedia Environment. *New Media & Society*, 17 (9), 1513–1529.

Rhodes, D., et al., 2016. 'Safe Schools Review Findings: Experts Respond'. *The Conversation*, 18 March. Available from: https://theconversation.com/safe-schools-review-findings-experts-respond-56425 [Accessed 29 May 2017].

Richards, C., et al., 2016. Non-binary or Genderqueer Genders. *International Review of Psychiatry*, 28 (1), 95–102.

Robinson, K., et al., 2014. *Growing Up Queer: Issues Facing Young Australians Who Are Gender Variant and Sexuality Diverse*. Melbourne, VIC: Young and Well Cooperative Research Centre.

Russell, S. T., 2002. Queer in America: Citizenship for Sexual Minority Youth. *Applied Developmental Science*, 6 (4), 258–263.

Russell, S. T., Clarke, T. J., and Clary, J., 2009. Are Teens "Post Gay"? Contemporary Adolescents' Sexual Identity Labels. *Journal of Youth and Adolescence*, 38 (7), 884–890.

Safi, M., 2015. Sydney School Received No Complaints from Parents about Gayby Baby film. *The Guardian*, 26 August. Available from: www.theguardian.com/world/2015/aug/26/sydney-school-received-no-complaints-from-parents-about-gayby-baby-film

Sensis Social Media Report, 2016. *How Australian People and Businesses Are Using Social Media* [online]. Available from: www.sensis.com.au/asset/PDFdirectory/Sensis_Social_Media_Report_2016.PDF [Accessed 26 May 2016].

Smith, E., et al., 2014. *From Blues to Rainbows: The Mental Health and Well-Being of Gender Diverse and Transgender Young People in Australia*. Melbourne, VIC: The Australian Research Centre in Sex, Health and Society, La Trobe University.

Turkle, S., 1995. *Life on the Screen*. New York, NY: Simon and Schuster.

Vivienne, S., 2016. *Digital Identity and Everyday Activism: Sharing Private Stories with Networked Publics*. London and New York, NY: Palgrave Macmillan.

Vivienne, S., 2017. "I Will Not Hate Myself Because You Cannot Accept Me": Problematizing Empowerment and Gender-diverse Selfies. *Popular Communication*, 15 (2), 126–140.

Wakeford, N., 2000 [1997]. Cyberqueer. In: D. Bell and B. M. Kennedy, eds. *The Cybercultures Reader*. Abingdon: Routledge, 401–415.

Wilchins, R., 2017. Is Trans Over? *The Advocate* [US News & Commentary], 13 June. Available from: www.advocate.com/transgender/2017/6/13/trans-over [Accessed 14 June 2017].

Chapter 11

Taking off the risk goggles

Exploring the intersection of young people's sexual and digital citizenship in sexual health promotion

Kath Albury and Paul Byron

Introduction

This chapter offers findings and observations from a series of workshops conducted with 77 health and education professionals in Sydney and Brisbane in 2015 (Albury and Byron 2015). It considers the implications of the diverse 'hot button' issues identified by participants as key concerns (or hurdles) for them in their work with young people. These included adult difficulties in understanding or 'translating' young people's contemporary digital media practices; adult concerns regarding young people's production and consumption of sexual content (specifically sexting and pornography); and frustration at a perceived lack of 'best practice' guidance and resources to help them better understand digital communication technologies.

The project[1] we worked on, which helped to generate the findings we discuss here, extends our research on young people and sexting in Australia (Albury et al. 2013) and young people's media use and sexuality education (Albury 2013), and builds upon our past investigations of young people's engagement (or lack thereof) with health promotion and sexuality education materials (Byron et al. 2013). As with those earlier studies, we consider how adult professionals (in this case, health and education workers) comprehend and engage with young people's digital media cultures. Unlike much research in this area that seeks to question and/or 'correct' young people's media and learning practices, our focus is on the relevance, impact and limitations of sexuality education and health promotion approaches.

The workshops we conducted were conceived as an experiment aimed at opening up an interdisciplinary conversation around the ways 'best practice' approaches to understanding digital media are currently defined in the space of sexual health education and health promotion. In this chapter we seek to reframe common 'risk-based' understandings of young people's media practices by offering alternative approaches drawn from the disciplines of media and cultural studies. It should be noted that we do not dismiss the real harms experienced by both adults and young people who encounter bullying, abuse and/or coercion in digital environments. Nor do we claim that our reflections on the four workshops we will describe are generalisable to all settings and contexts – they represent specific conversations with particular groups of sexual health educators. Rather, we seek to broaden discussion of the interplay of digital media and sexuality beyond a singular focus on risk. In particular, we propose a discursive model for reframing young people's digital practices as forms of participatory culture (Jenkins et al. 2016), and/or acts of digital and sexual citizenship (McCosker et al. 2016). That is, we suggest a rights-based understanding of young people's digital practices that recognises digital participation as both a mode of individual self-expression and self-formation, and a co-created site for negotiating and contesting collective values and identities. To do so, we will first explore recent theorisations of young people's citizenship in the digital age, before unpacking the 'hot button' issues presented by adult educators in our workshops. We will conclude by proposing alternative models for understanding digital media practices that acknowledge young people's rights to digital participation and self-representation.

Participation, rights and digital/sexual citizenship

While the notion of young people's rights to protection from sexual coercion and abuse is uncontroversial within Australian sexuality education policy and practice, as Evans et al. note (2009) young people's sexual agency is not well understood or supported. As a result, sexuality education (particularly as it is de-livered in secondary schools) seldom frames young people's claims to citizenship in terms of their *positive* rights to sexual self-expression or sexual citizenship. As Ken Plummer argues, rights and responsibilities are not simply given but 'have to be invented through human activities, and built into notions of communities, citizenship and identities' (1995, p. 150). In her interrogation of the concept of 'sexual rights', Rosalind Petchesky notes that within human rights discourse, sexual rights are most often framed in negative terms. That is, young people's negative rights, or 'freedoms from' unwanted sexual experiences are widely sup-ported, but their positive rights, or 'freedoms to' sexual expression and sexual experience, are far more problematic (Petchesky 2000).

Despite this relative absence of a 'sexual citizenship' framework in sexuality education more broadly, there is an emerging language of 'digital citizenship' being applied to young people's participation in online and mobile-mediated spaces, particularly in educational content that seeks to address online bullying and harassment (including behaviours relating to sexting and pornography). For example, the Alannah and Madeline Foundation's e-Smart program of-fers a 'Digital Licence' program through which young people can assert their citizenship (see www.digitallicence.com.au/). However, while the notion of 'digital citizenship' has significant traction in Australian educational contexts (see McCosker et al. 2016), the intersection of sexual citizenship and digital citizenship has not been articulated in either sexuality education and sexual health promotion or in 'cybersafety' education policy and practice. We are in-terested in how this kind of intersecting citizenship might be understood in the context of sexuality education and sexual health promotion, and how the concept of 'participatory culture' (Jenkins et al. 2016) might offer a way into this understanding.

To tease these questions out, we must consider the ways that forms of citizenship might be expressed (and claimed) via participation in digital spaces. When introducing their edited collection addressing 'acts of citizenship', Isin and Neilsen note that while multiple forms of citizenship are now emerging (e.g. environmental, sexual, cosmopolitan, consumer) these are not afforded legal status, and consequently are not formally associated with specific rights or obligations (2008, p. 1). The authors consequently propose a shift in the way that citizenship is currently conceived and investigated. They note that even where citizenship is framed in terms of 'status or practice' (2008, p. 2), the focus tends to be on singular or collective *human subjects*, rather on their collective *practices*. As the authors state, the focus here is primarily on 'the doer rather than the deed' (2008, p. 2). Isin and Neilsen propose a subtle but important shift in focus, from citizens-subjects to the acts and deeds through which citizenship is collectively and individually produced, claimed and recognised. Acts of citizenship are not simply political (in a regulatory or legislative sense), they argue, 'but also ethical (as in courageous), cultural (as in religious), sexual (as in pleasurable) and social (as in affiliative)' (2008, p. 2). They conclude that understanding citizenship as constituted through 'practices', 'acts' or 'deeds' requires an understanding of citizenship as 'simultaneously political, ethical and aesthetic' (2008, p. 4).

Perhaps unsurprisingly, the concept of 'acts of citizenship' is valuable for researchers, activists and artists seeking to interrogate social media practices (Burns 2015, Kuntsman 2015, 2017). For example, Adi Kuntsman's work on 'selfie citizenship' positions the practice of taking and sharing digital self-portraits (or selfies), and associated hashtags, comments and paratexts, as an act of citizenship that is both visual phenomena and network phenomena at the 'intersection of visual iconographies and social practices, political contexts and computer algorithms' (2015, n.p.). Like other social media researchers (such as Lasén 2004, Hjorth and Lim 2012) Kuntsman considers how these acts of self-representation and sociability can also be practices of intimacy, and a means of 'breaking down existing categories of belonging' that 'offer new forms of solidarity' (2015, n.p).

In their exploration of the potentials (and limitations) of the notion of digital citizenship, McCosker and colleagues observe that while this form of citizenship is increasingly invoked in the fields of education and public policy (particularly in relation to children and young people), 'expectations of young people, educators, social service providers and government authorities are framed around "the appropriate use of technology" rather than recognising or promoting digital participation as an act of citizenship' (2016, p. 1). Appropriateness, in this context, does not infer agency in terms of appropriate rights and responsibilities but is implicitly framed in terms of risk-management – that is, managing potential hazards such as bullying, data-breaches or 'overshares' in online spaces. In this context 'the notion of digital citizenship is [primarily] invoked negatively to address problems, with much less attention given to the promises of creative culture and alternative modes of participation' (McCosker et al. 2016, p. 1). Drawing on the work of Isin and Ruppert (2015) McCosker et al. conclude that digital citizenship is not shaped by the avoidance of 'risky' online practices but 'comes into being through digital acts and rights claims and through the varied and often resistant responses to the restrictions and allowances of participation' (2016, p. 2).

This understanding evokes Ken Plummer's framework for 'intimate citizenship', as a mode of citizenship relating to sexual practice, as well as gender and sexual identities (1995). In Plummer's terms, these modes of citizenship are constituted through a recognition that 'rights and responsibilities are not "natural" or "inalienable" but have to be invented through human activities, and built into notions of communities, citizenship and identities' (1995, p. 150). As Weeks (1998) suggests, sexual citizenship (which he aligns with Plummer's model of intimate citizenship) challenges Western traditions that seek to enforce clear boundaries between public acts and identities, and those that are – or 'should be' – private. As Weeks puts it,

> the sexual citizen ... makes a claim to transcend the limits of the personal sphere by going public, but the going public is, in a necessary but paradoxical move, about protecting the possibilities of private life and private choice in a more inclusive society.
>
> (1998, p. 37)

Similarly, acts of digital citizenship (including selfies) may trouble theoretical and practical frameworks that align young people's practices of sexed and gendered self-representation as inappropriate for public space and public view, and therefore inherently risky.

Like McCosker and colleagues, we acknowledge that acts of sexual and digital citizenship – including selfies and other digital practices – are not inherently 'free' spaces for young people. Rather, they can be seen as 'fluid interface[s] that connect control mechanisms with people and practices even within the most intimate of cultural contexts', offering new opportunities for adult surveillance and repressive regulation even as they erode boundaries between the public and private (McCosker et al. 2016, pp. 1–2). In this context, we ask how digital participation may be understood as an 'act of citizenship', and how this can be applied to practices of sexuality education and sexual health promotion. In other words, how can we best understand the intersection of sexual and digital citizenship? And what does this offer to current research, health promotion and sexuality education practices? More specifically, how might an understanding of diverse media practices within young people's sexual cultures facilitate service provision that better meets young people's needs? To consider the value of a sexual and digital citizenship approach to young people's media practices, we will first share some findings from the work we undertook, and contextualise these in order to propose some future directions for research, policy and practice.

About the workshops

The workshops we led were adapted from two existing Creative Commons courses, both grounded in participatory and practice-based approaches to media studies (Albury 2009, Senft et al. 2014). Through a partnership with Family Planning New South Wales and True[2] we invited health promotion officers, teachers and other interested professionals to participate in a three-hour set of activities entitled 'Rethinking Media and Sexuality Education'. Our partners provided venues for the workshops and invited members of their staff and broader community networks. Four workshops were conducted (two in each location), involving 77 participants. Most were health promoters (32%), followed by healthcare providers (14%), counsellors or youth social/support workers (14%) and community educators (14%). Other participants included secondary school teachers, education and welfare students, and public servants in the field of educational policy.

At the beginning of the workshop we asked participants to name their 'hot button' issues relating to young people and digital/social media. These were recorded on a whiteboard to be revisited at the end of the workshop. The most common issues and concerns raised related to:

- Difficulties in understanding young people's digital media practices, exacerbated by generational differences and news media 'moral panics'. Here, the perceived gap between young people's experiences of digital culture and adult anxieties regarding new technologies was seen to result in miscommunication between parents, educators and young people.
- Concerns about young people's peer-to-peer information cultures, and the proliferation of informal sources of information in relation to sex and relationships within digital media. Sexting and pornography emerged as key issues here, with concern regarding both relevant laws, and a lack of clarity regarding their potential impacts on young people's sexualities and sexual relationships. In this case, adult distrust of young people's peer-to-peer practices of media production and distribution led to missed opportunities for meaningful engagement with young people's informal sexual learning environments.
- Concerns regarding a lack of evidence with respect to 'best practice' – primarily in terms of engaging with young people on issues of pornography, sexting, digital media and screen-based practices but also in relation to adults' obligations under the law. This uncertainty regarding appropriate educational resources (and relevant legal and policy frameworks) undermined participants' confidence in their ability to facilitate high-quality sexuality education and health promotion activities with young people.

Following this introductory activity, participants were introduced to key media and cultural studies theories/concepts,[3] followed by workshop exercises focussed on digital media production practice. The workshops featured hands-on selfie exercises, adapted from the 'Sexuality, dating and gender' module of the Selfie Course (Senft et al. 2014). The first exercise invited participants to take a selfie (or digital self-portrait) that did not include their face but through which their friends would be able to identify them. In the second exercise, participants first engaged in a collaborative 'decoding' exercise in which they analysed three different images used as profile pictures on the dating app Tinder. They then worked in pairs to create dating app profile pictures that would entice a partner looking for 'marriage' (however that might be defined by the team). Following each exercise, the entire group reconvened to discuss the ease/difficulty of producing specific kinds of sexed and gendered self-representations via the selfie genre. Participants also reflected on their knowledge of various digital technologies (including camera phones) and apps and platforms such as Tinder and Instagram. Discussions also explored technical issues such as photo composition and lighting, and cultural and political understandings of how factors such as age, gender and sexual identity might impact media production and reception. As we discuss later, these activities were designed to encourage a conversation around shared understandings of what constitutes 'good' or 'bad' digital self-representation, and how this might change when different understandings of sex and gender were introduced as variables.

At the end of the workshop we asked participants to rate the workshop content and to speculate on the likelihood of these concepts or activities' being applied in participants' workplaces. We also invited the groups to express their preferences for future training and resources on these topics. The responses provided, and those in follow-up surveys, helped us not only to evaluate interest in the workshop content but also to consider the workplace and institutional barriers that professionals might encounter in their delivery of education and health promotion around 'hot button' issues, such as sexting. Before exploring the theoretical reasoning behind the workshops in more detail, we will first expand on the key issues raised in the four groups as a means of better understanding the ways that adult understanding (and misunderstanding) of young people's digital media practices might impact sexuality education and health promotion practice.

Difficulties in understanding digital media practices

As outlined in the previous section, workshop content did not offer participants specific solutions for 'problems' associated with young people's digital media cultures but sought to explore and discuss some of the key questions and anxieties faced by professionals working with young people, and to rethink these 'problems' through a critical approach informed by media studies, cultural theory and media practice. A common concern raised in all workshops was the difficulty experienced by adults seeking to understand young people's digital media practices, including their use of social media and mobile phones. Such concerns were expressed by participants themselves, in relation to their own work, but discussion often reflected on general difficulties faced by parents, teachers, and health and education professionals. Given the changing media environment, it was noted that professionals are grappling with how to factor new media practices into health and education agendas. Participants observed, however, that adult fears of emerging technology are not new, with some concerned that policy directives within schools and youth-focussed organisations were negatively influenced by popular 'moral panics' that focus on 'new technology as risk'.

Workshop participants suggested that for many adults and professionals, the 'new media' constitute 'new problems'. This was especially seen to be the case for professionals who began working in their fields prior to the emergence of smartphones, and the rise of social media platforms and practices. It was noted that generational differences can make adults more fearful of media practices that they did not directly experience and participate in as young people. There was a common concern regarding what might be understood as a lack of adult literacy in relation to digital media practices. For example, one participant described the impasse between the digital literacies of adults and young people as 'like speaking a different language'. Regarding young people, another participant asked, 'Do we think they've lost *our* skills of communication, or do we not know how to communicate with them?' Elsewhere, participants noted parents' tendency to distrust and blame technology yet juxtaposed this with schools' increasingly using technology in the classroom.

As noted earlier, workshop participants observed that journalistic 'moral panics' consistently shape their professional approaches to young people's digital media practices. Where service providers, parents and carers were primarily reliant on news reports for information regarding young people's activities, they tended to be both anxious and reactive in response. In group discussion, it was evident that where adults did not understand what young people were doing with digital and mobile media, it was difficult to communicate clearly and respectfully. Examples of concerns raised include the danger of social media 'exposure' and how this could affect young people's future, the potential effects of social media 'attention economies' (Marwick 2015), and the question of whether or not adults should regulate young people's 'screen time'.

Concerns about young people sourcing information from peers and other informal sources

Workshop participants both cited and expressed concerns regarding young people's sources of sexual information, and the level of influence and information provided by peers. Participants worried that they could not see or assess peer-to-peer communication via digital media. Consequently, anxiety regarding young people's 'sexting' practices (commonly understood as producing and sharing digital sexual images) and their consumption of pornography were raised in all four workshops. Several participants expressed uncertainty about how to address these topics with young people, given the lack of clarity around 'best practice'.

Pornography was more commonly discussed as something young people consume, although some concern was raised about whether young people are producing pornography. One participant raised the issue of 'porn addiction'. More commonly though, participants questioned the influence that pornography has on young people's ideas about sexuality and sexual relationships, and how this could influence what they believe to be 'normal'. While the focus on particular issues varied from group to group, it was notable that the potential effects of sexting and pornography on young people were raised in each workshop.

As is often the case in formal sexuality education settings (see Byron 2015), participants questioned not only the content of peer-to-peer communication (in terms of sharing sexually explicit material) but also the value of peer communication within social networking sites. These were primarily understood as 'negative' influences, as opposed to spaces that might potentially be supportive of young people's sexual health and well-being. This suggests that the problem of 'communication' for many adults who work in sexual health may result from a limited understanding of young people's media practices, as well as different generational styles and appropriations of media content and language.

Lack of 'best practice', up-to-date knowledge and workplace resourcing

Several participants sought resources and up-to-date information in their work roles to get a clearer sense of 'best practice' and latest evidence around the aforementioned issues. They also spoke of the frustration in finding reliable information, and the challenges of sorting through contradictory sources of evidence to seek practical guidelines (see Parkhurst 2017). This frustration is understandable given divergent disciplinary trajectories, particularly in studies of young people's use of sexually explicit media (McKee 2014). Participants were also uncertain of their mandatory reporting obligations in respect to digital technologies, with one group member complaining that their workplace training and protocol seemed more focussed on professional risks and the protection of staff and organisations, rather than protecting young people. In every workshop, there were stories of ongoing struggles to stay abreast of current legal obligations in this respect.

In each workshop, our participants also raised concerns regarding a lack of access to appropriate resources for addressing young people's use of digital media in sexuality and health education settings. Some expressed frustration in terms of not knowing where and how to source suitable resources, with the most up-to-date and useful information. One participant specifically mentioned their inability to find appropriate sex-positive resources to support their work with young people. Connections were drawn here between sexting and pornography including the legal conflation of 'underage sexting' with child pornography. One participant said they had read a lot about sexting and child pornography but found it difficult to know the most up-to-date laws, noting that in Australia these differ from state to state. Issues of consent arose in these discussions, including consent around sharing images and other media online (see Albury et al. 2013). Many participants were not only unsure as to how they should advise the young people they worked with but also uncertain of their own responsibilities should these issues arise in the workplace.

The 'hot button' issues outlined earlier will likely be familiar to most adults who work with young people. They highlight common anxieties regarding young people's uses of digital media, framing a range of practices (including producing and sharing images) as potentially risky or harmful. Workshop participants expressed frustration at the perceived 'gap' between young people's understandings and use of digital technologies, and the ways they themselves understood digital media practices. It was clear, however, that they were not *anti*-digital technologies – on the contrary, they wanted more information and resources to help them understand the role technologies might play in young people's lives. Crucially, participants did not favour abstinence messaging as a response to young people's mediated sexual cultures. Educators were critical of what one participant termed the 'stop intervention' (or risk-centred approach) but expressed frustration regarding a shortage of alternative discourses or evidence-based frameworks they might apply in their professional settings. It was notable that even when participants invoked personal or workplace policies affirming young people's sexual autonomy, discourses of rights and/or citizenship were not applied to media usage. Where a risk focus is applied to young people's media practices (and or sexual practices) there is an implication that young people intrinsically lack agency in these spaces. Such an approach fails to engage with the diverse ways in which young people engage in acts of sexual citizenship that promote safety (Byron and Hunt 2017).

Considering 'risk' as a barrier to the recognition of sexual citizenship

As Third et al. argue, education and policy approaches to young people's digital practices globally have tended to over-emphasise 'risk' as opposed to opportunity, thereby undermining children's and young people's rights to participation as set out in the UN Convention on the Rights of the Child (2014, p. 9). For young people, 'online opportunities and risks are interconnected' (Livingstone 2008, p. 397), so to only look at one side of this equation will generate a distorted account of digital media cultures. As Livingstone argues, 'what for an adult observer may seem risky, is for a teenager often precisely the opportunity that they seek' (2008, p. 397). Despite increasing critique, the 'risk paradigm' of adolescent health research is enduring (Michaud 2006). Its reach extends to public health policy and sexuality education, whereby a correlation of sexual health risks and 'media effect' can be found, and this is arguably 'framed by covert moralism' (Bale 2011, p. 304).

Livingstone and Görzig (2014) note that while risk is often conflated with harm, it is important to separate risk from harm when discussing young people's digital media practices, given that risk-taking is not necessarily harmful but is an important aspect of developing resilience. In her study of legal and education responses to teenage sexting, Nora Draper (2011) also highlights the dominance of risk frameworks, and the ways risk is unevenly gendered. Young women are primarily cast as risk subjects in discussion of sexting and this 'reflects a theme present during the emergence of earlier technologies' (Draper 2011, p. 227). This uneven application of technological *and* sexual risk is echoed by Nicola Döring (2014), who found that despite sexting being most commonly practiced among adults, 79% of the sexting literature she reviewed focussed on adolescent risk behaviour, most of which related to girls. Further to this, the online sexting campaigns she reviewed promote sexting abstinence and commonly 'engage in female victim blaming' (Döring 2014, n.p). She warns that

> academics, health care providers, educators, and public policy officials deal-
> ing with adolescent sexting need to engage in more meta-reflection of their
> different (sometimes very polarised) implicit and explicit norms regarding
> "healthy" and "normal" as opposed to "risky" and "deviant" adolescent
> sexualities.
>
> (Döring 2014, n.p.)

These tensions were reflected in our workshops, where participants noted ideo-logical tensions between personal or organisational support for young people's rights, and risk-based programmatic approaches that discourage all mediated sexual practices in the name of 'protection'.

We do not want to suggest that our workshop participants were in anyway misguided in terms of the issues they raised. On the contrary, the issues raised within the workshops are reflected throughout popular and academic literature addressing young people and digital media more broadly. While there is a con-siderable body of scholarly evidence acknowledging both risks and opportunities for young people using digital technologies (Livingstone 2008, Third et al. 2014), adult anxiety and lack of comfort with this space has, we suggest, produced a somewhat blinkered approach.

Where employees in risk-averse organisations are encouraged to focus solely on potential harms and 'negative impacts' of digital technology, they are, in effect, wearing goggles (or blinkers) that block other possible understandings of young people's practices and experiences. There is always the potential for risk or harm, yet quantitative and qualitative studies have demonstrated that young people's use of digital technology is an *ordinary* part of their everyday communication prac-tices (Harris 2014). Far from being perceived by young people as intrinsically risky/harmful, online and mobile media devices, platforms and applications are standard vehicles for self-presentation and representation, embedded within most relationships and friendships – both sexual and non-sexual (boyd 2014, Baym 2015). Where these quotidian practices of communication and/or self-expression are solely framed as 'risk behaviours' within health promotion or sexuality edu-cation practice, it is unsurprising that a 'communication gap' emerges between adult professionals and the young people they seek to support.

We suggest that professionals in this space might productively broaden their approach to digital technologies by removing their risk goggles. When the intersection of digital media, sexual identity and sexual expression is approached exclusively through the lens of risk, the only question that can be asked is 'what is digital media doing *to* young people (and how can we stop it)?' This question does not leave much space for recognising young people's agency and their sexual and digital citizenship. If we ask instead 'What are young people doing with mobile and online media? *How* are they doing it? With whom, and to what ends?', we are open to the possibility of recognising young people's digital practices as acts of citizenship. In the context of sexuality education and health promotion, this might also be seen as a 'strengths-based' or 'rights-based' approach. As outlined earlier, this approach would require sexual health educators and service providers to take a broader view of an evidence-base that extends beyond the disciplinary boundaries of public health research. Since the early-2000s, an emerging body of research in the fields of media and cultural studies has sought to understand the nuances of young people's online and mobile practices as they play out within specific settings and contexts (Ito et al. 2010). This literature, which frames media interactions as both social and relational in character, can be valuable to public health and education practitioners who wish to move beyond risk-based approaches so as to consider young people's digital citizenship.

From risk to participation

In a book-length critical reflection on their last decade of ethnographic digital media research, Henry Jenkins, Mizuto Ito and danah boyd explore young people's use of digital media as 'participatory culture' (Jenkins et al. 2016). While the researchers do not adopt an entirely unified approach to key questions (indeed, the book deliberately introduces agonistic dialogue around key terms such as 'participation'), they all reject a narrow focus on 'technology as risk' or 'media effects'. As Ito explains, a media effects approach draws on methodologies developed in fields such as experimental psychology, and seeks to assign measurable effects to variable 'doses' of specific kinds of media content (Jenkins et al. 2016, p. 92). Media effects research does not seek to understand the social or cultural context of media content and, more importantly, does not seek to explore the ways that *participation* in media practices (such as producing, sharing or commenting on selfies) might be valuable to young people on an individual and/or collective level (2016, p. 92).

In contrast, the authors apply the lens of 'participatory culture' as a means of understanding participation in such practices as forms of situated learning (Lave and Wenger 2009), as personal and collective practices of identity formation, and as practices of civic engagement and citizenship. Crucially, they caution against conflating participation with use of specific technologies (such as mobile phones) or platforms (such as Instagram). For the authors, participation has more to do with *shared* cultures than with the use of particular technologies, platforms or devices (Jenkins et al. 2016, p. 11). These shared cultures need not be 'resistant', or explicitly linked to marginalised identities or subcultural affinities – they can be 'ordinary' (for example, participation in Instagram hashtagging or selfie practices). Importantly, the authors note that participatory cultures are not always positive, and do not necessarily 'make the world a better place' (2016, p. 11). For example, boyd and Jenkins note that young people's production and sharing of digital pro-ana (anorexia) how-to guides could not be considered positive or pro-social in a broader context but still meet their criteria for participatory culture (2016, p. 11). This suggests that sexuality educators and health promotion professionals who deploy such concepts within their professional practice can adopt a broad lens, acknowledging young people's rights to participation in digital and sexual cultures without dismissing potential harms associated with online and offline sexual behaviours.

Conclusion

The 'selfie' activities we encouraged workshop participants to undertake did not directly address initial concerns regarding young people's use of media technologies, and did not seek to offer definitions of positive or negative impacts or effects. Instead, they encouraged direct participation in cultural practices (taking selfies) that invited health professionals to reflect on their own use of technology, and their practices of sexed and gendered self-representation. This approach was highly valued by participants, with more than half suggesting that they could directly apply this approach within their own workplaces. This suggests to us that the notion of participatory culture can offer a less risk-focussed means of engaging with key issues associated with digital practices, particularly where sexuality educators and health promotion staff are familiar with broader approaches to understanding 'media as practice' (Couldry 2012, Albury 2013). Where adult professionals acknowledge the value that these activities can have for young people, and how these activities relate to shared sexual (or social) cultures, it may become easier to open up supportive conversations with young people rather than simply advocating 'stop' interventions.

For Plummer, the question of who has 'access (or not) to representations' (particularly self-representation and acts of story-telling) is critical for understanding the ways in which intimate citizenships are both performed and recognised (1995, p. 150). Similarly, in her discussion of the concept of *sexual* citizenship, Petchesky observes that the ability to fully take pleasure in and ownership of one's sexual body, identity and subjectivity is dependent on collective recognition of a range of 'ethical principles … enabling conditions and material resources' (2000, p. 97). These include (but are not limited to) freedom from abuse or coercion *and* recognition of positive rights (or freedoms) in relation to personhood and autonomy. These frameworks and discussions are not new, nor controversial, but are yet to be applied in public health and education responses to young people's sexual and digital practices.

In this chapter, we have suggested that by expanding the current risk-focussed view of young people's digital practices, sexuality educators and health promotion professionals can better understand young people's mediated sexual cultures, and bridge the perceived 'communication gap'. Further, by broadening both individual and organisational understandings of what might count as 'best-practice' to encompass research conducted in the fields of media and cultural studies, a possibility emerges for more dialogic responses to 'controversial' issues such as sexting, or the consumption and sharing of sexually explicit media. By shifting away from a blinkered focus on risk, educators and sexual health promotion professionals can not only foster greater engagement with the participatory aspects of digital cultures but also benefit from an increased recognition of young people's competencies in sourcing, producing, engaging with, and sharing digital media content (Byron 2015). By reframing young people as not only the vulnerable subjects of media effects but media producers (Hasinoff 2012) and curators (Robards 2014), educators and health professionals can expand their understanding of the diverse range of opportunities and risks that young people negotiate in their mediated lives. Finally, by adopting an understanding of digital practices as acts of citizenship grounded in a participatory culture, we suggest that individual and organisations can begin to develop new ways of recognising young people's right to self-expression in digital spaces as forms of sexual citizenship.

Notes

1 The project was entitled the *Rethinking Media and Sexuality Education* research project and was approved by the UNSW Sydney Human Research Ethics Committee (HC15294).
2 Formerly known as Family Planning Queensland.
3 In Albury and Byron (2015), we outline key theoretical approaches as follows:

Encoding/Decoding (Hall 1972)

Hall suggests three models of possible audience interpretation: the dominant or hegemonic model (in which audiences do not significantly challenge media content), the negotiated model (in which audiences may agree with many aspects of the messaging they watch/listen to but still take exception to others), and the resistant model (in which audiences understand the content of the media they watch/listen to but still reject the messaging outright because it conflicts with their pre-existing beliefs and values). Hall's framework is valuable for thinking through the range of ways that diverse individuals and groups might respond quite differently to the same media content.

Circuit of Culture (du Gay et al. 2013 [1997])

The 'circuit of culture' was initially developed as a pedagogical tool for studying the use of media and technology as cultural practices. Du Gay and colleagues propose that aspects of media culture and practice (which the authors define as representation, identity, consumption, production and regulation) are interrelated. This framework suggests that media can be empirically studied and understood through a range of different lenses, at both the level of individual use and collective practice.

Media as Practice (Couldry 2012)

Couldry's framework describes various forms of interactions with digital media in neutral terms, as functional practices, rather than ascribing a psychological motive. It is useful for thinking about media as something we 'do' rather than something that is done to us. Couldry's taxonomy of media practices includes searching and search enabling, showing and being shown, presencing, archiving and complex media-related practices (which include keeping up with the news and commentary, keeping all channels open via continuous connectivity and screening out) (2012, pp. 49–57).

References

Albury, K., 2009. *Media and Sexuality*, One-day module for International 'Short Course in Critical Sexuality Theory and Research Methodologies', for the Ford Foundation and the International Association for the Study of Sexuality, Culture and Society (IASSCS).

Albury, K., 2013. Young People, Media and Sexual Learning: Rethinking Representation. *Sex Education*, 13 (1), s32–s44.

Albury, K. and Byron, P., 2015. *Rethinking Media and Sexuality Education: Research Report*, November 2015. Sydney: University of New South Wales (UNSW).

Albury, K., et al., 2013. *Young People and Sexting in Australia: Ethics, Representation and the Law*, April 2013. Sydney: ARC Centre for Creative Industries and Innovation/Journalism and Media Research Centre, UNSW.

Bale, C., 2011. Raunch or Romance? Framing and Interpreting the Relationship between Sexualized Culture and Young People's Sexual Health. *Sex Education*, 11 (3), 303–313.

Baym, N., 2015. *Personal Connections in the Digital Age* (2nd ed.). London: Polity.

boyd, d., 2014. *It's Complicated: The Social Lives of Networked Teens*. New Haven: Yale University Press.

Burns, A., 2015. Selfie Citizenship: The Political Uses of Personal Social Media Photography. *Medium*. Available from: https://medium.com/@AnneLBurns/selfie-citizenship-the-political-uses-of-personal-social-media-photography-8e91bbf71cba#.xaxyqdwbo [Accessed 30 January 2017].

Byron, P., 2015. Troubling Expertise: Social Media and Young People's Sexual Health. *Communication Research and Practice*, 1 (4), 322–334.

Byron, P., Evers, C., and Albury, K., 2013. 'It Would be Weird to Have that on Facebook': Young People's Use of Social Media and the Risk of Sharing Sexual Health Information. *Reproductive Health Matters*, 21 (41), 35–44.

Byron, P. and Hunt, J., 2017. 'That Happened to Me too': Young People's Informal Knowledge of Diverse Genders and Sexualities. *Sex Education*, 71 (3), 1–14.

Couldry, N., 2012. *Media, Society, World: Social Theory and Digital Media Practice*. London: Polity.

Döring, N., 2014. Consensual Sexting among Adolescents: Risk Prevention through Abstinence Education or Safer Sexting? *Cyberpsychology*, 8 (1). Available from: https://cyberpsychology.eu/article/view/4303/3352.

Draper, N. R. A., 2011. Is Your Teen at Risk? Discourses of Adolescent Sexting in United States Television News. *Journal of Children and Media*, 6 (2), 221–236.

Du Gay, P., et al., 2013. *Doing Cultural Studies: The Story of the Sony Walkman* (2nd ed.). London: Sage.

Evans, S. P., Krogh, C., and Carmody, M., 2009. Time to Get Cracking: The Challenge of Developing Best Practice in Australian Sexual Assault Prevention Education.

ACSSA Issues Paper, 11. Melbourne: Australian Centre for the Study of Sexual Assault, Australian Institute of Family Studies.

Hall, S., 1972. Encoding/Decoding. *Culture, Media, Language: Working Papers in Cultural Studies*, 79, 128–138.

Harris, A. J., 2014. Understanding the World of Digital Youth. In: F. M. Saleh, A. J. Grudzinskas, and A. Judge, eds. *Adolescent Sexual Behavior in the Digital Age: Considerations for Clinicians, Legal Professionals, and Educators.* New York, NY: Oxford University Press, 24–42.

Hasinoff, A., 2012. Sexting as Media Production: Rethinking Social Media and Sexuality. *New Media & Society*, 15 (4), 449–465. doi: 10.1177/1461444812459171.

Hjorth, L. and Lim, S. S., 2012. Mobile Intimacy in an Age of Affective Mobile Media. *Feminist Media Studies*, 12 (4), 477–484.

Isin, E. F. and Nielsen, G., 2008. Introduction. In: E. F. Isin and G. Neilsen, eds. *Acts of Citizenship*. London and New York, NY: Zed Books, 1–12.

Isin, E. F and Ruppert, E., 2015. *Being Digital Citizens*. London and New York, NY: Rowman and Littlefield International.

Ito, M., et al., 2010. *Hanging Out, Messing Around, and Geeking Out: Kids Living and Learning with New Media*. Cambridge, MA: The MIT Press.

Jenkins, H., Ito, M., and boyd, d. 2016. *Participatory Culture in a Networked Era*. London: Polity.

Kuntsman, A., 2015. *Acts of Selfie Citizenship*. Available from: https://vimeo.com/135043645 [Accessed 30 January 2017].

Kuntsman, A., 2017. *Selfie Citizenship*. London: Palgrave.

Lasén, A., 2004. Affective Technologies—Emotions and Mobile Phones. *Receiver, Vodaphone*, 11. Available from: www.academia.edu/472410/Affective_Technologies._Emotions_and_Mobile_Phones. [Accessed 30 January 2017].

Lave, J. and Wenger, E., 2009 [1991]. *Situated Learning: Legitimate Peripheral Participation*. New York, NY: Cambridge University Press.

Livingstone, S., 2008. Taking Risky Opportunities in Youthful Content Creation: Teenagers' Use of Social Networking Sites for Intimacy, Privacy and Self-expression. *New Media & Society*, 10 (3), 393–411.

Livingstone, S. and Görzig, A., 2014. When Adolescents Receive Sexual Messages on the Internet: Explaining Experiences of Risk and Harm. *Computers in Human Behavior*, 33, 8–15.

Marwick, A. E., 2015. Instafame: Luxury Selfies in the Attention Economy. *Public Culture*, 27 (175), 137–160.

McCosker, A., Vivienne, S., and Johns, A., 2016. Introduction: Beyond Freedom and Control? In: A. McCosker, S. Vivienne, and A. Johns, eds. *Negotiating Digital Citizenship: Control, Contest and Culture*. London/New York, NY: Roman and Littlefield international, 1–18.

McKee, A., 2014. Humanities and Social Scientific Research Methods in Porn Studies. *Porn Studies*, 1 (1–2), 53–63.

Michaud, P-A., 2006. Adolescents and Risks: Why Not Change Our Paradigm? *Journal of Adolescent Health*, 38 (5), 481–483.

Parkhurst, J., 2017. *The Politics of Evidence: From Evidence-Based Policy to the Governance of Evidence*. Oxon: Routledge.

Petchesky, R. P., 2000. Sexual Rights: Inventing a Concept, Mapping an International Practice. In: R. Parker, R. G. Barbosa, and P. Aggleton, eds. *Framing the Sexual Subject: The Politics of Gender, Sexuality and Power*. Berkeley: University of California Press, 81–103.

Plummer, K., 1995. *Telling Sexual Stories: Power, Change and Social Worlds*. London and New York, NY: Routledge.

Robards, B., 2014. Mediating Experiences of 'Growing Up' on Facebook's Timeline: Privacy, Ephemerality and the Reflexive Project of Self. In: A. Bennett and B. Robards, eds. *Mediated Youth Cultures: The Internet, Belonging and New Cultural Configurations*. Hampshire: Palgrave Macmillan.

Senft, T., et al., 2014. Sexuality, Dating and Gender, *Studying Selfies: A Critical Approach*. Available from: www.selfieresearchers.com/week-four-sexuality-dating-gender/ [Accessed 30 January 2017].

Third, A., et al., 2014. *Children's Rights in the Digital Age: A Download from Children around the World*. Melbourne: Young and Well Cooperative Research Centre.

Weeks, J., 1998. The Sexual Citizen. *Theory, Culture & Society*, 15 (3), 35–52.

Chapter 12

Queer youth refugees and the pursuit of the happy object

Documentary, technology and vulnerability

Christopher Pullen

The recent refugee crisis in Europe has been highlighted by key televisual documentary texts such as *Exodus: Our Journey Through Europe* (BBC 2016, UK), which make visible the representation of those perishing in the Mediterranean Sea. Televisual, cinematic and on-line documentaries often frame the vulnerability of refugees, largely focusing on the exploits of illegal people traffickers who use unsuitable and over-crowded vessels. Very little attention has, however, been afforded to the plight of queer youth refugees among this number. Despite this, one exception is *Exiled: Europe's Gay Refugees* (Channel 4 2016, UK) featuring 19-year-old Rami, a Syrian refugee now living in Cologne in Germany. In a key sequence, Rami is depicted as listening to the mobile phone on speaker, whilst in conversation with fellow queer youth refugees who are still living 'in transit' in Turkey. Rami is told news of his friend Mohammed:

> When we heard he had died [and he was murdered] we could not believe it. Please God nobody should die this way. Twenty times he was stabbed. Twenty times with a knife. He was stabbed twenty times then they beheaded him. They had tried to rape him. We are in a very dangerous situation. Nobody is helping us.

Mohammed does not perish at sea, his body to be found on the Mediterranean shoreline in the manner that worldwide media attention has rightly been afforded to the tragic death of refugee children (WSJ 2017); he is simply exterminated, with no one to recall this to the world but for Rami who uses his mobile phone as a tool of witness, in attempting to argue for the meaning and value of his beloved friend.

Lesbian, gay, bisexual, transgender and queer (LGBTQ) youth are largely absent within popular discourse on the refugee crisis. Where they are represented, their potential for sexual citizenship is mostly framed through their relationship to mobile communication technologies. A sense of absence, or missing presence pervades, in situating the queer youth refugee as failing to achieve authentic citizenship, rather relying on mediation through technology. This chapter explores the problematic representation of queer youth refugees, almost seemingly 'ghost-like' or absent within the mainstream spectrum of the refugee community and the mainstream media, denying normative and liberal representations of LGBTQ youth as sexual citizens with equality. I examine the vulnerable presence of queer youth in *Exiled* (2016) and *Hunted: The War Against Gays in Russia* (Channel 4 2014, UK), with the latter focussing on 'proto refugee' queer youth in Russia, who may be considered refugees in their own inhospitable homeland. Legislation banning the 'propaganda of homosexuality among minors' in Russia, which passed in 2013, has significantly altered the life chances of queer youth in that country (Pullen 2014). LGBTQ queer youth in Russia as 'proto-refugees' similar to refugees dispersed from their homeland, construct new modes of sexual citizenship, enabled by the mobility of modern technology. As John Urry (2007, p. 50) states '[I]n a mobile world there are extensive and intricate connections between physical travel and modes of communication and these form new fluidities that are difficult to stabilize'. Queer citizens in Russia engage in the liberating potential of online media to make new social connections in developing their sexual citizenship. However, whilst they may challenge ideologies, form alliances and make new partnerships, at the same time there is a lack of stability and relative vulnerability. This has led not only to the rise of homophobic vigilante groups, as discussed in *Hunted*, but also, in the case of the Russian republic of Chechnya, to the authorities launching an anti-gay campaign, which in 2017 led to their 'rounding up dozens of men suspected of being homosexual', involving three murders (Guardian 2017).

In this chapter, I explore a number of case studies that frame the documentary content, at the same time considering the potential of individuals to document the meaning of their lives as social actors, in challenging the notion of the authentic documented citizen. I examine the extreme vulnerability of queer refugee youth, and proto refugee youth, in relation to 'UndocuQueer' movement in the USA (UndocuQueer 2017), which, I argue, offers an idealistic social justice model of civil rights for queer citizens. In addition I consider the experiences of queer youths in Iran, framing the impact of queer activist Arsham Parsi and representations within the documentaries *Out in Iran: Inside Iran's Secret Gay World* (CBC 2007, Canada) and *A Jihad for Love* (Parvez Sharma 2007, USA). In each of these texts, I explore the significance of online media and documentary performativity (Pullen 2007, Pullen and Cooper 2010), considering the ambivalent use of technology. At the same time I foreground the potential of the 'autobiographical self' (Pullen 2016), whereby queer youth refugees frame aspects of intimacy, vulnerability and self-reflexivity in defining powerful new narratives of change. I examine the representation of queer youth developing their identity as sexual citizens, enabled through the mobility offered by new online technologies. Forming part of what Anthony Giddens (1991) terms as 'disembedding mechanisms', through which modern technology frees the individual from the hold of the local, there is a focus on 'lived time' or experiential time, rather than time focussed on local labour or local identity, in a rejection of physical local space. As Giddens affirms,

> [T]he severance of time from space does not mean that these henceforth become mutually alien aspects of human social organisation. On the

contrary: it provides the very basis for their recombination in the ways that coordinate social activities without necessarily reference to the particularities of place.

(p. 17)

I argue that queer youth as refugees and proto refugees reject a sense of local space in forming new modes of sexual citizenship and that this may be considered part of a wider 'queer diaspora' (Patton and Sánchez Eppler 2000, Gopinath 2005). The notion of the 'queer diaspora' involves a response to histories of colonial, ethical, racial, homophobic and transphobic oppression, through queer individuals forming a mobile sense of citizenship.

The social mobility of online media as a tool to emancipate individuals from the 'hold of the local' frames the potential of the Queer Diaspora as an enabling force of possibility and resistance, in forming new modes of sexual citizenship. As part of this, I argue that the performative potential of queer youth refugees offer a transnational prospect, 'not defined by national borders, societies and determinations, but by the possibilities that exist within the diverse constitution of [the queer diaspora, framing] the personal, the intimate, and the experiential' (Pullen 2012a, p. 16). Mobile communication technologies offer the potential for new models of citizenship based on mobility free from the hold of the local, and the dominant hierarchical form. Queer youth refugees may be considered vulnerable, but at the same time they are icons of agency and interaction that stimulate new ways of theorising sexual citizenship as mobile and not fixed in any place.

The queer body, citizenship and pursuit of the happy object

The queer 'refugee' body is not only represented as vulnerable in an inhospitable homeland or vulnerable en route to some imagined better place, but also often remains vulnerable even when a new homeland is found. For queer youth refugees, aspects of vulnerability are complex. Although queer youth might identify with libertarian notions of sexual citizenship, that appear to be 'privatised, deradicalised, de-eroticised and *confined* in all senses of the word: kept in place, policed, limited' (Bell and Binnie 2000, p. 3), through attachment to the nation state, potentially there are social networks of support, resistance and even legislation that might support the notion of the queer citizen. As Jeffrey Weeks (2000, p. 191) states, 'The 'moment of citizenship' is precisely this moment towards inclusion, towards redefining the polity to incorporate fully those that have felt excluded'. For queer youth refugees, aspects of exclusion and inclusion are fluid concepts, founded not on citizenship in relation to the nation state but rather through an intimation of citizenship framed within the modes of technological communication. Hence although there is the potential for the queer youth refugee to produce sexual citizenship in the manner of 'intimate citizenship' (Plummer 2003), in the presentation of intimate narrative that frames the democratic ideal, this is problematic as the queer youth refugee is a mobile sexual citizen, unfixed in abode. Vulnerability is specifically apparent for queer youth refugees, in their doubly abject situation as devalued in comparison to queer youth that may be 'authentic citizens', and through the fact that their sexual citizenship is acted out though technology, and is reliant on this form.

For queer youth refugees the performance and representation of technology, offers a complex relationship to life chances and the search for the 'happy object', in working towards citizenship. As Sara Ahmed (2010, p. 21) argues,

> Happiness involves affect (to be happy is to be affected by something), intentionality (to be happy is to be happy about something), and evaluation or judgement (to be happy about something makes something good). If happiness creates its objects, then such objects are passed around, accumulating positive affective value as social goods.

For refugee queer youth then, the search for the happy object might involve the affective potential of making social connections and finding a new place for home, enabled through new online technologies.

The search for the 'happy object' of finding new community and social/sexual partners by proto refugee queer youths is, however, depicted in *Hunted* as complex and problematic. Without the protection of law enforcers, groups of thugs target vulnerable queer youth with impunity; queer youth are literally hunted as 'fair game' by perpetrators accessing them primarily through queer dating apps. Mobile communication technologies here not only offer the means to entrap those that wish to find freedom or liberty as they pursue the 'happy object', but are also figured in framing the vulnerability of queer youth by the documentary producers. For example, 23-year-old Iraqi refugee Mustapha is represented in *Exiled* as using dating apps to find sex work as he has little support from the community in Germany (discussed later). Whilst the documentary producer empathises with his situation, greater focus is given to the constitution of his possible sex work than to his abject vulnerability in failing to achieve ownership of the 'happy object' of staying in Europe.

Maria Stehle (2016, p. 106) advises in exploring the representation of migrants attempting to arrive in Europe in search of happiness:

> It is neither the search itself nor the unhappy effects, but rather the ambivalences that arise from both the searches themselves and the unhappiness they produce that open up avenues for an alternative set of imaginings.

In this way, whilst technology is represented as clearly framing the means for the refugee to achieve happiness, alternative imaginings are presented. For example in *Exiled* although online smartphone technology is represented as the means to follow safe pathways through GPS, find safe connections and build communities, the refugees' vulnerability is simultaneously represented as co-present in the context of these enabling technologies. This is apparent where a high financial commitment is needed to own and maintain such technology, suggesting refugees could be vulnerable to robbery. Also queer youth refugees might be vulnerable to predators by being drawn into sex work that itself is enabled by the technology of dating apps. The pursuit of happiness through the aid of technology, hence, is complex when read in these documentary examples.

UndocuQueer and queer diaspora

However, if we consider the rise of the 'UndocuQueer' movement in the USA, happiness might more clearly defined, relative to a social justice ideology, that addresses 'real world processes of inequality, such as racism and homophobia, that disrupt civic participation' (Teunis and Gilbert 2007, p. 2) for minority groups. The 'UndocuQueer' movement and the '1.5-generation' (not quite second generation) in the USA, includes 'undocumented immigrants who are politically active on issues of immigration and same-sex sexuality [often signifying] those who emigrate before adolescence' (Seif 2014, p. 90). As Hinda Seif reports, citing the influence of activists Tania Unzueta and Julio Salgado, the movement started in 2010:

> This new strategy for the immigrant rights movement … gave voice to and made visible people who had been objectified as "illegal aliens". … Used with tactics such as voter mobilizations and sit-ins inspired by the U.S. civil rights movement, this humanization of undocumented youth was highly effective.
>
> (Seif 2014, p. 88)

Undocumented queer youth in the USA play a major part in mediating the discourse of the queer migrant and the refugee, evident in their ability to produce content that speaks personally about their aspirations and their life chances in finding a new home in the USA, often arriving from Latin America. This, I argue, is contextual to the discourse of mainstream documentaries such as *Hunted* and *Exiled*, where similarly technology and social networking are foregrounded in producing, or critiquing, notions of sexual citizenship and the 'promise of happiness' (Ahmed 2010).

The desire to achieve happiness through social justice is particularly evident in the online video entitled 'UndocuQueer Manifesto' produced by United We Dream (2017), where a diverse range of queer youth offer affirmative visions:

> Our love and queerness and our transitions, have travelled through mountains, rivers, deserts and oceans, and settled in the hearts of open minds. We

are all different people with different names, cultures, bodies, desires, roads and different life philosophies, invested in working collectively towards the liberation of our dreams. … We seek to bring an end to the violence within our communities and families. … If you believe in social justice, then what makes us different than you?

(YouTube 2017a)

Offering a youth-centred focus, which frames a range of contributors of diverse sexual identity and racial backgrounds, the documentary reflects the aspirations of young queer undocumented citizens, advocating a social justice model that might be accommodating to all. This does not only include positive statements on integration, such as

What makes me a fierce "UndocuQueer", is my determination and my active pursuit of my higher education … My whole life I have been wanting to be a member of the military, and the fact that I am undocumented deprives me from that opportunity.

(YouTube 2017b)

There are also direct challenges to established authority. For example in a video entitled 'BREAK THE CAGE: STOP Detaining & Abusing LGBTQ Immigrants', rather than a positive upbeat message with personal statements as 'talking head' representations, we are presented with menacing music, with text-based content. Central within this is the statement by Joclyn Mendoza, transgender leader with United We Dream,

We are put into gay 'Pods' and solitary confinement for being LGBTQ while in immigration detention. We demand that President Obama and DHS secretary Jeh Johnson end human rights violations.

(YouTube 2017c)

Oscillating between testaments of assimilation regarding academia and the military, in contrast to abjections of political discontent, multivalent levels of engagement are inherent in defining a 'queer diaspora'.

In considering the notion of queer diaspora, Gayatari Gopinath (2005, p. 11) tells us that

Suturing 'queer' to 'diaspora'.… recuperates those desires, practices, and subjectivities that are rendered impossible and unimaginable within conventional diasporic and nationalist imaginaries. A consideration of queerness, in other words, becomes a way to challenge nationalist ideologies by restoring the impure, inauthentic, non-reproductive potential of the notion of diaspora. The concept of the queer diaspora enables a simultaneous critique of heterosexuality and the nation form while exploding the binary oppositions between nation and diaspora, heterosexuality and homosexuality, original and copy.

In this sense, then, while the work of the 'UndocuQueer' movement advocates a social justice model that might seem closely meshed to assimilationist contexts of nationality, the concept of the queer diaspora presents an inherent direct political challenge to the primacy of authentic documentation. This challenge is enabled through personal interactions with new technologies, such as the use of social networking, appearances within online video, and interactions with smartphone technology, offering some documentary veracity as bearing witness.

Documentary, autobiographical self and witness

Although documentary frames the dominant heterocentric anthropological voice of the mainstream, involving 'the encoding of history in documents' (Rabinowitz 1994, p. 18), inevitably outsiders or those that may be 'undocumented' offers some subcultural potential in writing themselves into history. By producing an autobiographical self, based on intimacy and vulnerability (Pullen 2016), LGBTQ youth within the queer diaspora challenge their 'undocumented status', questioning notions of proper history and authentic documentation. As Gayatri Gopinath (2005, p. 4) tells us,

> Queer diasporic cultural forms and practices point to submerged histories of racist and colonial violence that continue to resonate in the present and that make themselves felt through bodily desire. It is through the queer diasporic body that these histories are brought into the present; it is also through the queer diasporic body that their legacies are imaginatively contested and transformed.

Although there is an 'anthropological unconsciousness' within documentary form, which Bill Nichols suggests prioritises 'whiteness, maleness, [the] body of the observer, the experimental [and the] canonical conventions of western narrative' (Nichols 1994, p. 65), 'undocumented' queer youth subvert these normative ways of viewing, through personally framing histories of racial and homo-/transphobic oppression.

Such queer diasporic performances that frame the autobiographical self involve

> Testimonials [that] are first person, oral more than literary, personal more than theatrical. Such work explores the personal as political at the level of textual self-representation, as well as at the level of lived experience.
>
> (Nichols 1994, p. 8)

Lived experience, I argue, is related in reference not only to the performance of the 'undocumented' documentary subject but also to the ability to share the experience in terms of witness as a physical body connected to the event, involving as Rodger Hallas (2009, p. 11) attests: '[t]o witness requires one's physical presence at the event. To *bear witness* (to testify) to that event also requires the physical presence of the self same witness at the moment of enunciation'. There is a sense of reciprocity in this process in bearing witness to trauma that affirms the 'magnitude of the event'. The parties involved that bear witness in some ways relive the event, reflecting their personal emotions not only as autobiographical subjects sharing feelings and responses but also in establishing the significance of the event. For Rami, for example, on hearing the news of Mohammed's tragic murder (discussed earlier), he is a witness not only to the event itself but to news of the event; this itself is made more vivid by the means in which he represents himself. By allowing himself to be represented as hearing the news of the murder of a beloved friend on speaker setting on a mobile phone, rather than presenting himself as presenting the news, he makes himself vulnerable – seemingly a traumatic victim himself. Such a representation of vulnerability, offers a powerful documentary vision of witness and feeling, framing the loss of life chances and responses to such loss.

However, as I argue in the next section, diverse layers of agency may be apparent in defining new opportunities for social justice by bearing witness within documentary form.

Queer youth refugees in Iran[1]

In 2005, Iran was the focus of international attention, when two young men, Mahmoud Asgari, aged 17, and Ayaz Marhoni, aged 18, were publicly hanged in the Edalat (Justice) Square of the town of Mashhad in north-east Iran, found guilty of homosexual acts. Disturbing images of the two young men were disseminated online, initially represented as blindfolded, with ropes around their necks just before execution, and then represented with their bodies swinging from the rope at the end of a crane. We are told that 'prior to their execution, the teenagers were held in prison for 14 months and severely beaten with 228 lashes' (Gay Orbit 2006), later they were tried under Islamic Sharia law, then sentenced to death.

Although Brain Whitaker (2006) reveals countries such as Jordan and Saudi Arabia are equally as punitive, Iran has become a central focus for its severe oppression of queer lives, despite official denial of the existence of gay men and lesbians in the country (CNN 2008).[2] Parvez Sharma's *A Jihad for Love* and Farid Haerinejad's *Out in Iran* are documentary texts that exposed the hidden life stories of queer citizens in Iran; they also suggested that rather than shameful, many were adherent to religious order, and many were starting a gay civil rights movement in the country.

In 2004, at age 24, Arsham Parsi started a revolutionary website called Iranian Queer Organisation while he was still living in Iran. At the time of writing he remains an activist, now running The Iranian Railroad for Queer Refugees.

Parsi tells us in his autobiographical account *Exiled for Love: The Journey of an Iranian Queer Activist* (2015, p. 13) that

> I was fourteen when I discovered who I was. And, in that same moment I found out that I could be punished by death [under the prescribed punishments within Sharia Law]. Being thrown from the top of a tall building. Being cut in half by a sword. Hanging. Stoning. [Sharia Law] described in great detail all of these methods of execution and encouraged punishments for homosexuality. ... I became obsessed about the idea of being stoned to death. I thought about it constantly: while I was at school, at home with my family, and especially when I lay alone in my bed at night.

As a youth he was troubled by his queer identification, feeling like an abject outsider that could lawfully be eliminated at any time. Although he identified himself as a 'sexual citizen' making connections with a wider community where he felt he might fit in, living in a nation state where queer citizenship is denied, he considered himself as an abject subject, liable to be persecuted or erased. Such oppression, however, involves complex relations to wider society, as an US human rights speaker tells us in *Out in Iran*:

> Most morals cases, sexual offences cases in Iran are tried in closed sessions, information doesn't leak out of the courtroom. Because of stigma and shame families and friends of the accused don't want to talk.

Hence few people involve themselves in a challenge to the status quo for fear of association and moral judgement.

Despite this, as Parsi grew up he started feeling more confident regarding his identity, after seeing positive representations of queer life online. However he also became galvanised into action when two of his queer friends committed suicide:

> Their deaths galvanized him to begin a gay and lesbian support group, conducted furtively and electronically, consisting largely of articles on gay-related subjects from English language sources. The enterprise grew to include six separate electronic magazines.

(Stephens 2007)

The Iranian Queer Organisation website was hosted in Norway (Homan 2008), achieving a membership of 5,000 Iranian users, whilst disseminating positive messages concerning gay and lesbian identity, and warning of oppression and torture perpetrated against homosexuals in Iran. However Parsi was considered a threat by the authorities in Iran, leading him to leave the country in fear for his life, later taking refuge in Turkey (discussed later) before achieving refugee status in Canada.

While we discover in Farid Haerinejad's documentary *Out in Iran*, that Mani Zaniar continued Arsham Parsi's activist work in Iran, with Zaniar telling us,

> The only important thing is that someday I could walk and breathe freely in this country. And get to choose the one I love and live with him freely. To have the same rights as other citizens: to have the right to legal marriage, to have the right to adopt a child. These are very basic things. It's not extraordinary at all. … Right now its hope that's all.

Zaniar, like Parsi, cannot remain in Iran because his participation in *Out in Iran* makes him vulnerable. Such a focus on an unspeakable and untenable life is apparent in Parvez Sharma's documentary *A Jihad for Love*.

Filmed over five and a half years in 12 countries and in nine languages, Parvez Sharma's *A Jihad for Love* was an enduring and large-scale project, where Sharma 'seeks to reclaim the Islamic concept of a greater Jihad', which, whilst it is often associated with war, may be interpreted as 'an inner struggle' or 'to strive in the path of God'. Parvez not only explores the lives of many queer citizens adherent to the Islamic faith but also he focusses on many refugees living outside their homeland; central within this is the representation of queer youth activist Arsham Parsi before he gained asylum in Canada, alongside other refugees.

In a pivotal sequence in *Jihad for Love* Arsham and Payam along with Amir and Mojtaba whose identities are concealed, are represented as living 'in transit' in Turkey through applying to the United Nations High Commissioner for Refugees (UNHCR). They seem like a family kinship group in the manner of Kath Weston's (1991) concept of 'families we choose', making home altogether in a relatively makeshift and squalid flat in central Turkey. Payam tells us,

> Even though we have left Iran we still don't feel safe. Arsham and I wish Amir and Mojtaba weren't afraid to show their faces [in this documentary]. Fear has followed us from Iran to Turkey. They're afraid for their families' safety [should their identities be found out at home]. … Turkey doesn't grant refugee status to Iranian refugees. Were only allowed to stay until the UNHCR decides our cases. If we win our cases we will have to leave Turkey. If we lose we will be sent back to Iran.

This fragile kinship family unit awaits the outcomes of their respective cases brought to the UNHCR. During this time, the 'family' group travel by bus to a hillside overlooking a city, they lie on the ground in close quarters as animals huddle together to settle in for the night appreciating the warmth of their bodies. They discuss a wedding video that Mojtaba and his partner had produced, which unfortunately was taken by the police in Iran, and which could have been used to provide evidence in Mojtaba's case to the UNHCR in affirming his queer status as a refugee – now uncertainty pervades.

A Jihad for Love frames the trial of the queer youth refugee, revealing the un-just status at home as much as the troubling journey ahead and the uncertain prospect of reaching a new home. Central within this is not only the significance of bearing witness to the events that have unfolded, involving accounts of the past, the experience of the moment and hopes for the future but also that such testaments relate to the affective possibility of happiness or the resolution of such fears, where contentment may be found in the arrival at new places. However, as Ahmed (2010) tells us, for the migrant there is a complex relationship to the achievement of happiness. The 'melancholy migrant, [is] the one who refuses to participate in the national game' (p. 142), seeming as 'a rather ghostly figure, haunting contemporary culture as a… hurtful reminder of racism' (p. 148) em-bodying 'the persistence of histories (of racism) that cannot be wished away by happiness' (p. 159). For the queer refugee, the achievement of the happy object, arriving or to stay in Europe or America, or to be officially documented as an authentic citizen, is doubly abject engaging not only with histories of racism, but also those of homophobia, and the extreme violence exerted upon the queer body.

Violence and abject melancholia

While the iconic murders of Mahmoud Asgari (aged 17) and Ayaz Marhoni (aged 18) in Iran in 2005 (discussed earlier), offer a vivid representation of the ultimate vulnerability of the queer body, I argue that the documentaries *Hunted* and *Exiled* contextualise to the contemporary use of personal media technology, in framing new subtle contexts of vulnerability in the production of sexual citizenship. At the same time there are concerns with regards to documentary ethics, such as in the recording of the vulnerability of the queer youth refugee.

In both *Exiled* and *Hunted* smartphone technology and, particularly, the use of social networking apps seem to offer liberation in the ability to make friends and form communities of resistance or empowerment. There are, however, also moral imperatives and dangers in using these technologies. The Middle Eastern refugee has little means of support and potentially is encouraged to find sex work enabled by the use of technology in order to survive. The Russian 'undocumented' queer youth tries to escape from oppression by using dating apps to find partners and friends but is easily caught or trapped by punishing individuals, posing with false identities.

In the documentary *Hunted* vigilante groups are represented as searching for gay men to target. In a key sequence after the film-makers have gained access to a vigilante group[3] based in St Petersburg, we are told that 'this is a regular Sunday pastime' and that the 'network is active in over 30 Russian cities, and continually uploads [videos to the internet of] vicious assaults and humiliating interviews with their victims'. The vigilante group use online social networking to make contact with a victim, who is brought back to the flat, unaware that this was an entrapment.

Whilst the producers are discouraged from filming the assault, the producers tell us that 'there are 13 men spoiling for a fight' directed by a female leader of the vigilante group called Katia. In what makes for very uncomfortable viewing, we are advised that the film producers 'fight their way back into the room' hoping to limit the extent of the assault on the individual. After a period in which the camera fails to clearly focus on what is taking place, all we see are shifting figures milling about the room in a menacing manner, with the sound of the victim painfully growling as if subject to extreme restraint. As the camera moves forward we see the victim depicted as on a bed, initially with a larger, violent figure towering over him, punching at his body, while later two men sit on either side of the victim, rigorously holding him down. In this oppressive context, we get the impression that the assailants find some physically charged sexual pleasure in this assault as much as this appears as a retribution for some imagined crime.

Whilst the victim is still visibly struggling, group leader Katia attempts to get the 'interview' to be uploaded online for humiliation. Katia asks absurd questions, including 'You don't want to talk to a pretty girl?', 'Shall I give you a massage?', then, laughing, 'You Faggot!' Later he is warned, 'You are not going anywhere till you have answered my questions'.

Although the documentary makers blur the face of the victim to protect his identity, he appears to be a young gay man under the age of 20. He is questioned relentlessly about sexual practice, in a humiliating and taunting manner. Near the end of the 'interview' Katia asks what will happen if his face is shown online; the victim attests that he will lose his job, and the vigilante group laughs with extreme pleasure and satisfaction, followed by a comment from one of the group, 'Shall we piss on him?'. While this does not take place he is humiliated further, filmed being made to dance holding cans in a childlike manner, accompanied by simplistic music. After this he is told to 'piss off' in what was an assault that lasted for over an hour. The documentary makers advise us, 'We left with him to offer assistance and support. He asked us not to contact the police'.

Although there is intent to communicate a very specific message about belonging, inclusion, danger and risk in this horrifying account, contentious ethical imperatives are apparent in filming this assault. Linda Williams points out that there is 'no perfect ethical solution to the question of documentary intervention' (1999, p. 188). This raises questions such as 'What is an ethically appropriate response of a documentarian faced with human misery? [and] What is the documentarian's commitment to the truth of a situation as weighted against his or her subjective entanglement within?' (p. 176). We experience a potential ambivalence; in considering the ethical care of the victim as an individual, in contrast with the ethical imperative of broadcasting the assault for the common good of society – to protect others. Such contention is similarly evident in *Exiled*, where Mustapha is represented as unable to make a living in Cologne, Germany, and he is forced to consider engaging in sex work to make money.

Documentary maker Shaunagh Connaire visits Mustapha who had left a refugee camp in Germany then found a flat in Cologne, but now has to move out, as he has little income. Connaire tells us that 'two years ago Mustapha was studying archaeology at university [in Iraq], but Isis took control of his hometown, so he fled to Germany'. However Mustapha does not find life in Germany as he expected:

> I was in a camp for six months, it was the worst time of my whole life. Men attacked me they punched me and they bruised my face. They tried to have sex with me. They said horrible things, the words were worse than the beating, [calling me]: faggot, freak, worthless, immoral [and] humourless. … Instead of returning to the camp, I'd prefer to go back to Iraq. Perhaps Iraq was better than the days at the camp.

A focus is made upon the vulnerability of his identity not only as a potential academic, who presumably had a promising career back in Iraq, until the arrival of Isis, but also even in Europe where he believed that he could be given shelter and comfort, that he is now a target of abuse, reduced to the status of an abject outsider. As Maria Stehle (2016, p. 108) tells us,

> Europe is both, the evil culprit and the happy object that always remains out of reach. For the Europeans, Europe emerges as a contradictory concept: a space to be protected against an influx of unwanted and undocumented people and a space that fails to offer protection to, for example, refugees.

Although Mustapha might seem to meet the cultural expectations of a desirable European citizen by being an aspiring academic, he fails to find a better life in Germany, and his life goals are reduced, now seeming as an abject melancholic migrant.

Such tension is further evident when Conairre meets up with Mustapha, a few days later, in an area she describes as 'Cologne's very very vibrant gay scene'. She wanders through a bustling street filled with social revellers, seeming to enjoy a warm summer's evening. Conairre finds Mustapha, standing alone within the crowd. She asks him what he will do now that he has left his flat. Although he receives benefit payments, he is unable to find a place to live and is 'willing to do *anything* to avoid returning to a refugee camp', suggesting that he will engage in 'survival sex' as a vulnerable homeless youth without financial support (Hein 2011). Mustapha tells Connaire,

> Because I'll be homeless soon, I have to prepare to sell my body so I can sleep in a bed. I am not the only refugee to do this. A lot of refugees do this.

Connaire moves closer to him as he is sat down, whilst he scrolls through a gay dating app on his mobile phone. Mustapha finds a possible client, advising that as a refugee he will receive little money for sex work, but at least it will be some income. When Mustapha agrees to meet up with a potential client using his mobile phone, Connaire responds as if disturbed and upset with 'Oh gosh!', then asks if she can see a photo. Mustapha reveals that this person does not have a photo, and Connaire sums up, 'So you don't know what this guy looks like, or how old he is'.

Whilst we find out that the possible client is likely aged 43, the scene ends with Mustapha and Connaire looking down at the glowing mobile phone screen, with the knowledge that Mustapha will likely sell his body for sex, as there is nothing else for him to do.

A sense of melancholia pervades, yet frames the notion of continued hope. Despite likely embarking in sex work, Mustapha holds on to the dream of living in Europe, whatever the costs. However, as Ahmed (2010, p. 189) points out,

> Hope could be described as a stubborn attachment to a lost object, which stops the subject from 'moving on'. Hope can even form a function of melancholia, as a way of holding on to something that has gone, even if hope feels quite different as a relationship to that something.

In this sense Mustapha is represented as remaining hopeful, even where the punitive costs are high. Mustapha's dream of finding happiness in Europe seems to be failing, but the documentary makers want to focus on his journey of hopefulness, rather than necessarily on the price that must be paid to achieve the goal of living in Europe. Mustapha is constructed as the abject melancholic refugee who is vulnerable and needing care, represented as literally needing to sell himself, in order to take control and retain the lost project of the happy object.

Despite this, we never find out what took place after Mustapha's final scene in *Exiled*, whether he did embark on sex work, or not. While other figures in the documentary, such as Rami (discussed earlier), who seems to find a place to live where he is settled, and Bashar, an ex-Iraqi pop star who is resilient in defining his queer identity and appears optimistic, both affirm their potential to become sexual citizens, the representation of Mustapha is incomplete, seeming almost forgotten. Mustapha remains a ghostly figure, as the audience are denied closure of his documentary narrative, seeming to fail in the project of becoming a citizen.

Conclusion

Queer youth refugees and proto refugees, on the trail to finding a new homeland or trapped within a homeland, appear as ghostly figures, suspended in time and seeming to exist as outside time. They appear within documentary form as transitory figures disconnected from models of authentic citizenship yet are vivid apparitions of sexual citizenship through the means of online technology. The courageous and highly political documentary performers discussed in this chapter offer testaments of survival, seeming to live in the present day as if among us as wholly life affirming. Arsham Parsi's work at age 24 in forming a civil rights movement for queer youth in Iran utilising online media; Rami's and Mustapha's exhibitions of vulnerability in bearing witness within the mainstream documentary *Exiled*, at the ages of 19 and 23, respectively; and the various online video testaments of queer youth forming part of the UndocuQueer movement reveal an incredible strength and determination. At the same time whilst the unidentified male queer youth victim in *Hunted* seems to possess no identity, in fact his strength and resolve are vivid, demonstrated in his ability to survive the assault. It is this ability to move forward, survive and fight another day that is central in estimating the potential of the queer youth refugee to claim their status as a sexual citizen.

Technology not only plays a role in our ability to gain access to these stories and enable a sense of citizenship but also represents a character in the stories that are told. Queer youth refuges, through utilising online new media and smartphone technology, potentially find the means to build community, make social connections, and are assured of routes or directions. The character of technology as a tool of access *and* storytelling, not only offers scope revealing new dimensions to a wider society, but also it offers a point of identification for personal reflection. For example the representations of both Rami and Mustapha as utilising the smartphone, in the former to hear news of a friend who we find has been murdered, and in the latter to meet sexual clients in order to pay his way, frames the significance of testimony, bearing witness in their demonstration of survival.

Queer youth refugees not only demonstrate the ability to survive but also frame the incomprehensible loss, encouraging us to take action. Our knowledge of Rami's friend Mohammed who was beheaded in an assault, alongside Mahmoud Asgari and Ayaz Marhoni, who were hanged as punishment for homosexual acts, reveal the extreme punitive action exerted upon those within the queer diaspora. Our task in this respect must be to not look away and to sustain the gaze, bearing witness as part of this spectrum. As witnesses ourselves to the incomprehensible stories of punishment, vulnerability, endurance and resolve, we have the potential to not only draw attention to the plight and determination of the queer youth refugee as an abject sexual citizen but also to integrate ourselves as agents for change in modifying and sharing our citizenship ideals.

Notes

1   This section includes some edited and updated content originally published in Pullen (2012b).
2   President Mahmoud Ahmadinejad also denied the existence of the Holocaust.
3   The group is called 'Occupy Pedophilia', which the documentary producer tells us is named in this manner 'as with many Russians the group connects Pedophilia with homosexuality'.

References

Ahmed, S., 2010. *The Search for Happiness.* Durham, NC: Duke University Press.
Bell, D. and Binnie, J., 2000. *The Sexual Citizen.* Cambridge: Polity Press.
CNN, 2008. Ahmadinejad speaks; outrage and controversy follow. *CNN*, 24 September. Available from: http://edition.cnn.com/2007/US/09/24/us.iran/index.html [Accessed 8 July 2008].
Gay Orbit, 2006. *Iranian Gay Youths Hanged.* Posted by: Michael, 21 July 2005. Available from: http://gayorbit.net/?p=2459 [Accessed 11 October 2006].

Giddens, A., 1991. *Modernity and Self Identity: Self and Society in the late Modern Age*. Cambridge: Polity Press.

Gopinath, S., 2005. *Impossible Desires: Queer Diasporas and South Asian Public Cultures*. Durham, NC: Duke University Press.

Guardian, 2017. Chechen Police 'have Rounded up more than 100 Suspected Gay Men'. *Guardian*, 2 April. Available from: www.theguardian.com/world/2017/apr/02/chechen-police-rounded-up-100-gay-men-report-russian-newspaper-chechnya [Accessed 6 May 2017].

Hallas, R., 2009. *Reframing Bodies: AIDS, Bearing Witness, and the Queer Moving Image*. Durham, NC: Duke University Press.

Hein, L.C., 2011. Survival Strategies of Male Homeless Adolescents. *Journal of The American Psychiatric Nurses Association*, 17 (4), 274–282.

Homan, 2008. 'Fighting for Tomorrow', An Interview with Arsham Parsi, by Afdhere Jama. Available from: www.homanla.org/New/Arsham_oct06.htm [Accessed 20 July 2008].

Nichols, B., 1994. *Blurred Boundaries: Questions of Meaning in Contemporary Culture*. Bloomington: Indiana University Press.

Parsi, A., 2015. *Exiled for Love: The Journey of an Iranian Queer*. Nova Scotia: Fernwood Publishing.

Patton, C. and Sánchez Eppler, B., eds, 2000. *Queer Diasporas*. Durham, NC: Duke University Press.

Plummer, K., 2003. *Intimate Citizenship: Private Decisions and Public Dialogues*. Washington, DC: University of Washington Press.

Pullen, C., 2007. *Documenting Gay Men: Identity and Performance in Reality Television and Documentary Film*. Jefferson, NC: McFarland.

Pullen, C., 2012a. Introduction. In: C. Pullen, ed. *LGBT Transnational Identity and the Media*. Basingstoke. Palgrave MacMillan, 1–20.

Pullen, C., 2012b. *Gay Identity, New Storytelling and the Media*. Basingstoke: Palgrave MacMillan.

Pullen, C., 2014. Introduction. In: C. Pullen, ed. *Queer Youth and Media Cultures*. Basingstoke: Palgrave MacMillan, 1–15.

Pullen, C., 2016. *Pedro Zamora, Sexuality and AIDS Education: The Autobiographical Self, Activism and The Real World*. New York, NY: Cambria Press.

Pullen, C. and Cooper, M., eds. 2010. *LGBT Identity and Online New Media*. London: Routledge.

Rabinowitz, P., 1994. *They Must be Represented: The Politics of Documentary*. New York, NY: Verso.

Seif, H., 2014. "Coming Out of the Shadows" and "Undocuqueer" Undocumented Immigrants Transforming Sexuality Discourse and Activism. *Journal of Language and Sexuality*, 3 (1), 87–120.

Stehle, M., 2016. 'Happy Object' Europe? The Search for Europe in Essayistic Documentary Films. *Studies in European Cinema*, 13 (2), 105–118.

Stephens, B., 2007. The Queerest Denial: Ahmadinejad Says There Are No Gays in Iran. *Opinion Journal*. Tuesday, October 2, 2007. Available from: http://opinionjournal.com/columnists/bstephens/?id=110010679 [Accessed 15 February 2008].

Teunis, N. and Gilbert, H., 2007. Introduction: The Analysis of Sexual inequality. In: N., Teunis and G. Herdt, eds. *Sexual Inequalities and Social Justice*. Berkeley: University of California Press, 1–30.

UndocuQueer, 2017. *Equality Archive: UndocuQueer Movement*. Available from: https://equalityarchive.com/issues/UndocuQueer-movement/ [Accessed 12 April 2017].

United We Dream, 2017. *Immigrant Youth Building a Movement for Justice*. Available from: https://unitedwedream.org/about/projects/quip/ [Accessed 12 April 2017].

Urry, J., 2007. *Mobilities*. Cambridge: Polity Press.

Weeks, J., 2000. *Making Sexual History*. Cambridge: Polity Press.

Weston, K., 1991. *Families We Choose: Lesbians, Gays, Kinship*. New York, NY: Columbia University Press.

Whitaker, B., 2006. *Unspeakable Love: Gay and Lesbian Life in the Middle East*. London: Saqi.

Williams, L., 1999. The Ethics of Intervention: Dennis O'Rourke's The Good Woman of Bancock. In: J. M. Gaines and M. Renov, eds. *Collecting Visible Evidence*. Minneapolis: University of Minnesota Press, 176–189.

WSJ, 2017. Image of Drowned Syrian Boy Echoes Around World. *Wall Street Journal*, [3 September, 2015]. Available from: www.wsj.com/articles/image-of-syrian-boy-washed-up-on-beach-hits-hard-1441282847 [Accessed 1 May 2107].

YouTube, 2017a. *UndocuQueer Manifesto*. Available from: www.youtube.com/watch?v=ANlKTdTWp4s&feature=youtu.be [Accessed 12 April 2017].

YouTube, 2017b. *Undocuqueer Video*. Available from: www.youtube.com/watch?v=_9XDe4FT4ec [Accessed 12 April 2017].

YouTube, 2017c. *BREAK THE CAGE: STOP Detaining & Abusing LGBTQ Immigrants*. Available from: www.youtube.com/watch?v=Npfnx7gfqgw [Accessed 12 April 2017].

Section 5

Work

Chapter 13

Young LGBTQ teachers

Work and sexual citizenship in contradictory times

Tania Ferfolja

Introduction

Schools are highly conservative and heteronormative institutions that have a history as problematic sites for lesbian, gay, bisexual, trans* and queer (LGBTQ) students and teachers. This conservatism derives partly from a tradition of surveillance that required of teachers 'a higher expectation of conforming to social norms than the average citizen' (Kahn and Gorski 2016, p. 15). As Piddocke, Romulo and Manley-Casimir (1997, p. 13) argued two decades ago, 'The teacher interprets and applies curricula and can divert curricula from their intended purposes. Consequently, those who would control education must control the behaviour of the teacher'. This discourse still dominates. Teachers engaged by state and religious institutions are required to create future subjects who uphold particular social and ethical standards. Being *in loco parentis*, teachers are under surveillance; they are expected to be role models who mirror or even transcend the constructed morality of the general population; a population that deems that the only appropriate adult (and child) citizen reflects the normative subjectivities of being cis-gendered and heterosexual.

Such a view is strongly institutionalised in Australian schools. Policy, curriculum, pedagogy and practices as well as unwritten rules and procedures discursively constitute and reinforce the normalisation and superiority of cis-gendered and heterosexual subjectivities; gender and sexuality diversity is largely silenced and made invisible. This is inarguably problematic when broader sociocultural, legislative and political discourses in relation to gender and sexuality diversity are becoming increasingly equitable in Australia and across other Western societies. Despite this, heteronormativity remains a dominating feature of schools and its influence is buoyed by conservative lobbyists and politicians who make visibility of such diversity a potential liability for teachers.

Such institutional marginalisation creates tensions for LGBTQ young people who have grown up in a society more liberal than in previous generations and who embark on a career cloaked in heteronormative conservatism. Yet, no known research specifically examines the experiences of these young teachers at this critical, historical juncture. Although working within heteronormative contexts that predominantly exclude or ignore such citizens, this chapter illustrates how some young LGBTQ teachers enact their power, negotiate their subjectivity and make themselves visible in certain contexts within their school communities.

Background

Gender and sexuality diversity in schools

The topic of LGBTQ subjectivities in school has been a burgeoning focus for academic examination over the last three decades; however, the bulk of scholarship has concentrated on the experiences of students (Kahn and Gorski 2016). Such literature overwhelmingly evidences the ongoing harassment and discrimination experienced by many young people and the consequences of such experiences for social, emotional, academic and life outcomes (see for example Hillier et al. 2010, Guasp 2012, Kosciw et al. 2014, Ullman 2015, Kahn and Gorski 2016). By comparison, relatively little has been published about LGBTQ *teachers*, and that which has been undertaken tends to focus on general workplace climate and experiences (Griffin 1992, Khayatt 1992, Kissen 1996, Ferfolja 1998, 2005, Evans 2002, Lugg 2006, Jackson 2007, Gray 2013, Ferfolja and Stavrou 2015, Wright and Smith 2015, Gray et al. 2016), policy (Jones et al. 2014) and more recently on the impact of marriage equality laws on their professional subjectivities (Neary 2017, Neary et al. 2017). What has been clearly established in the literature is that LGBTQ teachers have experienced, and continue to experience, various forms of marginalisation, harassment and discrimination, both overt and covert, by their employing institutions as well as their colleagues, students and schooling communities (Callaghan 2007, Ferfolja 2009, Rudoe 2010, Ferfolja and Hopkins 2013, Wright and Smith 2015).

In effect, such research illustrates that LGBTQ teachers have been excluded as both sexual and school citizens – omitted from being visible, heard or able to draw on their private selves in their professional lives. This stands in stark contrast to their heterosexual colleagues whose cis-gendered and cis-sexual status is omnipresent both materially and discursively, constituted in, through and by the institution, and where their heterosexuality privileges them as citizens (Richardson 2017). Conceptualisations of citizenship are broad and contested, but of importance to this discussion is the notion that citizenship should include *full* membership in a community – where the community is the school; a commitment to the values and ideals of that community; access to civic, social and political rights (Dejaeghere 2008); and a sense of belonging.

It is little wonder that LGBTQ individuals are marginalised as citizens, considering how discourse – that is, broadly speaking, what is articulable about a community, practice or thing – embodies 'meaning and social relationships' and 'constitutes both subjectivity and power relations' (Ball 1990, p. 2). Discourses have their power in sociopolitical and cultural institutions (Weedon 1987), including education, although they may be resisted and challenged. Subjectivity, constituted in discourse, is fluid and contextual yet simultaneously policed.

Transgressions of what is constructed as subjectively 'normal' are disciplined (Foucault 1978). Thus, historically, dominant discourses about LGBTQ teachers have positioned them as abnormal, sick, hypersexual, predatory and as possessing a sexual proclivity for children (Callaghan 2007, Rudoe 2010). As a result, many teachers have experienced discrimination and harassment, have been dismissed from, or overlooked for, employment and passed over for particular roles and pro-motion (Callaghan 2007, Ferfolja 2009, Ferfolja and Hopkins 2013). Many have had to hide or manage their sexuality to avoid exposure or have been compelled to negotiate their professional identities to pass as heterosexual or to conceal their sexuality in some way (Griffin 1992, Jackson 2006, Ferfolja and Hopkins 2013, Gray 2013, Neary 2017), or they have fore-fronted different aspects of their subjectivity, such as being a parent (and therefore heteronormalised), to enable fuller access to and within the profession (Ferfolja 2014). Under these conditions, it would be difficult for LGBTQ teachers to experience an unfettered sense of belonging in a school community. Feelings of integration are further complicated by the conflicted and contradictory landscape in which teachers work.

Insights into the Australian context

In Australia, discrimination based on sexual orientation in employment, goods and service provision has been legislated against since the mid-1980s. Additional legislative amendments aimed at greater equity of access passed in the first decade of the twenty-first century. Political activism by LGBTQ organisations, groups and individuals, coupled with visibility in the media and popular cul-ture, have resulted in long-awaited progress towards a more equitable society for these communities. These developments, however, are not reflected in schools. As Kahn and Gorski (2016) astutely point out, schools do not necessarily change in accordance with sociocultural shifts. Additionally, legislative change and pro-tective employment provisions can only provide limited security for people (Jones et al. 2014) and do not guarantee that discrimination will not occur; after all, discrimination can be enacted in intangible ways.

However, discrimination is not always intangible. LGBTQ teachers work against a complex backdrop of increasing visibility but also a legacy of public moral panics pertaining to the inclusion in education of gender-and-sexuality-diversity-related content, which has been used recurrently for political expediency and wedge-politicking during the last decade. For example, in 2005, a teacher employing an empathy exercise with a year 9 class that related to being lesbian or gay, caused a media and political uproar. The then NSW State Education min-ister banned the use of the materials for being 'inappropriate'. According to the NSW Teachers' Federation, the lesson concerned complied with Departmental guidelines and had been available on the Department's website for a period of 12 months prior (Welch 2005, see also Ferfolja 2013).

Similarly, in 2015, an Australian, award-winning documentary, Gayby Baby, was to be viewed by students in NSW secondary schools on Wear It Purple Day.[1]

The film examined the experiences of children living in lesbian-and-gay-headed families. Despite media reports claiming there were no parental complaints to the school centrally involved with the initiative (Safi 2015), the then Minister for Education banned the viewing during school hours, claiming that it was 'not part of the curriculum' (McDougall 2015), a view easily contested. Once again, this was in response to a relatively few vocal individuals who used conservative politicians and media to support their agenda.

Most recently, an initiative called the Safe Schools Coalition Victoria, which originated in that state, aimed to create safe and inclusive schools for LGBTQ students and families. The success of this initiative resulted in it being available to the nation's primary and secondary schools under the name Safe Schools Coalition Australia (SSCA). Schools could choose, or not, to sign up to SSCA, with the only formal requirement being the Principal's commitment to creating a homo/transphobia-free schools. However, a public backlash ensued, led by some right-wing politicians, conservative media and religious groups. The attack resulted in the Australian federal government calling a review and subsequently rescinding the funding for SSCA. Several state governments then withdrew the programme from schools, except in Victoria, where it has been removed from the control of the developers and will be subsumed into Department initiatives, and the Australian Capital Territory (ACT), which, reportedly, will be soon launching the 'ACT's answer to Safe Schools' (Baker 2017 but see also Law 2017 for a detailed review of the SSCA moral panic).

These examples illustrate a history of public political meddling that reinforces discourses that construct gender-and-sexuality-related content as inappropriate in school education; by extension, this negatively marks the lives of LGBTQ students, teachers and families and hinders progress towards greater societal understanding through education. These interferences are made by conservative politicians, journalists and others for a media moment, yet they are hackneyed practices that continue to be reused for political expediency and personal publicity at the expense of the marginalised. LGBTQ people are also citizens of the nation, and such approaches evidence public institutions attacking their citizens by demeaning their social contribution and their rights to be visible, heard and catered for. Such public moral panics coupled with silences around gender and sexuality diversity in schools, partly the legacy of such attacks, mark and defame LGBTQ individuals rendering them as non-citizens in school communities. It is against this landscape that the young teachers whose voices contribute to this chapter have embarked on their careers.

The study

Six young adults launching or soon to embark on their teaching career volunteered to participate in this small-scale qualitative study examining the experiences of young LGBTQ teachers. The participants were informed about the research through snowballing and through a Facebook post (not posted by the author). The participants, four men and two women, were all in their early to mid-20s, with one identifying as queer (Sean), one identifying as lesbian (Bonnie) and four identifying as gay (Richard, Tony, Marla and Jake). All had been teaching between three months and three years, except for Bonnie, a trainee teacher in her final year of an undergraduate teaching degree. Three participants were high school trained and three were primary school trained. For ease of discussion in this chapter, all will be referred to as 'teachers'. Five participants taught in suburbs of the Greater Sydney area and in state-controlled schools, which are legally bound by anti-discrimination legislation (private religious schools are not); of these, three were working in the inner west, a highly-diverse area with a visible LGBTQ population; one was working in the western suburbs and another was working in a semi-rural location – both of which are generally considered conservative regions. The sixth, Jake, taught in an elite, religiously-affiliated boys school transitioning to coeducational; however, his data has been excluded from this discussion because he was the only teacher from a private, religious non-Sydney school.

The interviews, conducted online, were semi-structured in nature which enabled fluidity in the exchange between researcher and researched and ensured a more natural, easy dialogue. Questions addressed demographic information as well as perceived challenges, visibility, pedagogy/practice and identity performance in relation to their LGBTQ subjectivity and in light of the current sociopolitical context. The interviews lasted up to 55 minutes, were digitally recorded via the online conferencing platform Zoom and transcribed by the author. To protect the confidentiality of the participants, pseudonyms and discontinuous narratives are used throughout (Khayatt 1992). This is to ensure participant voices are in the historical record without rendering them vulnerable (Leavy 2007). The transcriptions were imported into Nvivo for data management where they were coded thematically (Saldana 2009). These were then recoded to establish more nuanced sub-themes that related to the sociocultural and political discourses that constitute subjective experience (Ezzy 2002). The themes discussed in the remainder of this chapter focus on the prevailing nature of heteronormativity in their schooling cultures, their negotiations of it, and the ways in which these teachers created spaces to establish themselves as visible subjects.

Cultures of heteronormativity

Participants in this study variously expressed how they felt welcome at their schools. As interviews developed, however, noticeable tensions and complexities surfaced in relation to the prevailing heteronormativity of their workplaces. These tensions were not always tangible, but participants hinted at an unease about the status, representation, understanding and ultimately inclusion of gender and sexuality diversity in their schools. For instance, there was a belief that reflected the popular rhetoric that schools in certain regions of Sydney with a highly diverse and liberal demographic would be more open to gender and sexuality diversity. Bonnie, who taught in the inner west of the city, known for its high LGBTQ population, pointed out that although she mostly kept her sexuality quiet, she did not 'think it would be an issue' in this locale; that is, that her lesbian subjectivity would be accepted by the school.

> I think especially in the inner city I don't think I'll have any problems with teachers except for having to come out with everyone when you say partner and you then have to clarify that it's not a man. I think after that they're fine. ... I think the schools themselves, especially in the inner city should be fine.
>
> (Bonnie)

Marla who was in a casual position in an inner west school experienced similar collegial exchanges with respect to her relationships.

> One of the school admin officers and a couple of the infants' school teachers, some of them are a bit more chatty, and I've just mentioned in passing that I'm dating a [names occupation] and the school admin officer did say, 'So where is he working?' and not that I had a problem with it, but it's like, 'Oh *she's* working at X' and she was fine afterwards.
>
> (Marla – her emphasis)

Two important issues are apparent here. The first, is that in these schools, being LGBTQ is explicitly articulable and therefore made visible; that is, participants spoke of their sexuality diversity with relative confidence without experiencing retribution. Greater social awareness has undoubtedly contributed to this scenario, as *historically* such honesty with colleagues may well have resulted in negative consequences (Ferfolja 1998, 2005, 2009). However, and somewhat contradictorily, these extracts simultaneously illustrate the pervasive heteronormative culture present in these same schools. Teachers, as representatives of the institution, continue to assume their colleagues are heterosexual. Rich (1980/1993) coined this phenomenon as 'compulsory heterosexuality' nearly 40 years ago. Despite the locale and broader social recognition of gender and sexuality diversities, heteronormalising assumptions by school staff prevail.

Participants spoke of other instances of heteronormativity in their inner west schools. For instance, Marla seemed uneasy about staff ignorance in relation to LGBTQ people and their lives.

> I did have a discussion with the librarian ... even though she has her own religious views, she's quite open. 'How do gay people choose who's going to have the baby?' It's obviously a planned decision most of the time.
>
> (Marla)

This extract raises a complex tension. Although there appears greater comfort in broaching such topics in informal conversation than in the past, and although it is important that people ask questions to self-educate, the degree of naivety is concerning, particularly when coming from someone who is 'quite open' and working in an area known for its high LGBTQ population. The omnipresence of heteronormativity was also mentioned by Bonnie who voiced how her heterosexual colleagues were dismissive of the needs of LGBTQ-headed families. This was despite the school's liberal locale and her colleague's explicit knowledge that gender- and sexuality-diverse families attended the school. There was, reportedly, no concern about the need for inclusion of these families in school activities and one could argue they were actively perceived and constructed as non-citizens – made invisible and denied presence by heteronormative teacher citizens.

> The ... teachers are like, 'They have two mums' - it sounds like a novelty kind of thing. I just don't think they understand... I don't think they know how to react. ... It's not seen as 'normal' or the 'same-but-different'. ... Even when I go as far as saying maybe we should be a bit more careful around Mother's Day or how we talk about it ... they're like, 'Oh no, because most people have this' [i.e. opposite gendered parents]. It's very heteronormative.
>
> (Bonnie)

Sean, communicated a prevailing heteronormativity by pointing to the lack of everyday visibility of gender and sexuality diversity in his inner west school, except in one corridor where LGBTQ-friendly posters were displayed. This corridor led to the teachers' restroom which the only known trans* student was permitted to use; interestingly, other students were not permitted in that corridor. As Sean summed up, 'So to me the only notable, demonstrative support for queerness in the school seems to be for him'. The school did, however, engage in 'Wear It Purple' on the one day of the year this celebration is held.

These workplaces and sites of learning, according to the participants, overwhelmingly catered for the normative heterosexual subject who constituted the school citizen. There was little, if any, inclusion through representation, understanding or embracing of LGBTQ people in curriculum or practice. Visibility of diverse genders/sexualities was limited temporally and spatially and this did not go unnoticed by these neophyte teachers who were still 'finding their feet' in the world of teaching, as the next section illuminates.

Fallout from heteronormative cultures

The prevailing heteronormativity demonstrated by the exclusion and invisibility of gender and sexuality diversity in the everyday, coupled with recent public hysteria in relation to such diversity being included in schools (and perhaps a lack of explicit direction in syllabus documentation, see Ullman and Ferfolja 2014), generally resulted in participants being careful about references to gender and sexuality diversity in their classrooms, despite their openness with colleagues. Marla, Bonnie, Tony and Sean all thought the conservative social climate, exemplified by recent moral panics, had impacted what teachers felt they could say or do in relation to gender and sexuality diversity. Bonnie commented that even teacher education courses had 'become a bit more sensitive'.

Marla expressed concern that she did not want to be seen as 'pushing an agenda' or expressing in the classroom a politic of diversity that beyond schools is now mainstream, legally legitimated and reflected in popular culture; such fears also, unfortunately, reflect historical research findings extending back two decades (Ferfolja 1998).

> I was just showing them some [CD covers] and I put up one on David Bowie... And one of the kids asked me, why does he look like a girl? ... And I didn't know how much to really say. ...The only thing that I pretty much said was, you know what? All actors, musicians ... they all wear makeup whether they're on TV or in photos. I just cut through it like that and I felt that was the only way that I could be true to my beliefs and not seem like I was pushing an agenda in any shape or form... So I guess, in some senses it [i.e. recent moral panic] does affect how I teach ...It's definitely there that I worry that people or parents would assume that I'm trying to push an agenda by discussing things like that.
>
> (Marla)

Similarly, Richard stated,

> I've never brought in gay perspectives. I think I touched on it once. This conversation came up that a girl can't have a girlfriend. So we had a brief discussion about that, but then I kind of skimmed past it because I wasn't sure how deep I could go into it.
>
> (Richard)

The personal impact of the recent moral panics was eloquently reflected upon by Tony, a teacher in his third year, who, as a highly politicised, visible and 'out' gay teacher, felt the impact of the sociopolitical regression:

> What the recent political climate did, especially around Safe Schools, or in my experience, was when you were confident and when you felt able to push forward in a few different steps, suddenly that got pushed backwards, and there was this glimmer in my career of what change could look like and what could be done in a school and I think the recent political climate has really stepped that back. ... There was never the expectation that I would receive homophobia or face challenges from the system per se, in doing quite minor things or even in just existing as openly gay in the school context. But I always thought there would be support from the system if you did and I think

recently, because of the whole Safe Schools thing, nobody even in the system wants to touch LGBTQ issues because of the political fear around it.

(Tony)

These extracts point to the surveillance these young teachers experienced and the negotiations they were compelled to make. Engaged in the everyday require-ments of the profession, they were cognisant of the silences, invisibility and exclu-sions towards gender and sexuality diversity created by and beyond the school. Their schools discursively maintained a heteronormative boundary-marking of what constituted the normalised subject and, at times, the participants felt obliged to reflect these dominant schooling discourses, becoming complicit in heteronormalising practices. Surveillance and the threat of perceived punish-ment (Foucault 1978) if they breached heteronormative values obliged them to be evasive; this consequentially reinforced discourses that conflicted with their positionality, values and expectations as LGBTQ subjects. The fallout from the schools' heteronormative cultures and broader political interferences impacted their teaching practice, professional experiences and perceptions of what is/is not possible.

Creating resistant spaces within the heteronormative

In many ways, the school culture and the attendant behaviours, attitudes and manner in which participants engaged with the profession reflect historical find-ings of marginalisation; it seems that despite some increased interpersonal colle-gial acceptance little has changed for LGBTQ teachers at work. This is, however, not to suggest that these young teachers are powerless in their diversity; power operates at all levels (Foucault 1978) and participants demonstrated their power through a variety of means. One way of doing this was through their resolve for normalisation and their rejection of heteronormative assumptions and practices of the self when with colleagues. Although, they tended to forefront their teacher subjectivity through discourses of professionalism and excellence (Ferfolja and Hopkins 2013), what became clear during the interviews was how these young teachers variously rejected silencing about themselves and demonstrated an in-tention to challenge heteronormative assumptions and normalise diversity when deemed possible. For example, both Marla and Sean rejected the need to label themselves under particular gender and sexuality categories.

I'm not completely open about it but I don't think I hide it. That would be the best way to describe it. … I'd like to say it's one of the least interesting things about me. It could be any label, photographer, feminist, gay – I don't like any of those labels as certain expectations then get placed on you. … I just want to be known as Marla and that's really it.

(Marla)

> It's very jarring to me [telling people of his sexuality diversity]. It's kind of very Catholic guilty and I grew up very Catholic and I just don't like the conversation and so I just kind of let that sit there and let people come up with their own decisions.
>
> (Sean)

As Sean suggests, the process of having 'the conversation' conjures notions of the Foucauldian (1978) confessional where, in an unequal power relationship, the 'offender' discloses their transgression to a (heterosexual) authority, relieving themselves of a burden and seeking atonement. In so doing, the heterosexual subject becomes both entitled and exalted through the right to approve or condemn the confessor's LGBTQ subjectivity. By selectively resisting the coming out discourse through non-engagement, or normalisation in everyday conversations, or by minimising one's LGBTQ subjectivity, Marla and Sean sought to reject the subjugated position of confessor, revoking the power bestowed upon the heteronormative subject by normalising their own subjectivities through non-participation in what has become akin to a revelatory tradition. As Sean pointed out, 'people are used to that idea of a coming out process' which constitutes and maintains a privileging of the heteronormative; both Sean and Marla challenged this tradition.

Bonnie corrected people when heteronormative assumptions were made about her sexuality. As a trainee teacher, she was at a considerable power disadvantage in the institution. Her openness may have been detrimental to her teaching practice experience and outcomes as she was at the mercy of the staff culture. However, by choosing to articulate her sexuality, she challenged heteronormative assumptions and sought to position herself as an equal in the exchange.

> If I'm on [teaching practice] … you know, you sit in the staffroom and you talk about what you did on the weekends and I'd say my partner … and when they say oh he or whatever, then I say, well actually she, that kind of thing. I don't necessarily go out and say, 'Hey everyone I'm gay', but if it comes up I don't hide it. … I guess I'm very open with who I am, and I'm not going to be someone who will stay closeted in my job.
>
> (Bonnie)

Tony reclaimed his power in the classroom by removing conjecture about his sexuality and positioning himself firmly as a gay teacher within the school.

> So in my first year, the advice of my colleagues was to create that teacher … persona that was not gay, and to not let the students know: 'Do not come out to the students. Shut down that conversation and that question at all costs'. … So obviously the kids did ask the questions and the questions kept coming and whenever I would put up that block that was a green light to them that this is something that we could continue to attack and should

continue to attack. … Because all that didn't work and because I was feeling safer in my second year, a change of head teacher and the positive political climate I suppose, I felt more comfortable to come out … So I did that. I came out and that was all fine. There has not been any homophobic abuse from the students that I teach since I just said, this is who and this is what I am.

(Tony)

By articulating his sexuality, Tony disarmed student conjecture but not to seek approval via a confessional. Power, for the students, lay in Tony's silences and deflections which reinforced the notion that being gay was something to hide; a subjectivity that required policing and punishment through harassment and abuse. Tony's consequent articulation of 'this is who and this is what I am' and subsequent performances of 'campness' which were 'fantastic' for his 'pedagogy and classroom practice', resulted in a 'sense of ownership of me from the kids and the parents who've witnessed that'. Tony rejected colleagues' recommendations to self-silence. This rejection normalised being gay as a real and possible subjective location for the teacher subject. By doing so, Tony became a part of the school in the eyes of some, even though his subjective performances conflicted with the approach desired and articulated by some school authorities. Unfortunately, space limitations preclude further discussion, but suffice it to say that Tony's visibility enabled him to find work as an engaged, committed and more effective teacher.

Conclusion

Schools remain highly heteronormative institutions and, as the accounts of these young teachers illustrate, they continue to silence and marginalise LGBTQ subjectivities. Although some change is apparent in terms of discussions about diversity with (select) colleagues, invisibility still largely prevails as school values and ideals fail to include gender and sexuality diversity. Despite the fact that participants felt welcomed in their schools, there were tensions and complexities in their narratives that demonstrate their schools have considerable work to do to become inclusive workplaces for LGBTQ teachers as well as inclusive educational sites for *all* students and families. The heartening factor in participant narratives was their resistance to be silent and invisible particularly with colleagues and that they possessed a firm resolve to challenge heteronormative assumptions about who they were and how they should engage their LGBTQ status.

For true inclusion to occur that enables the embracing of all school citizens, those whose responsibility it is to lead education at the highest levels, such as Departments of Education and state and federal governments, need to take a stronger stand to ensure the visibility and voice of LGBTQ subjects in learning and teaching. Young teachers need to see themselves reflected in their places of work; otherwise they remain on the outside in conflicted and contradictory spaces. As Sean eloquently explained with respect to his feelings of belonging to the school community,

> In terms of my queerness, honestly not at all. As far as I'm aware I'm the only LGBTQI identifying teacher at the school. It's interesting. ...Younger teachers may be asking me about my personal life a bit more, or making a comment about someone being attractive, but it's a queer teacher being led into the fold rather than a sense that I'm able to speak to another queer teacher and identify with that. ... I've one friend who was also made permanent at the exact time as me ... and she identifies as female and lesbian and so that's been really great. I have that kind of sense of belonging in this broader collegial sense, but not, not in school. No.

Note

1 Wear It Purple is a student-led, not-for-profit organisation that seeks to create a world 'in which every young person can thrive, irrelevant of sex, sexuality or gender identity' (see www.wearitpurple.org/about).

References

Baker, E., 2017. ACT Education Minister Yvette Berry Cautions Schools on Same-Sex Marriage. *The Canberra Times.* September 21. Available at: www.canberratimes.com.au/act-news/act-education-minister-yvette-berry-cautions-schools-on-samesex-marriage-20170920-gyl17m.html [Accessed 3 October 2017].

Ball, S. J., 1990. Introducing Monsieur Foucault. In: S. J. Ball, ed. *Foucault and Education. Disciplines and Knowledge.* London: Routledge, 1–8.

Callaghan, T., 2007. *That's So Gay.* Saarbrücken: VDM Verlag.

Dejaeghere, J. G., 2008. Citizenship as Privilege and Power: Australian Educators' Lived Experiences as Citizens. *Comparative Education Review,* 52 (3), 357–380.

Evans, K., 2002. *Negotiating the Self: Identity, Sexuality, and Emotion in Learning to Teach.* New York, NY: Routledge.

Ezzy, D., 2002. *Qualitative Analysis. Practice and Innovation.* NSW: Allen & Unwin.

Ferfolja, T., 1998. Australian Lesbian Teachers. A Reflection of Homophobic Harassment of High School Teachers in New South Wales Government Schools. *Gender and Education,* 10 (4), 401–415.

Ferfolja, T., 2005. Institutional Silence: Experiences of Australian Lesbian Teachers Working in Catholic High Schools. *Journal of Gay and Lesbian Issues in Education,* 2 (3), 51–66.

Ferfolja, T., 2009. Lesbian Teachers, Harassment and the Workplace. *Teaching and Teacher Education,* 26 (3), 408–414.

Ferfolja, T., 2013. Sexual Diversity, Discrimination and 'Homosexuality Policy' in New South Wales' Government Schools. *Sex Education,* 13 (2), 159–171.

Ferfolja, T., 2014. Reframing Queer Teacher Subjects; Neither in Nor Out but Present. In: A. Harris and E.M. Gray, eds. *Queer Teachers, Identity and Performativity.* London: Palgrave Macmillan, 29–44.

Ferfolja, T. and Hopkins, L., 2013. The Complexities of Workplace Experience for Lesbian and Gay Teachers. *Critical Studies in Education*, 54 (3), 311–324.

Ferfolja, T. and Stavrou, E., 2015. Workplace Experiences of Australian Lesbian and Gay Teachers: Findings from a National Survey. *Canadian Journal of Educational Administration and Policy*, 173, 113–138.

Foucault, M., 1978. *The History of Sexuality. Volume 1: An Introduction.* R. Hurley, Trans. New York, NY: Vintage Books.

Gray, E. M., 2013. Coming Out as a Lesbian, Gay or Bisexual Teacher: Negotiating Private and Professional Worlds. *Sex Education*, 13 (6), 702–714.

Gray, E. M., Harris, A., and Jones, T., 2016. Australian LGBTQ Teachers, Exclusionary Spaces and Points of Interruption. *Sexualities*, 19 (3), 286–303.

Griffin, P., 1992. From Hiding Out to Coming Out: Empowering Lesbian and Gay Educators. *Journal of Homosexuality*, 2 (3/4), 167–195.

Guasp, A., 2012. *The School Report. The Experiences of Gay Young People in Britain's Schools in 2012.* Stonewall. University of Cambridge Centre for family Research. Available from: www.stonewall.org.uk/sites/default/files/The_School_Report__2012_.pdf [Accessed 20 July 2017].

Hillier, L., et al., 2010. *Writing Themselves in 3: The Third National Report on the Sexuality, Health and Well-being of Same Sex Attracted Young People.* Wodonga: Australian Research Centre in Sex, Health and Society, La Trobe University.

Jackson, J., 2007. *Unmasking Identities: An Exploration of the Lives of Gay and Lesbian Teachers.* Lanham, MD: Lexington Books.

Jackson, J. M., 2006. Removing the Masks: Considerations by Gay and Lesbian Teachers When Negotiating the Closet Door, *Journal of Poverty*, 10 (2), 27–52.

Jones, T., Gray, E., and Harris, A., 2014. GLBTIQ Teachers in Australian Education Policy: Protections, Suspicions, and Restrictions. *Sex Education*, 14 (3), 358–353.

Kahn, M. and Gorski, P. C., 2016. The Gendered and Heterosexist Evolution of the Teacher Exemplar in the United States: Equity Implications for LGBTQ and Gender Nonconforming Teachers. *International Journal of Multicultural Education*, 18 (2), 15–39.

Khayatt, M. D., 1992. *Lesbian Teachers. An Invisible Presence.* Albany: State University of New York Press.

Kissen, R. M., 1996. *The Last Closet. The Real Lives of Lesbian and Gay Teachers.* Portsmouth, NH: Heinemann.

Kosciw, J. G., et al., 2014. *The 2013 National School Climate Survey: The Experiences of Lesbian, Gay, Bisexual and Transgender Youth in Our Nation's Schools.* New York, NY: GLSEN.

Law, B., 2017. Moral Panic 101. Equality, Acceptance and the Safe Schools Scandal. *Quarterly Essay*, 67.

Leavy, P. L., 2007. Feminist Postmodernism and Poststructuralism. In: S. N. Hesse-Biber and P. L. Leavy, eds. *Feminist Research Practice.* Thousand Oaks, CA: Sage, 83–108.

Lugg, C. A., 2006. Thinking about Sodomy: Public Schools, Legal Panopticons, and Queers. *Educational Policy*, 20 (1), 35–58.

McDougall, B., 2015. Burwood Girls High School: Anger Over Gay Parenting Documentary 'Gayby Baby'. *The Daily Telegraph*, 25 August. Available from: www.dailytelegraph.com.au/news/nsw/burwood-girls-high-school-anger-over-gay-parenting-documentary-gayby-baby/news-story/3833febe90f5df2f19ea16ab3a8c5245 [Accessed November 2015].

Neary, A., 2017. Lesbian, Gay and Bisexual Teachers' Ambivalent Relations with Parents and Students While Entering into a Civil Partnership. *Irish Educational Studies*, 36 (1), 57–72.

Neary, A., Gray, B., and O'Sullivan, M., 2017. Lesbian, Gay and Bisexual Teachers' Negotiations of Civil Partnership and Schools: Ambivalent Attachments to Religion and Secularism. *Discourse: Studies in the Cultural Politics of Education* [online]. doi:10.1080/01596306.2016.1276432.

Piddocke, S., Romulo, M., and Manley-Casimir, M., 1997. *Teachers in Trouble: An Exploration of the Normative Character of Teaching.* Toronto, Canada: University of Toronto Press.

Rich, A., 1980/1993. Compulsory Heterosexuality and Lesbian Existence. In: H. Abelove, M. Barale, and D. Halperin eds. *Lesbian and Gay Studies Reader.* New York, NY: Routledge, 227–254.

Richardson, D., 2017. Rethinking Sexual Citizenship. *Sociology,* 51 (2), 208–224.

Rudoe, N., 2010. Lesbian Teachers' Identity, Power and the Public/Private Boundary. *Sex Education,* 10 (1), 23–36.

Safi, M., 2015. Sydney School Received No Complaints from Parents about Gaby Baby Film. *The Guardian,* 26 August. Available from: www.theguardian.com/world/2015/aug/26/sydney-school-received-no-complaints-from-parents-about-gayby-baby-film [Accessed 18 July 2017].

Saldana, J., 2009. *The Coding Manual for Qualitative Researchers.* Phoenix, AZ: Sage Publications.

Ullman, J., 2015. *Free to Be?: Exploring the Schooling Experiences of Australia's Sexuality and Gender Diverse Secondary School Students.* Penrith: Centre for Educational Research, Western Sydney University.

Ullman, J. and Ferfolja, T., 2014. Bureaucratic Constructions of Sexual Diversity: Sensitive', 'Controversial' and Silencing. *Teaching Education* [online]. Available from: www-tandfonline-com.ezproxy.uws.edu.au/doi/abs/10.1080/10476210.2014.959487.

Weedon, C., 1987. *Feminist Practice and Poststructuralist Theory.* Oxford: Blackwell.

Welch, D., 2005. Let's Talk about It. *Sydney Morning Herald,* 11 June. Available from: www.smh.com.au/ news/Employment-News/Lets-talk-about-it/2005/06/10/1118347577924.html

Wright, T. E. and Smith, N. J., 2015. A Safer Place? LGBT Educators, School Climate, and Implications for Administrators. *The Educational Forum,* 79 (4), 394–407.

Chapter 14

Gay, famous and working hard on YouTube

Influencers, queer microcelebrity publics and discursive activism

Crystal Abidin and Rob Cover

Introduction

Influencers are everyday, ordinary Internet users who accumulate a relatively large public following on blogs and social media, principally through the textual and visual narration of their personal lives and lifestyles. Subsequent to their emergence in the early-2000s, Influencers have progressed from hobbyist home-based webcamming and desktop publishing to extremely lucrative full-time careers. They engage with their followers in digital and physical spaces, and monetise their following by integrating 'advertorials' into their blog or social media posts. In the context of monetising their everyday lives and earning a living through digital activity, micro-celebrity Influencers perform a new form of labour commensurate with the digital turn in neo-liberal economies. So viable and attractive are their activities that a new industry has grown up rapidly, with followers intensifying in brand loyalty to their favourites, wannabe Influencers attempting to mimic successful exemplars, and businesses clamouring to tap into the following of these notable icons. Influencers capitalise on their high visibility in digital spaces to propel themselves into other mainstream media industries including television, cinema, music, publishing and fashion.

Many Influencers are also engaging in social justice ecologies, using the 'work' of their lifestyle narratives and platforms to personalise and promote causes pertaining to politics and lesbian, gay, bisexual, trans and queer (LGBTQ) advocacy. These queer Influencers are important nodes in LGBTQ networks online, especially as they have become ambassadors for various queer-related community and corporate services, amplifying crucial health and well-being messages as informal sexuality educators, and continuing to foster a sense of community and loyalty among their young followers. Within a framework of sexual citizenship, the emerging relationship between new forms of labour and new forms of sexuality are unsurprising. Indeed, as Bell and Binnie (2006, p. 869) have pointed out, contemporary citizenship models produce identity within models of both rights and responsibilities, the latter of which is modelled on responsibilities for labour.

While Influencers are now established across social media platforms and old/new media, much of their content is based on the 'vlogging' framework developed on YouTube in the mid-2000s. Queer Influencers on YouTube, however, operate with distinct cultural repertoires and community vernacular. In instituting and enacting the narrative tropes of queer confessions – such as coming out, struggling with depression or self-harm, the processes of transitioning, confirming a relationship, or announcing a breakup – queer Influencers on YouTube tend to adopt the stance of responsibility, care and advocacy when addressing young followers, especially those they imagine to be closeted, struggling or looking for guidance.

In this chapter, we draw on digital ethnography to produce a content analysis of a gay-identifying Australian YouTube Influencer, Troye Sivan, as an exemplar, focussed on how he used initially his status as an Influencer creating digital content to promote discursive queer support, and how he constituted and utilised queer networks of microcelebrity in a form that simultaneously undertook work for both a rights-based activism and for his career.

Queer networks on YouTube

Every social media platform has a specific repertoire of normative usage and a dominant form of cultural content shaped by the architecture of the platform, key nodes who are often highly prolific and influential users, and the cultural norms of the masses of users. Researchers have studied such normative forms and functions as 'platform vernaculars', or a 'unique combination of styles, grammars, and logics' as a dominant 'genre of communication' (Gibbs et al. 2015, p. 257). Platform vernaculars are co-created through their 'logics of architecture and use' (Gibbs et al. 2015, p. 255), 'mediated practices and communicative habits of users', 'ongoing interactions between platforms and users', and migration across various social media (Gibbs et al. 2015, p. 257). Within each specific social media platform are also various cultures of users, some dominant, some mainstream, and others marginal or underground. Each subculture may practice their own genre of content production and communicative intimacies (Abidin 2015), creating and sustaining specific community 'norms' that emerge from interactive engagement and collaborative participation among users themselves (García-Rapp and Roca-Cuberes 2017).

As the reactions from ordinary viewers, prolific Influencers and YouTube as a corporation evidence, YouTube is undeniably an important space for queer young people to congregate, produce and consume content, look to queer Influencers as role-models and key opinion-makers, develop queer networks that carry across various social media, and foster community beliefs and norms. In this vein, then, YouTube operates as a setting for the performance of particular kinds of sexual citizenship that blur the boundaries between labour, identity, sexuality, rights, justice and consumption.

YouTube Influencers such as Troye Sivan play the role of opinion-maker who can craft discursive networks around themselves as the instigative node. By using a personal voice that is 'engaging and... controversially honest' (Abidin 2017b, p. 502), queer Influencers may present as 'an authoritative yet approachable identity' (Johnston 2017, p. 76), and treat taboo topics with 'intimacy and insight' through personal disclosure (Abidin 2017b, p. 504). Such narrative strategies, wherein sexual literacies are intricately tied into a 'personal journey' rather than the cold facts of queer support agencies, effectively ride on the Influencers' charisma to engage young audiences (Abidin 2017b, p. 504). Furthermore, many Influencers give in to the allure of 'sex bait' or the 'use of sex talk as bait to increase reader-ship and sustain their readers' accessibility and intimacy to their blog persona' (Abidin 2017b, p. 500), and in so doing they inevitably provide new spaces of conversation around minority gender and sexual literacies.

By voluntarily disclosing highly private, personal and privileged information to their community, such viewers allow their collective vulnerability to constitute a queer public, comprising 'the conjoint pleasure of self-disclosure and sharing' (Cover and Prosser 2013, p. 84) in which young people are encouraged into this safe space to seek 'solidarity, support, and engagement' from others (Green et al. 2015, p. 709) through a 'sense of communitarian responsibility' (Cover and Prosser 2013, p. 84). These comment sections then serve as subcultural spaces in which like-minded queer youth offer support and advice to each other (Abidin 2017b, p. 504), and closeted queer youth learn about an accepting public commu-nity for whom these conversations can unfold in a safe space.

Followers are also encouraged to vlog and share personal experiences, using the queer Influencer's narrative or style as a template, thus increasing the volume of content addressing concerns of queer youth and replicating the visibility of queer support through YouTube's algorithmic recommendations and suggested videos. In the same way a 'network of interlinked blog posts on a shared topic' becomes more 'politically significant' than 'the individual blog post' (Shaw 2012, p. 375) in blogging networks; on YouTube the comments section represents the 'aggregation of individual experiences' and thus creates 'a database of experi-ences' that other queer youth can harness. As such, it is the 'day-to-day inter-linkage and exchange' between users in a networked community that make the medium political (Shaw 2012, p. 375), in a practice that Mazanderani et al. (2013, p. 424) term '"people power" advocacy'.

Troye Sivan

The vast majority of queer discursive videos on YouTube today borrow on the legacy of the *It Gets Better* network of videos, focussed on the production and shar-ing of content that is in the recognisable form of coming out narratives, personal histories, stories of struggle and vulnerability, and eventual acceptance and sta-bility. Pioneers of the *It Gets Better* movement, gay couple Dan Savage and Terry Miller responded to the spate of sexuality-related youth suicide media reports in October 2010 (Cover 2012a) by uploading the first *It Gets Better* video on YouTube in September 2010, recounting their struggles as closeted gay teenagers in school, how they came out to their friends and family, how they were gradually accepted by a community of friends and family, how they found love in each other, their experiences of coupling and parenting, and the progress of a life that 'got better' (Gal et al. 2016, pp. 1698–1699) after their schooling years. The eventual resolution in this 'social drama' (Turner 1975) was the couple's ability to successfully form a normative family unit through coupling and parenting, and their capacity to successfully participate in adult life through building careers and maintaining a network of friends. As such, participation in the queer publics of coming out on YouTube re-enacts a queer young person's sense of belonging to 'the political, the individual and the social' (Cover and Prosser 2013, p. 84).

In his study of gay and lesbian YouTube celebrities' coming out vlogs, media studies scholar Michael Lovelock argues that coming out vlogs 'make legible a normative gay youth subject position which is shaped by the specific tropes, conventions and commercial rationale of YouTube fame itself' (2017, p. 87), thus institutionalising 'particular scripts of coming out' to the point of becoming 'cliché' (2017, p. 88). Lovelock argues that YouTube celebrity has 'its own regime of entrepreneurialism, self-branding and the commodification of the 'authentic' self' (2017, p. 88). However, equating successful YouTube celebrity to an authentic self (in the singular) seems applicable mostly to the genre of confessional vlogs on YouTube and is an over-generalisation of the diverse ecology of microcelebrity and Internet celebrity genres and formats on YouTube which respond to the complex and competing demands of narrative, labour, content creation, microcelebrity and social justice norms.

Influencers on YouTube base their performance on 'an architecture of "anchor" material and "filler" material' wherein the former is the mainstay of thematic content production and the latter complementary output to foster interactions and intimacies with audiences (Abidin 2017a, p. 4). For instance, YouTubers known for producing excellent music covers (anchor) may occasionally indulge followers in Q&As, giveaways or vlog confessions (filler). Indeed, some YouTubers may peddle entirely in anchor content, choosing to publish only their gameplay (such as VanossGaming), makeup tutorials or humorous skits, to name a few, without crafting a behind-the-scenes or back-end persona to engage with followers (Abidin 2016, 2017a). YouTubers who adopt this strategy are thus evaluated by followers less on any authentic disclosure and more on the excellence and professionalism of their content. However, for queer Influencers, the distinction between anchor and filler content is not so clear, given that the bulk of their content is premised on the narration of their lifestyles and personal lives. Often, branded content is so interwoven into their personal narratives that it becomes difficult to demarcate commercial and non-commercial messages. As such, their social, cultural and economic value is complexly intertwined with their performance of self-disclosure, in which personal flaws, vulnerability and taboo discourses are volunteered in exchange for relatability from viewers.

Troye Sivan is originally from South Africa but lives in Perth, Western Australia, with his family. Born in 1995, he was talent-spotted as a child for having a beautiful singing voice and performed at numerous events. Although like many Influencers Sivan manages a host of digital estates, this chapter will focus on his two YouTube channels and particularly on a purposive sampling of nine videos on his personal channel to illustrate some key arguments related to the intersection of sexual citizenship and the work of digital content creation.

Sivan began his YouTube channel @TroyeSivan18 at age 12 in 2007 and had produced more than 140 videos by August 2017. A notable turning point in the types and forms of content he produced took place in 2013 when Sivan came out in a milestone vlog as gay. Around the same time, Sivan was talent scouted by music label EMI Australia and introduced a second channel, @TroyeSivanVEVO, managed by the US-based video hosting corporation VEVO, which promotes official music videos and content from Warner Music Group, Sony Music Entertainment and Universal Music Group. This second channel has produced over 40 videos as of August 2017. Subsequent to conducting digital participant observation and immersion on his channel and since 2011, it is discernible that his digital content at that site can be organised across three categories or types, each of which will be addressed in the following: (1) personal vlogs, in which Sivan addresses his viewers in first-person dialogue format; (2) brand collaborations, in which Sivan shares queer and sexuality-related content sponsored and paid for by clients; and (3) Influencer collaborations, in which Sivan appears alongside other prominent (queer) YouTube Influencers in his content in a bid to share their reach and mutually expand their networks.

Personal vlogs

The most significant personal vlog for this study is Sivan's milestone coming out video titled 'Coming Out', which has accumulated over 7,500,000 views (Sivan 2013). In his preamble, Sivan tells viewers, 'this is probably the most nervous I've ever been in my entire life' and that he came out to his family on this date three years before in 2010. He proceeds to tell viewers,

> and on August 7, 2013, I want *you guys* to know that I am gay. It feels kinda weird to have to announce it like this on the internet, but um I feel like a lot of you guys are like real, genuine friends of mine, and I share everything with the internet, I share every aspect of my life with the internet. And um, whether or not this is a good thing, I don't know, but this is not something that I am ashamed of. It's not something that anyone should have to be ashamed of.
>
> (Sivan 2013)

Here, Sivan adopts a homonormative discourse grounded in essentialist approaches to sexuality that are recognisable to audiences for the purposes of belonging and community citizenship. He describes how he had always felt 'different' when he was younger, how he had intrinsically 'always known' that he was 'different', and shared the revelation of how he first came out to his best friend at age 14-and-a-half. Sivan narrates that he was 'genuinely not ready' to accept himself and, while speculating that he might have been bisexual, turned to his laptop for answers (Sivan 2013). At this juncture, he asserts his impetus and intentions for producing the coming out video:

> The majority of the reason why I'm doing this today is because I hope that people like 14-year-old Troye are going to find this video, because I watched pretty much every coming out video on YouTube [...] I watched it between 14-and-the-half and 15, and those coming out videos, and those people on YouTube, those brave brave brave people on YouTube, without them I don't know where I'd be, I don't know, I genuinely don't know what I would have done because um, yeah it just kinda showed me that it's okay. There's people out there living healthy happy lives who are absolutely fine, and they happen to be gay as well.
>
> (Sivan 2013)

Sivan wraps up the video with a message of encouragement to young viewers who may be closeted:

> I'm also here to say that my message is that it can be good right from the start. You know, you could have a completely smooth smooth sail out of the closet. Though this video has probably been the hardest video to make, that I've ever made, I hope that nothing will change. I'm going to leave my email address in the down bar, so you guys can contact me with any questions or queries. And I'm also going to put a whole lot of resources for young gay teens in the description that um, the kind of resources that helped me out when I was a scared little 14-year-old. I love you guys so much. Seriously, I do, I really do.
>
> (Sivan 2013)

The video description points to queer resources, such as links to The Trevor Project, Trevor Space, HRC, Minus18 and GLAAD (formerly the Gay & Lesbian Alliance Against Defamation, a media monitoring organisation in the United States of America). In this context, the labour of digital content creation is synonymous with both the performance of sexual identity through a recognisable coming out video and community-articulated justice through the provision of advice, support and resources that – potentially – his viewership may not necessarily have sought to access elsewhere.

A second personal vlog of note is titled 'DO I HAVE A BOYFRIEND?' and has accumulated over 4,900,000 views (Sivan 2015a). Sivan is captured talking to the camera responding to questions, screen-grabbed and displayed on the screen, accumulated from the #asktroye hashtag on Twitter. Of the dozen or so questions addressed, two in particular relate overly to Sivan's sexuality. The first was

'#asktroye What was it like having to play a sexually successful straight guy in the Spud films? Also, will there be more of them?'

To this, Sivan responds,

> It was weird. I mean, I have, believe it or not, actually kissed more girls in my life than boys. I think it's never not weird to kiss someone on camera in front of like fifty other people. You do it a bunch of times, you have to stop half way through cos they have to fix like, a light, [background track stops for impact] maybe there was one time where one of you used too much tongue.
>
> (Sivan 2015a)

The second question was '@troyesivan #AskTroye how do you feel about equal marriage rights in the U.S.?!' In the video, Sivan appears visibly excited, getting up from his chair and waving his arms in the air:

> As a young LGBT person I would just like to say thank you, thank you, thank you, thank you, thank you, to everyone who has ever ever fought for this cause, because my life as an LGBT person who doesn't even live in America, but I just know this is gonna have a knock-on effect, this is a huge huge huge step, from my point of view I just wanna say thank you so so so much. Love wins! [mock waving a flag on camera] This is a pride flag, it's invisible, you can't see it, but it's here! [sic]
>
> (Sivan 2015a)

Notable across both of these examples, then, is the production of content that articulates a sexual citizenship through belonging within a rights-based that reproduces a particular set of normativities (Johnston 2017, pp. 160–161). Here, sexual citizenship is represented through the 'work' of engaging with a particular liberal-humanist framework of political and social change while simultaneously grounding that political engagement through an articulation of the individualised, personal narrative.

Brand collaborations

Collaborations between Influencers and brands/organisations, much like Influencer/Influencer collaborations described later, are instances in which the 'work' of queer microcelebrities is integrated, reflecting the networked approach to new forms of labour in an online setting. Collaboration implies working together, but it also produces mutual outcomes that might include an increased viewership for the Influencer but at the same time an increased attentiveness to a social, political or commercial artefact. In this context, the social networking formation that constitutes identity performances in mutual relationality (Cover 2012b) is extended to the formation in which Influencer identity is an act of *work* that is consciously and creatively produced in mutual relationality with others who also labour for the digital attention afforded by identity as brand.

In an example of brand collaboration content production, in partnership with Paper Magazine and Google, Sivan recounts his first experience at a pride parade years ago. Titled 'My First Pride Parade', the video has accumulated over 544,000 views (Sivan 2017). As he performs a voice-over, Sivan is observed in various locations, such as a darkroom with rainbow light falling on his face, being out in the streets among pride flags or dancing with the pride flag in a photography studio. He summarises his first memory of pride as such:

> There is some sort of like kinship amongst the LGBT people that is actually indescribable to me. Everyone should go to pride, I think. The electricity that's in the air, for me at least that was as life-changing moment. Plus it's really really really fun. Being surrounded by people who are just like you, as crazy as you, maybe even crazier than you, it's like electrifying. I've never felt anything like it. There is a community in the world you who love and support you absolutely and unconditionally.
>
> (Sivan 2017)

The second brand collaboration titled 'How To Have Sex. Safely!' features Sivan promoting Durex condoms while educating his young audience (Sivan 2015b). The video has accumulated over 1,500,000 views and was the second episode of his series 'Awkward conversations with Troye' (Sivan 2015b). The video description carried typical Influencer tropes in which outbound links to sponsors were archived. In this particular advertorial, Sivan placed URLs to Durex Australia's Facebook page and website, with the text 'Get your hands on the goods right here' (Sivan 2015b). In his preamble, Sivan explains his motivations for this advertorial:

> Upon reading your comments in my last video, one of the most common questions was, what seems like quite an obvious one to some of you but to other people it's like, I have no idea… basically it's how do you have safe sex. What does the word safe sex mean? And so I turned to personal knowledge and the internet, and this is what I found.
>
> (Sivan 2015b)

Providing entertainment value and retaining audience attention, Sivan uses both humour (blowing up a condom) and shares safe sex tips while it deflates. In these few minutes, Sivan lectures young people on a variety of safe sex topics, including why they should use condoms, what condoms are made of, how much they cost, how to purchase discreetly avoiding embarrassment and important techniques for their safe use (Sivan 2015b).

In the vein of Influencer commerce, Sivan prompts viewers to leave feedback and promotes his sponsor once more:

> I hope you guys like this video. If you have any questions or comments or anything like that, please use the comments section below. The idea behind

these videos is they spark conversation and educate you guys while I also educate myself. Again this series is made possible by the people over at Durex. The link to their website is in the description box below. They have a bunch of information about safe sex and condoms and all of that. We survived! You didn't have to talk to your parents about it! You didn't have to talk to your friends about it! Thank me later!

(Sivan 2015b)

The third brand collaboration is also in partnership with Durex, as evidenced by the video description and Sivan's allusions to his work with them. Titled 'Is It Easier To Get AIDS If You're Gay?', and having accumulated over 1,300,000 views, the video takes the format of Sivan clearing up 'misconceptions about HIV and AIDS' by responding to Google auto-complete queries (Sivan 2015c). Through a series of questions, he informs viewers what HIV is and how it harms the body, how the HIV endemic started, misconceptions about how HIV was thought to be 'gay cancer' and what scientists have learned since then, how HIV is transmitted, how condoms used 'properly, consistently, and correctly' can help to prevent HIV, and whether condoms have expiration dates and why (Sivan 2015c). At the end of his mini-lecture, Sivan visibly expresses some discomfort and awkwardness at his own candour, and exaggeratedly takes deep breaths to celebrate his successful tackling of a tricky issue.

Brand collaborations have been carefully selected. One way in which to think about the work of collaborating with a brand is to understand it not only as a form of endorsement (of a production or an idea or a health warning) but as that which actively reinforces the existing brand of the self. Here, labour is directed towards the self-production of status as an Influencer in ways which speak not to the individual but to a recognisable sexual identity – in this case, an LGBTQ male reinforced by an older connectivity with HIV, AIDS and safe-sex education practices.

Influencer collaborations

As part of the relational work activated through mutually beneficial collaboration, Sivan collaborates with several other YouTube Influencers of all genders and sexualities. Although other collaborators differ from for-profit and not-for-profit organisational brands, there is a shared sense of work across YouTubers who undertake specific labour to cross-promote each other. The work, however, is often framed within affective, domestic and intimate performances that on the surface disavow the work setting of cross-promotion and shared creative production. This is particularly the case for work among male YouTube Influencers who are straight, out-queer or ambiguous-queer.

The first Influencer collaboration is with American YouTube Influencer Tyler Oakley, who is also openly gay. In 'Face Painting with #Troyler (ft Tyler Oakley)', with over 460,000 views, Sivan and Oakley attempt the 'Not my arms' YouTube challenge, in which one person completes basic tasks, such as putting on makeup or eating food, by using the arms of a second person who is sitting behind them (Sivan 2014a). Oakley tells viewers that the challenge is in celebration of 'Valentine's Day', to which Sivan says they will be 'painting each other's face with cute Valentine's Day stuff' (Sivan 2014a). The video shows them setting up in what looks to be Oakley's living room.

While negotiating the baggy t-shirt they are about to share, Sivan slips his arms under Oakley's as the latter giggles hysterically from being ticklish. In the moments in which they paint each other's faces, both men are seen touching each other's faces, pausing for brief cuddles, sharing intense glares, blowing warm breaths down each other's neck, playfully pinching nipples and holding hands. At one point, Oakley tells Sivan, 'Hey your face is so soft' as Sivan looks at him lovingly. Their giggles eventually lead to the duo falling off the chair and outside the frame (Sivan 2014a). As part of the collaboration, Sivan ends the clip by telling viewers,

> We also made a video over on Tyler's channel… I mean, we collab-ed a couple of months ago, so I guess you should also watch that while you're at it, which you can click… here to see, and that is it.
>
> (Sivan 2014a)

A second Influencer collaboration features UK-based Marcus Butler. In '7 Second Challenge with Marcus Butler!', which has accumulated over 4,500,000 views, Sivan and Butler dare each other to 'do shit in 7 seconds', such as answer quizzes or complete dares (Sivan 2014b). Having recently ended a prolific heterosexual relationship with fellow English YouTube Influencer Niomi Smart, Butler is assumed to be straight. Yet in the preamble, Sivan contrasts his smaller-frame and feminine masculinity against Butler's buff and rugged physique with the quip 'and I'm wearing a sports jersey today feeling hella masculine and shit' (Sivan 2014b).

As they partake in the challenge, in the heat of excitement, Butler tells Sivan to 'feel my heart', at which Sivan places his hand over Butler's chest and playfully gropes him over his tight t-shirt (Sivan 2014b). Such intimate body language continues throughout the video across a range of challenges and activities from removing shirts to shared touch during push-ups. Like other Influencer collaborations, the video ends with Sivan encouraging his viewers to subscribe to Butler: 'Seriously though, Marcus is one of my favourite people in the world. And I love his videos, so please please go subscribe' (Sivan 2014b).

The third Influencer collaboration is with South African YouTube Influencer Blessing Xaba; he is one of the few non-white Influencers to appear on Sivan's collaborations. In 'PAINTING WITH BLESSING' viewed over 1,100,000 times, the openly gay Xaba and Sivan set out to make pieces of art for Sivan's bedroom (Sivan 2014c). The video comprises sped-up footage of the men negotiating paint cans and canvas boards, while painting and (at times) dancing. They are also seen assisting each other with various tasks, interspliced with behind-the-scenes footage of the duo goofing around (Sivan 2014c).

In all three of the Influencer collaboration cases, a performance of identity is produced through a particular kind of community relationality, although in its (often fictionalised) narratives they speak to the kinds of domesticity that are most closely aligned with the privatised nature of sexual citizenship: bedrooms, homes, coupled relationships, intimate friendships. Unlike the earlier brand collaborations that involve a connection with public affairs issues and sexual health advice resources, these latter collaborations produce content that both relates and reinforces the domestic, everydayness of non-heteronormative sexual identities.

It is also in these moments that trust is fostered between Influencers and viewers, and the former becomes an 'agony aunt to a niche market' about the everyday practicalities and philosophical complexities of queer everyday life, from relationships to sexual health (Abidin 2017b, p. 504). This is especially important as the preambles in the vlogs of queer Influencers tend to position a large segment of viewers as queer young people, many of whom they presume to be closeted, struggling or looking for guidance, akin to the framing of the *It Gets Better* legacy of videos. Unlike the *It Gets Better* resources, however, this advisory role, which includes interactive feedback, questions, dialogue and engagement across multiple platforms (Cover 2012b) provides another nuanced, contemporary work-role for the queer Influencer.

Queer microcelebrity publics

Understanding and making sense of queer microcelebrity Influencers and the ways in which their public role can be read as a form of work within a sexual citizenship framework obliges us to return to the history of contemporary digital/visual queer communication. In its Web 2.0 setting, queer vlogging remains governed by the norms of the YouTube 'coming out' video. To investigate the narrative structure of coming out stories, Cover and Prosser (2013) studied memorial accounts and contemporary coming out narratives. They argue that although the genre has changed throughout history, 'core elements and key ideas' in the rhetorical cycle among young queer men include (1) feelings of isolation or loneliness as a young boy, (2) self-perceiving as masculine but as not meeting expectations of hegemonic or hyper-masculinity, (3) having always known one is gay as a child but not necessarily knowing the name for it, (4) a moment of bravery in either a first sexual encounter or in disclosing and confessing a non-heteronormative sexual identity, and (5) typically coming to a sense of belonging to a community or online community or through a coupled relationship (Cover and Prosser 2013, p. 85). However, they argue that coming out narratives for queer persons must not be read as either linear or truncated in the age of the Internet (p. 86).

Morris and Anderson, likewise, argue that the 'Generation' of 'contemporary male youth' is characterised by more 'inclusive masculinities and attitudes'; the use of technological devices to share resources, visible affect and perform 'emotional care work' on social media; and the use of technology to 'consume large amounts of pornography [resulting in] liberal perspectives towards sexual diversity' (2015, p. 1203). At the intersection of a cultural studies approach to coming out narratives (Cover and Prosser 2013) and the sociological approach to male youth sexuality practices in digital spaces (Morris and Anderson 2015), a framework is warranted for discerning a more graduated and extended cycle of coming out narratives for queer Influencers on YouTube who sit at the intersection of queer publics and microcelebrity publics.

The queer Influencer framework of digital content for sexual belonging, as related in the Troye Sivan examples, can be understood to be based on the form of digital coming out narrative, but offering a differentiated and graduated self-reflexivity while simultaneously positioning the coming out story as simultaneously a 'personal' account and a 'work practice' that undertakes labour which both earns for the brand and performs a service for that brand's public. 'Ordinary' coming out does not, in other words, involve the labour of (paid) digital content creation, the latter of which comes to subsume the former in contemporary queer communication. Where Cover and Prosser (2013) uncovered a narrative that commenced with describing feelings of isolation and loneliness in youth, Influencers' accounts of queer microcelebrity articulate isolation in relation to the distinction between school (sometimes as 'real life') and digital spaces (for example, friends on Tumblr and YouTube). Reading this through the lens of 'networked work', school becomes the site as the posited as *prior* to working life, while online activities are *post-school* in the sense that they are self-consciously performed as labour. Rather than being seen as 'typically coming to a sense of belonging to a community or online community or through a coupled relationship' (Cover and Prosser 2013, p. 85), Influencers acknowledge receiving affirmation from their followers and their fellow YouTube Influencers as a general sign of acceptance, and the coming out experience is subsequently enshrined as inspirational by the YouTube community, followers and sometimes the press more generally. In that context, an Influencer's corpus of materials undertake further labour in the sense that it operates as a resource. While coming out is not a singular act but one that is constituted in the persistent need for public repetition, the coming out of the Influencer is one which does a different kind of further labour: the Influencer takes on new public responsibilities as an out queer subject, typically through a more public discourse of one's personal, private and domestic gendered and sexual life as a form of discursive activism, while simultaneously taking on queer-celebratory or queer-targeted brand sponsorship work, promoting mental, social, physical and sexual health and support-seeking.

The processes of self-disclosure which operate on the one hand as a contemporary and digital form of cultural capital among the network of queer Influencers through collective branding, and on the other as economic capital with potential clients and sponsors through an expansion of their marketable personae, present a model of self-disclosure that shifts from the earlier coming out videos. In other words, the 'mediated coming out' of queer Influencers contribute in converting their 'non-normative sexualities into commercially lucrative labour within the YouTube celebrity economy' (Lovelock 2017, pp. 98–99), wherein their queer identities are a 'potential resource' for a 'successful self-brand' (Lovelock 2017, p. 100). As such, their coming out narratives are more graduated and extended, including extensive padding and preparation to create anticipation, milking the peak of attention cycles to extend their shelf life and cultivate more viable digital estates, and long-tail closure and aftercare to conscientiously wrap up a season of self-branding and transit into the next.

Conclusion

A consideration of queer Influencers who use and engage with YouTube is significant at this time, given their role in responding to concerns over how queer content is moderated. In March 2017, YouTube changed its algorithms to render queer content on its platform 'invisible', by categorising videos with queer content under 'restricted mode' (Hunt 2017). As such, videos with queer content and by queer Influencers no longer appeared on the landing page and did not rank during search queries. A public dialogue with YouTube occurred online across a number of platforms. Prominent queer Influencers on YouTube – including UK-based Rowan Ellis, who is married to her lesbian partner (Shu 2017), and US-based Tyler Oakley, who identifies as gay (Associated Press 2017) – have also used their prolific social media platforms to call out YouTube for its relegation of queer content as non-normative, with positive agreement from the video platform company. Their actions demonstrate the kind of role played by Influencers in queer community activities and the intersection of that work between the personal concern of ensuring their content is available and the community concern of ensuring equal citizenship in digital worlds.

As more closeted queer Influencers come out and more straight Influencers play with queer bait, queer vlog content is snowballing on YouTube. Yet, despite the vast array of genders, sexualities and family structures, the demographic representation of such (quasi-)queer Influencers still appears to be predominantly cisgender, White and (serial) monogamous, resulting in the 'further entrench[ment]' of micro-minorities and groups experiencing intersectional marginality (Peters 2011, p. 207). However, for the most part, a large portion of the pressure exerted upon Influencers comes from clients and sponsors, many of whom are keen and quick to capitalise on moves towards liberalism, greater diversity and thus an expanding consumer market. Queer Influencers on YouTube thus 'reconcil[e] gay and lesbian sexualities with neoliberal-capitalist ideologies of self-sufficiency, entrepreneurialism and individual enterprise, in ways that do not challenge the normativity of heterosexuality or the emotional costs to gay and lesbian life which this entails' (Lovelock 2017, p. 99).

However, is all queer visibility on the internet good, productive or safe visibility? It appears not. A recent article from technology and culture magazine *The Verge* reports that vlogs of transgender YouTubers cataloguing their transition were data-scraped by an art and research project known as HRT Transgender Dataset. In this instance, 'before and after HRT' faces were collected as 'biometric data' and used to train 'facial recognition software' to read faces. Although these YouTube videos were publicly available, not all individuals were contacted to provide consent to be included in the dataset (Vincent 2017). Transgender vloggers interviewed by *The Verge* reveal that such mechanisms 'may make them a target' in social spaces where they may be closeted (Vincent 2017). As such, queer Influencers who voluntarily practice self-disclosure (Abidin 2013) and communicative intimacies (Abidin 2015) as a parasocial strategy to engage followers ultimately risk public surveillance and vulnerability even while fostering and maintaining safe spaces for their followers to participate in discursive activism. In that context, the model of sexual citizenship labour that queer Influencers embody is not necessarily a model that should be deployed for all queer citizens.

References

Abidin, C., 2013. Cyber-BFFs: Assessing Women's 'Perceived Interconnectedness' in Singapore's Commercial Lifestyle Blog Industry. *Global Media Journal Australian Edition*, 7 (1).

Abidin, C., 2015. Communicative ❤ Intimacies: Influencers and Perceived Interconnectedness. *Ada: A Journal of Gender, New Media, & Technology*, 8.

Abidin, C., 2016. "Aren't These Just Young, Rich Women Doing Vain Things Online?": Influencer Selfies as Subversive Frivolity. *Social Media + Society*, 2 (2), 1–17.

Abidin, C., 2017a. #familygoals: Family Influencers, Calibrated Amateurism, and Justifying Young Digital Labour. *Social Media + Society*, 3 (2), 1–15.

Abidin, C., 2017b. Sex Bait: Sex Talk on Commercial Blogs as Informal Sexuality Education. In: L. Allen and M. L. Rasmussen, eds. *Palgrave Handbook of Sexuality Education*. London: Palgrave Macmillan, 493–508.

Associated Press, 2017. YouTube Reverses Some Restrictions on LGBT-Themed Content Following Uproar. *The Telegraph*, 21 March. Available from: www.telegraph.co.uk/technology/2017/03/21/youtube-reverses-restrictions-gay-themed-content-following-uproar/

Bell, D. and Binnie, J., 2006. Geographies of Sexual Citizenship. *Political Geography*, 25 (8), 869–873.

Cover, R., 2012a. *Queer Youth Suicide, Culture and Identity: Unliveable Lives?* London and New York: Routledge.

Cover, R., 2012b. Performing and Undoing Identity Online: Social Networking, Identity Theories and the Incompatibility of Online Profiles and Friendship Regimes. *Convergence*, 18 (2), 177–193.

Cover, R. and Prosser, R., 2013. Memorial Accounts: Queer Young Men, Identity and Contemporary Coming Out Narratives Online. *Australian Feminist Studies*, 28 (75), 81–94.

Gal, N., Shifman, L., and Kampf, Z., 2016. 'It Gets Better': Internet Memes and the Construction of Collective Identity. *New Media & Society*, 18 (8), 1698–1714.

García-Rapp, F. and Roca-Cuberes, C., 2017. Being an Online Celebrity: Norms and Expectations of YouTube's Beauty Community. *First Monday*, 22 (7).

Gibbs, M., et al., 2015. #Funeral and Instagram: Death, Social Media, and Platform Vernacular. *Information, Communication & Society*, 18 (3), 255–268.

Green, M., Bobrowicz, A., and Ang, C. S., 2015. The Lesbian, Gay, Bisexual and Transgender Community Online: Discussions of Bullying and Self-disclosure in YouTube Videos. *Behaviour & Information Technology*, 34 (7), 704–712.

Hunt, E., 2017. LGBT Community Anger over YouTube Restrictions Which Make Their Videos Invisible. *The Guardian*, 20 March. Available from: www.theguardian.com/technology/2017/mar/20/lgbt-community-anger-over-youtube-restrictions-which-make-their-videos-invisible

Johnston, J., 2017. Subscribing to Sex Edutainment: Sex Education, Online Video, and the YouTube Star. *Television & New Media*, 18 (1), 76–92.

Lovelock, M., 2017. 'Is Every YouTuber Going to Make a Coming Out Video Eventually?': YouTube Celebrity Video Bloggers and Lesbian and Gay Identity. *Celebrity Studies*, 8 (1), 87–103.

Mazanderani, F., O'Neill, B., and Powell, J., 2013. 'People Power' or 'Pester Power'? YouTube as a Forum for the Generation of Evidence and Patient Advocacy. *Patient Education and Counseling*, 93, 420–425.

Morris, M. and Anderson, E., 2015. 'Charlie Is So Cool Like': Authenticity, Popularity and Inclusive Masculinity on YouTube. *Sociology*, 49 (6), 1200–1217.

Peters, W., 2011. Pink Dollars, White Collars: Queer as Folk, Valuable Viewers, and the Price of Gay TV. *Critical Studies in Media Communication*, 28 (3), 193–212.

Shaw, F., 2012. HOTTEST 100 WOMEN: Cross-platform Discursive Activism in Feminist Blogging Networks. *Australian Feminist Studies*, 27 (74), 373–387.

Shu, C., 2017. YouTube Responds to Complaints that Its Restricted Mode Censors LGBT Videos. *TechCrunch.com*, 19 March. Available from: https://techcrunch.com/2017/03/19/youtube-lgbt-restricted-mode/

Sivan, T., 2013. Coming Out. *YouTube.com*, 7 August 2013. Available from: www.youtube.com/watch?v=JoL-MnXvK80

Sivan, T., 2014a. Face Painting with #Troyler (ft Tyler Oakley). *YouTube.com*, 14 February 2014. Available from: www.youtube.com/watch?v=iN-ciEkviRo

Sivan, T., 2014b. 7 Second Challenge with Marcus Butler! *YouTube.com*, 5 May 2014. Available from: www.youtube.com/watch?v=IaRTmpuoFY8

Sivan, T., 2014c. PAINTING WITH BLESSING. *YouTube.com*, 7 October 2014. Available from: www.youtube.com/watch?v=V9qM2iRkfGY

Sivan, T., 2015a. DO I HAVE A BOYFRIEND? *YouTube.com*, 28 June 2015. Available from: www.youtube.com/watch?v=-jlOUBH3ud4

Sivan, T., 2015b. How to Have Sex. Safely! *YouTube.com*, 17 October 2015. Available from: www.youtube.com/watch?v=K1TtnxaPRms

Sivan, T., 2015c. Is It Easier to Get AIDS if You're Gay? *YouTube.com*, 5 December 2015. Available from: www.youtube.com/watch?v=pNwiLU90TAc

Sivan, T., 2017. My First Pride Parade. *YouTube.com*, 27 June 2017. Available from: www.youtube.com/watch?v=yGn5e6WlmcE

Turner, V., 1975. *Dramas, Fields, and Metaphors: Symbolic Action in Human Society*. Ithaca, NY: Cornell University Press.

Vincent, J., 2017. Transgender YouTubers had their Videos Grabbed to Train Facial Recognition Software. *The Verge*, 22 August. Available from: www.theverge.com/2017/8/22/16180080/transgender-youtubers-ai-facial-recognition-dataset [Accessed 23 August 2017].

Chapter 15

Mediating aspirant religious-sexual futures

In God's hands?

Yvette Taylor

Introduction: youth futures, queer precarity and religions (un)certainty

This chapter explores the construction of vocational and familial futures in times of aspiring, post-welfare or crisis youth transitions, as mediated by sexual-religious identification. It draws on findings from a recent study, *Making Space for Queer Identifying Religious Youth*, which considers lesbian, gay, bisexual and transgender (LGBT) young people's constructions and experiences of religious-sexual fields, as typically separated and oppositional in everyday cultural imaginaries and sociolegal policy framings. By considering the intersectional relations of both sexuality and religion, the chapter highlights pragmatic and caring orientations including a 'calling' to religion as a site of present-future vocational and familial investment. I challenge the separation of religion and sexuality in youth transitions, and in notions of the 'times we're in' as compelling certain kinds of future-orientated aspirant (and secular) selves. The chapter hopes to contribute to theorising the intersection of sexuality and religion in further understanding the subversive – and conservative – potential of religious-sexual values and futures. Such orientations interface with aspects of 'getting by' and 'getting on' and at once re-inscribe and stretch normative vocational and familial choices. Citizenship claims centre around full recognition and legitimation in different social spheres, including, for example, the right to employment and social welfare protections, the right to family life and the right to religion. These citizenship protections are increasingly recognised in international 'Equalities' legislation, promising protection on key characteristics such as gender, sexuality, race, religion and age. Yet, religion and sexuality still collide in legislative and popular imaginations and realisations of citizenship status negotiated in an increasingly secular UK context, where the supposed decline of religion may be conflated with an increased entitlement to sexual citizenship for lesbian, gay, bisexual, trans and queer (LGBTQ) groups. Such a conflation sidelines the citizenship possibilities and realities negotiated and imagined by queer religious youth in imagining future forms of employment and family formations.

Generally, both religion and sexuality are under-investigated as influencing young peoples' vocational and familial futures. In terms of sexuality, young people find themselves awkwardly navigating a youth-at-risk discourse as well as a youth-as-sexually-liberated-and-free discourse (Rasmussen 2010, Yip and Page 2013, Taylor and Snowdon 2014a, Taylor et al. 2014). Ideas of risk pervade the category of youth more generally, witnessed in recent policy and political discourses (Allen and Taylor 2013). The discourse of 'aspiration' as a self-motivational tool that can propel young people into secure employment positions is increasingly promoted as policy and cultural cure for social-ills. Indeed being 'someone' who aspires in particular ways is becoming something of an imperative cutting across political discourse and tropes of aspiration and social mobility in modern-day societies (Evans 2010). This becoming 'someone' as a self-actualised and entitled subject is also apparent within celebrations of the 'world we've won' as LGBT groups realise sexual citizenship in the realms of family and working lives (Weeks 2007, McDermott 2011). Young people are increasingly positioned as now accessing a future, denied to previous LGBT generations. But the (secular) language of 'becoming' and 'citizenship' also centres an older LGBT 'sexual citizen' (as consumer, citizen, resident) and once again 'youth' slip out of this frame, constituting another intersectional gap in thinking about sexual citizenship. In 'arriving' in places of sexual citizenship, young people are often seen as the beneficiaries of previous generations' struggles but are simultaneously invisibilised as 'not yet' fully in the worlds of family and employment.

Within the field of youth studies, young people are often positioned as inhabiting a transitional stage, 'neither the first nor the last', in the life course, existing 'in transition' and 'as transition' (Jones 2009, p. 84). Within sexuality studies, work often disregards the religious aspects of LGBTQ lives or refers to religious associations only as negative, harmful or superficial (Yip 1997, Gross and Yip 2010). Yet various religious institutions and stances have articulated enormously complicated and contrary perspectives (Taylor and Snowdon 2014a). Locating young people in specific, changing times means being attentive to how they construct their personal and social identities, and possible futures.

Rather than viewing religion as another matter of individualised choice and lifestyle, which citizens are increasingly opting out of, Modood (2015) argues against secularism and for a positive role for religion in contemporary society, and for thinking about religion as a public, not just a private good. Indeed, in 'post-welfare' times of economic crisis, austerity and cutbacks, religious bodies and individuals have been asked to 'stand-in' and care for congregations and communities, arguably extending their collective and social capacities as key organisers of public good. Religion – both formal and otherwise – has also been considered as a site of social investment and return, as a buffer against isolation and risk and as a space for capital accumulation of both a social and material nature (Mellor 2010). The long-standing reality of religious spaces that 'provide' and 'care' for communities and congregants is arguably heightened in contemporary post-welfare times. This practice may increase the visibility and desirability of religious orientations, specifically for young people, as counter-normative, even activist and 'anti-capitalist'.

A sense of queer precarity – of not necessarily having access to the 'right kind' of normative future, as well as a sense of religious (un)certainty – of religious commitment potentially in doubt, mediated young people's becoming otherwise. This chapter aims to contribute to theorising the intersection of sexuality and religion, and to further understanding of the subversive and conservative potential of religious-sexual values and futures. There is scope to consider collective orientations and religious vocations, alongside a turn to individualisation and de-traditionalisation, whereby a 'calling' to religion as a site of present-future vocational investment may weave in alternative and conservative possibilities for young lives. Young people may actively conceive of alternatives to dominant exchange value relationships and structures of chrono-normative temporalities, as upwardly mobile, aspirant and becoming (Edelman 2004, Halberstam 2005, Love 2007). Here, both a sense of queer precarity – of not necessarily having access to the 'right kind' of normative futures – as well as a sense of religious (un)certainty – of religious commitment potentially in doubt – mediated young people's becoming otherwise.

The chapter is based on fieldwork with 38 respondents recruited across three UK sites, Newcastle, Manchester and London, liaising with key gatekeepers and using a snowballing method for what might be considered a 'hard to reach' group. The project adopted a mixed-method research design, consisting of individual face-to-face interviews, diaries and a mapping exercise (see Taylor 2015 for a fuller methods discussion). For the purposes of the study, young people were broadly defined as under-35 years, with the youngest respondent being 17 and the oldest being 34 years old (the mean age of respondents was 24 years old). Overall the project recruited a very middle-class sample, typical of sexualities research generally and often seen as symptomatic of 'hard to reach' groups (Taylor 2007). Most of the participants considered themselves to be white British, with only a few identifying as white Other, such as Greek Cypriot (1 interviewee), Spanish (1) and Italian (1). In terms of sex and gender identity 19 participants identified as female, 15 identified as male, two identified as gender-queer, one identified as gender-queer and transgender and one identified as transsexual female-to-male. According to self-ascription, the sexual identity of participants can be broadly categorised as gay (15 respondents), lesbian (13), bisexual (5), queer (4) and asexual (1).

Most participants self-identified with the denomination of their church: Church of England (6 participants), Methodist (3), Catholic (2), Quaker (2), Charismatic (1), Ecumenical (1) and Evangelical (1). Two participants identified as Unitarian but with Pagan and Buddhist leanings. Where churches were non-denominational, like the Metropolitan Community Church (MCC) (15 participants), some participants also identified with the denomination within which they had been brought up (Church of England, 3 participants; Catholic, 2; Greek Orthodox, 1; and Methodist, 1). Five other participants did not attend a church, attended a non-denominational church (other than MCC), did not know or did not identify with the denomination of their church.

This chapter considers religious-sexual futures in precarious times, and the pragmatic, alternative and conservative responses to these through imagined and intersecting 'work', 'church' and 'family' futures. It asks, how and in what ways are respondents' religious-sexual futures placed 'In God's hands'. The next section explores such uncertainty as part of the 'times we're in', and as a means of re-orientating youthful selves in compliant and resistant ways.

(Not) living by bread alone: optimism and (un) certainty

> Romans Chapter teaches that suffering produces endurance and endurance produces suffering ... 'Worry about nothing, but pray about everything'. It's about being able to ground ourselves in the scripture, all of our hopes and fears, for me as a Christian can be understood and comprehended better through contemplation. Ultimately, we have got God so what more should I really have to want. Jesus Christ teaches that we live by bread alone, that's how our life is. We shouldn't fear too much for worldly things but concentrate on God through Christ.
>
> (Andrew, 24)

The conditions of contemporary neo-liberalism arguably demand and shape a future-oriented, enterprising, capital accruing subject (Skeggs 2004), where capital is accrued in the person and generative of future value (Adkins 2012). The 'enterprising subject' compelled by competition, inequality and rational self-interest, is a particular kind of middle-class subject who can generate value by accruing more capital through their already normative biographies and trajectories, secured through existing social, cultural and economic resources (Taylor and Scurry 2011, Falconer and Taylor 2016).

Such a mode of being is also governed by a temporality that values reproductive maturity and wealth accumulation, setting up the 'future' as a particular achievement, a realisation of the right 'aspirations' at the right time. The linking of economic and reproductive worth compels some researchers to ask how non-normative identities might relate to alternative values and temporalities.

Studies of working-class groups highlight differences in 'becoming' otherwise, which are often mis-recognised as deficits, as not arriving in proper familial or vocational positions. Rather than displaying proprietorial orientations towards the future, working-class personhood can be viewed as protectionist rather than proprietorial (Skeggs 1997, Skeggs and Loveday 2012). Living in the here and now is manifest in a more pragmatic concern for 'getting by' and managing precarity rather than futurity, or 'getting on' (Taylor 2012, Mckenzie 2015). While *class* has been a dominant feature in the re-consideration of value, religion and sexuality can further unsettle conceptualisations of value-aspiration among queer religious youth, whereby a 'calling' may be seen as a form of religious-vocational 'care', mediated too by sexuality.

Researchers of gender and sexuality have theorised non-normative gender and sexual identities as subverting the normative life-course. 'Queer temporality' includes and arguably extends beyond gender and sexuality to articulate alternative ways of life, which do not conform to pressures to reproduce, and accumulate wealth. Queer theory, in troubling the reification of innate gender categories and the imperative of reproduction, aims to 'articulate an alternative vision of life, love and labour' (Halberstam 2005, p. 6), a different way of organising human sociality and a different orientation to futurity. In the 'clock time' of capitalism (Adkins 2009) certain time cycles (leisure, recreation, work, family, domesticity) and life stages (growing up, partnering, parenting, careers) are naturalised and internalised, reproducing heteronormative 'chrononormativity'. In questioning linear and homogenous time, room is arguably made for the transient, the fleeting, the contingent; for 'strange' temporalities, imaginative life schedules and even eccentric economic practices (Halberstam 2005).

Such alternative temporalities conjure different futures, where chance or untimeliness are key elements in a political effort to 'bring into existence futures that dislocate themselves from the dominant tendencies and forces of the present' (Grosz 2004, p. 14). Edelman (2004) and Halberstam (2005), for example, assert that queer subjects should embrace non-productivity and resist narratives of futurity explicitly bound in capitalist accumulation. However, this side-lines practical and pragmatic (im)possibilities, and the likely intersection of alternative *and* conservative possibilities in the same time and space, as subjects navigate broader social contexts. Specifically 'queer' times, prioritises and isolates 'queerness' above other locations, such as class (Taylor 2007, 2012, McDermott 2011). With this in mind, Renold (2008) argues that the emancipatory potential of such alternative narratives are at risk of being overstated with 'queer subversions' only sustainable from places of power, suggesting limited possibilities for the relatively powerless to subvert.

Conceptualisations of queer times risk reinforcing similar assumptions to those often evident in conceptualisations of religious identities, i.e. that their presumed status as exceptions to the mainstream exempts them from the social structural factors that constrain the lives of everybody else. Even so, religious institutions and practices also structure time, at micro and macro levels, from Weberian 'protestant ethics' and deferred gratification, through to Wilcox's (2009) consideration of religious lesbians and how straight-religious time impacts them. Mapping religion and sexuality together potentially avoids the prioritisation of any one of these differences, focussing instead on the situational specifics by which certain elements of one's identity become muted and, at another time, become heightened.

Many interviewees in this study spoke of the need to be flexible and adaptable to be securely placed in the job-market, to be at-the-ready; while for some this was articulated as a freeing of possibilities ('I am pretty flexible when it comes to the future, I am willing to let it take me where it wants', Julian, 20), others spoke more of this as a compulsory orientation, where 'today is today', and everyday immediacy replaces planning, accumulation and future-thinking:

> To be adaptable. The only chance is to be adaptable. I would like to have a bit more quietness and tranquillity and settled plans but how things are right now, be adaptable; be ready for whatever is coming … today is today. I've been worrying about the future hundreds of hours, what's going to happen with the cuts, what is happening with the job, are they going to keep me here or not; the future is not in my hands any more.
>
> (Jacob, 30)

Neo-liberal demands contrast with what can be considered value activity in Christian terms, such as, for example, prayer, contemplations and silence. The peculiarly neo-liberal challenges and conflicts, whereby life experience is imbued with the expectation of individual empowerment and adaptability but is actually characterised by powerlessness in the face of a future that seems pre-determined by external factors, was repeated across accounts of 'getting-on' and 'getting by'.

Some interviewees' aspirations were constructed against 'big business', corporate greed or some unspecific notion of capitalism in general and routine and day-to-day work specifically. In articulating against-the-grain options, others described pivotal moments and 'heart' changes in deciding what was important to them in life, re-orientating their future employment expectations. John discusses this later in terms of his sexual orientation facilitating a rethinking of normative success, graduate trajectories and vocational orientations. There is some ambivalence and hesitation here as John moves between what was once desired and a conflicting present, balancing 'social roles', materiality and 'feeling better'.

> My friend has started a graduate job … and is doing 8 to 8 and works Saturdays and it's a three year graduate training programme, and I consider her very successful because that's what I used to view successful as, very professional, it gives you status, it used to be a safe thing. And then all of a sudden I got really emotional and sort of, after I came out at 16, and reinterpreted what my view of success was, and for me it would be some role that provided me with an outlet to sort of express or help, like it became a very 'heart' decision as a career, and now I would pick something very vocational as opposed to before where I'd just pick something about money really, about status, but now I actually want to pick something that expresses or contributes to something. But I've got this conflicting, because I still would like to have a disposable income…
>
> (John, 21)

Like John, other interviewees situated their commitment to caring professions as important for their own sense of worth and social contribution, at the same time as being financially desirable. This was done by imagining themselves as one day inhabiting the more 'senior positions' (George, 23) in caring professions and by casting caring professions rather widely to include, for example, scientists, solicitors, counsellors, doctors, peacekeepers and ambassadors as those actively 'caring' for and contributing to society.

For example, Adrian (29) wanted to run his own charity and hoped 'to be a force for change really'. While imagining himself within the field of science, and pursing a PhD, Lesley (21) also spoke of the appeal to be active in politics, to do research, act as a human rights layer or have a future in ministry ('I want to change the world, I really do'). Rather than dismissing such ambitions as naïve youthful hopes, it is important to situate these as connecting sexuality and religion, where both these orientations create a space for collective change as desired. Such desires interface aspects of 'getting by' and 'getting on' and are at once alternative and conservative, re-inscribing and stretching normative vocational choices. Attending to these expressions means stretching ideas of sexual citizenship, whereby sexuality may not always be the primary motivation for queer religious youth in imagining their public-private futures.

Thomas (34) felt his future involved 'social work type stuff' at the interface of queer-religion 'around Christian LGBT type stuff':

> *I can speak as a Quaker and a gay man*, I've got these two experiences: I've got this experience of what it's like to have had all this prejudice, but I've survived it, and also being someone with faith in an increasingly secularizing world, and just show to people that it's normal.
>
> (Thomas, 34)

It is not necessarily the case that a religious identity includes a critique of capitalism, or any re-situating of value; nonetheless respondents made explicit connections between dissatisfaction with the lack of collective welfare, re-orientations towards these caring logics, critique of 'clock time' ('8 until 10 sort of thing') and salary/status accumulation ('to pick something that expresses'). Perhaps unsurprisingly, participants wanted to help the 'weak, needy and poor', rather than *being* 'weak, needy and poor' themselves. The balance between alternative and normative narratives and choices, involves aligning with recognisable neo-liberal identities for *themselves* whilst concurrently tackling the negative outcomes of neo-liberal capitalism for *others*. Such desires interface aspects of 'getting by' and 'getting on' and are at once alternative and conservative, re-inscribing and stretching normative vocational choices. This forces a challenge to the normative boundaries of citizenship, as involving a claim to recognition through distinct and still separated categories (as a sexual or religious subject, for example), and it stretches the ways these are (de)legitimised whereby queer religious youth may not always welcome inclusion within normative citizenship frames.

Church futures: religious optimism and (un)becoming

Many, if not all, interviewees had considered vocational roles within (various) churches, as sites of collective care and familial-type identities, whereby church community was seen – and questioned – as 'family'. These vocational desires were somewhat queer in themselves, stretching the language and usage of 'vocation' in most mainstream Christian circles, as typically reserved for ordained ministry. Stretched possibilities of 'vocational roles' included a much wider range of responsibilities in church, including 'ministerial roles' (as assumed to include both lay and ordained people) and non-stipendiary service. That these desires exist within marginalised gendered-queer presences within church vocations, and that young participants were framing these as wide and possible is significant (see Taylor and Snowdon 2014b) in relation to sexual citizenship, as mediated by rather than automatically opposed to religiosity.

Such considerations are also of interest in highlighting the intersection of the vocational and the familial in (queer) re-shapings of 'getting on' and 'getting by'. Many of the young participants had religious vocations in mind and were considering their possible future place in these fields, with and against a sense of inclusive practices and possibilities. Many participants considered if, for example, inclusive churches, such as the MCC founded in, by and for the LGBT community, would represent more pragmatic and comfortable locations while also being cautious that vocations within somewhat peripheral churches could render them economically precarious by virtue of their being unattached to traditional established churches. The viability of sexuality citizenship mediated by economic precarity, was felt here in relation to religious spaces and institutional existences.

Nonetheless many respondents frequently expressed future religious vocation as a 'calling'. The idea of a 'calling', as a specifically *religious* drive into the future does itself subvert some of the linear logics of educational attainment followed by employability, and the separation of the emotional private self, from a public rational and working self. But such 'callings' were also deflected and silenced in the context of hostile and emotive views regarding the public place of LGBT visibility in religious contexts. For example, Estelle (25) had initially planned a certain kind of religious future, going to university to study Theology, but her feelings of disconnect meant that she changed course after just two weeks (see Falconer and Taylor 2016). Imaginings of citizenship within church communities may be constrained by such disconnection, and so the aspirations and enactment for one form of religious belonging are at odds. Often religious orientations, possibilities and practicalities were in motion and were seen to be sites of future reconciliation, even when definite 'callings' and actualised pursuits of that future (such as in studying Theology) were interrupted and uncertain:

> Obviously I'm going to continue pursuing ordination ... I feel like I'm called to do. It's a very unfashionable term outside the Church to talk about

'calling' but 'vocation' is a much more socially acceptable term. Because a lot of MCC priests are non-stipendiary I will probably consider a chaplaincy career alongside that. I'm looking for a placement in higher education chaplaincy at the moment ... I do worry about not being able to find work, not just in the short term but actually even post ordination, will there be work in the Church for me? Will it be funded? Will I have to move, potentially move countries? But I think despite that I plan to continue working with MCC.

(Kelly, 26)

I'm currently undergoing a process with the local diocese and that is to discern my vocation as I feel drawn to the Priesthood. That's where I see myself heading and so far that is where I feel God is pointing me and really I have understood that sense of calling over a period of two and a half years. So I am on a journey of exploration and growth in order to take me to the next step.

(Andrew, 24)

Such pursuits, situated within a complex matrix of aspiration ('I think that is really what I want to do'), compulsion ('calling') and pragmatics ('Will it be funded?') are not likely to be recognised as 'queer'. Taking these accounts seriously means stretching the go-to parameters in describing LGBT youth trajectories as secular (Yip and Page 2013, Taylor and Snowdon 2014a):

My plans for the near future are to continue coming to the church, to this church, for worship, and to continue studying...I'm looking at doing Theology, so a completely pretty different direction from what I've been doing, but I'd like to, maybe at some point in the future, go and do a course on that. I'm not achieving spiritually what I need to achieve, not being able to give it the dedication and the commitment. That's my biggest fear, my dedication to my spiritual growth.

(Valerie, 28)

In the following, both Andrew and Claire express quite a paternalistic and a potentially somewhat patronising version of religious reach and relevance as 'challenging', 'gritty' and even comedic places are invoked as sites of need, care and investment. Andrew situates such cares locally within a 'return to nature' religious narrative, where investment is seen to reap the most benefits – for himself as a future minister and a larger disadvantaged community:

There is a TV series on at the moment, called Rev, with Tom Hollander. It's a comedy, but it is a very gritty comedy and that highlights, very accurately I would say, the Church's current role and experience from the perspective of a Parish Priest in a very challenging Parish ... I can see the challenges there and I can actually see the benefits that you could reap from that, being in a very rural environment looking at how we can preserve God's creation and how we can nurture it, as we were commanded to in the book of Genesis.

(Andrew 24)

Like Andrew, Claire located her religious growth and belonging, alongside a collective community development, yet the language of 'planting a Church' in a rural location arguably conveys potentially troubling links between self-change and community change echoing traditional 'mission' dimensions of religion. That said, Claire is specifically dwelling on the possibility of fostering an MCC in, for and by LGBT groups, potentially stretching 'conservative' dimensions of religion, towards an alternative imagination, potentially allowing for a more expansive understanding of sexual citizenship as also related to vocation and pastoral care within LGBT communities:

> We have talked about moving to – this is going to sound a bit crazy – but moving to [X]! Just because it's somewhere that we've found that we really like and we've been talking about how there needs to be more MCC churches in the UK. And we've been wondering, [partner] and I, if we could start a church somewhere, which is a really big thing. But we're just taking it one step at a time … I think everything we've learned from MCC, we can carry to the church.
>
> (Claire, 24)

Overall, and in the accounts provided earlier, religious hopes intersect aspects of 'getting by', where sexual-religious identities and presences sometimes do not easily sit together, felt as hostility, not belonging and as 'heart changes' compelling (future) reconciliation. Both Andrew and Claire identify the 'challenges' and 'benefits' of religious investment where, these combine resourced hopes to 'get on', to attain vocational roles within churches, and to imagine an inclusive elsewhere to be filled with queer religiosity. In turn, the narrative of easily 'getting on' is interrupted by queer precarity and religious uncertainty and by, for example, the routinised practice of dedication, abiding by scripture, spiritual growth and doubt – unhurried practices which arguably slow down the acceleration of neo-liberal times and forward motion of youthful 'becomings'. In current times of 'aspiring', 'post-welfare' or 'crisis' youth transitions, sexual-religious identification mediates the construction of vocational and familial futures, complicating private-public divides, where church may be cast as family and vice versa. Rethinking such public-private intersections allows a more nuanced negotiation of subversive and conservative futures, stepping away from the separation of religion and sexuality in legislative and popular imaginations and realisations of citizenship status.

Family futures: publics-privates

The right to a 'family life' has been a contested and celebrated point in sexualities research, with some scholars noting the 'world we've won' in securing LGBT sexual citizenship, including the right to same-sex marriage in many parts of the world (Weeks 2007). In some ways, this is seen to constitute a freedom and access to the future, withheld from previous LGBT generations. Such framing centres an older LGBT 'sexual citizen' (as consumer, citizen, resident) and once again 'youth' slip out of the frame, constituting another intersectional gap in thinking about family futures. The 'calling' to religion as a site of present-future vocational investment, highlights pragmatic and caring orientations, as well as deference to an ultimate authority ('...what God wanted me to do...'). These stretches and balances are also played out in respondents' articulations of family futures as a site of contested, classed and gendered reproductions (Taylor 2009, Mckenzie 2015).

In the accounts they provided, participants often highlighted supportive connectivities (Weeks et al. 2001), describing the potential of (religious) vocations and family lives, echoing research on class and gender relations (Mellor 2010). In different configurations of being, relating and valuing, caring has been seen as an essential way in which working-class groups – and particularly working-class mothers – live with others, often outside the norms of respectable heteronormativity (Skeggs 1997, Taylor 2009). Orientations towards immediacy rather than futurity can involve efforts to have a good time in bleak conditions, to make the best of limited circumstances and to rely on 'supportive connectivities' rather than 'self accumulation' (Skeggs 2004). Familial socialities can also involve the gift of attention over time as a distinct value (Skeggs and Loveday 2012), stretching heteronormative 'spacetimes' (Halberstam 2005, Love 2007).

However, many interviewees did hope for normative lives ('the suburban life'), situated alongside rather than departing from broader social expectations and pressures, so while Julian states, 'I am pretty flexible when it comes to the future, I am willing to let it take me where it wants', he nonetheless frames this flexibility via certain (homo)normativities:

> In my dad's last letter, his main worry has been that being gay has therefore voided my chance of a normal future and that is precisely the opposite of how I feel. I don't know whether it's optimistic to hope this but I have always been hoping for just a normal, have a relationship, maybe adopt a kid, own my own house, have a good job; it's always been fairly normal in my mind, in terms of the future. At the moment, in terms of the here and now, I am trying to work on my dad and trying to get him to see that this is what I want and hopefully that is possible.
>
> (Julian, 20)

Within the context of historical non-recognition and continued social injustice, it is feasible to rethink these everyday familial hopes as alternative (Weeks et al. 2001, Taylor 2009) in the way that feminist authors have sought to imbue working-class hopes with value. Stephen's account highlights the desirability of 'honesty' as a practice, place and identity ('a priest that is openly gay') where times and spaces do not collide:

> My for the future is I hope to get married, I hope to have that union blessed, I hope to become a priest but I hope to become a priest that is openly gay and can be honest about my relationship; it brings me nothing but love and

support and I just want to be open about that, really. I don't want to have to lie, or have my boyfriend at the back of the rectory somewhere, only allowed out on week-ends kind of thing. I think that's a real part of what I've been doing with 'Inclusive Church' and everything, is actually honesty.

(Stephen, 22)

In imaging family futures, respondents often made reference to the place of religion in their family lives, including, for example, via same-sex marriages and ceremonies ('I would like to do the boring settle down, kids possibly, that sort of settled life. And if the church could be involved in that, then great', Evelyn, 26):

I'd like a house, a car, children, I'd like to be able to provide for my children and I'd like to live forever with my wife. I'd like to be married. I'd like a nice job, I'd like to go on holidays once a year, and I'd like my children to be able to talk to me about anything and it would be nice if they could experience the same sort of religious experience as I have, but I wouldn't be fussed if they didn't. If they turned round to me and said, 'I'm straight and not a Christian' then I'd be like, 'That's fine. Do you love me? Excellent, that's good.'

(Nicola, 21)

Nicola's question seems to echo a central consideration in this chapter: on the one hand this centralisation of family-child-love may be seen as a particular refraction of the ethos of liberal acceptance, while on the other it can be understood as subversive and unsettling, intersecting religious-sexual identities in publics-private spheres and the forging of pragmatic *and* aspirant futures.

Conclusion

In this study, intersectional relations of sexuality and religion actively lead young people's aspirations towards pragmatic and caring orientations, and away from a self-accumulating subject able to 'get on' and 'get ahead'. This includes a 'calling' to religion as a site of present-future vocational investment, even as the gendering of these investments – and material realisations – remains a powerful constraint (Taylor and Snowdon 2014a). Here, religion can be queered as an inclusive practice and one which young LGBT people are not automatically excluded from in their future-orientations and pragmatic aspirations in 'getting-by'. Young people may actively conceive of alternatives to dominant exchange value relationships and structures of chrono-normative temporalities, as upwardly mobile, aspirant and becoming. Here, both a sense of queer precarity – of not necessarily having access to the 'right kind' of normative futures – as well as a sense of religious (un) certainty – of religious commitment potentially in doubt – mediates young people's becoming otherwise.

Religion and sexuality constitute significant fields of existence potentially challenging, resisting and responding to heteronormative neo-liberal capitalist forms of selfhood and futurity, interfacing 'getting by' and 'getting on' in vocational and familial choices. Queer theorisations on alternative values centre 'strange' temporalities and futurities: ways of relating to people that are not orientated around exchange and accumulation and imaginative uses of time that are not oriented around reproduction or productivity (Halberstam 2005). This represents a useful shattering of chrono-normative and 'clock time' logic (Adkins 2009) but it is also necessary to take account of the material contexts of such stretches and subversions. Overall, the chapter hopes to contribute to theorising the intersection of sexuality and religion, and to further understanding of the subversive potential of alternative values and 'futures'. This contribution may also work against the disciplinary division witnessed in the separation of 'youth studies', 'sexuality studies' and 'religious studies'.

In negotiating citizenship status within a UK context increasingly framed as secular, with the 'secular' often framed as positive and enabling to the realisation of sexual citizenship, this chapter challenges the separation and isolation of 'sexual citizenship' from other religion life experiences, practices and identities. That sexuality and religion *relate* in the negotiation of employment and family futures, as the often primary areas of citizenship inclusion, challenges this separation, stretching thinking beyond a simple normative/subversive binary in relating (non)normative lives and inclusion into the workplace and family as citizens.

References

Adkins, L., 2009. Sociological Futures: From Clock Time to Event Time. *Sociological Research Online*, 14, 1–5.

Adkins, L., 2012. Out of Work Or Out of Time? Rethinking Labor after the Financial Crisis. *South Atlantic Quarterly*, 111, 621–641.

Allen, K. and Taylor, Y., 2013. Placed Parenting, Locating Unrest: Failed Femininities, Troubled Mothers and Rioting Subjects. *Studies in the Maternal* [online] Special Issue on Austerity Parenting, 4 (2), 1–25. Available from: www.mamsie.bbk.ac.uk/articles/abstract/10.16995/sim.39/ [Accessed 2 January 2014].

Edelman, L., 2004. *No Future: Queer Theory and the Death Drive*. New York, NY: Duke University Press.

Evans, S., 2010. Becoming 'Somebody': Examining Class and Gender through Higher Education. In: Y. Taylor, ed., *Classed Intersections: Spaces, Selves, Knowledges*. Farnham: Ashgate, 99–119.

Falconer, E. and Taylor, Y., 2016. Negotiating Queer and Religious Identities in Higher Education: Queering 'Progression' in the 'University Experience'. *British Journal of the Sociology of Education*, 38 (6), 782–797.

Gross, M. and Yip, A. K., 2010. Living Spirituality and Sexuality: A Comparison of Lesbian, Gay and Bisexual Christians in France and Britain. *Social Compass*, 57 (1), 40–59.

Grosz, E., 2004. *The Nick of Time*. New York, NY: Duke University Press.

Halberstam, J., 2005. *In a Queer Time and Place*. New York: NYU Press.

Jones, G., 2009. *Youth*. Cambridge: Polity Press.

Love, H., 2007. *Feeling Backward: Loss and the Politics of Queer History*. Cambridge, MA: Harvard University Press.

McDermott, E., 2011. The World Some have Won: Sexuality, Class and Inequality. In: Y. Taylor, ed. Special Issue 'Sexuality and Class', *Sexualities* 14 (1), 63–78.

Mckenzie L., 2015. *Getting By: Estates, Class and Culture in Austerity Britain.* Bristol: Policy Press.

Mellor, J., 2010. The Significance of Bonding Capital: Class, Ethnicity, Faith and British Muslim Women's Routes to University. In: Y. Taylor, ed. *Classed Intersections: Spaces, Selves, Knowledges.* Farnham: Ashgate, 73–93.

Modood, T., 2015. State-Religion Connections and Multicultural Citizenship. In: J. L. Cohen and C. Laborde, eds. *Religion, Secularism, and Constitutional Democracy.* New York, NY: Columbia University Press, 182–203.

Rasmussen, M. L., 2010. Secularism, Religion and 'Progressive' Sex Education. *Sexualities*, 13 (6), 699–712.

Renold, E., 2008. Queering Masculinity: Re-theorising Contemporary Tomboyism in the Schizoid Space of Innocent/Heterosexualized Young Femininities. *Girlhood Studies*, 1 (2), 129–151.

Skeggs, B., 1997. *Formations of Class and Gender.* London: SAGE.

Skeggs, B., 2004. *Class, Self, Culture.* London: Routledge.

Skeggs, B. and Loveday, V., 2012. Struggles for Value: Value Practices, Injustice, Judgment, Affect and the Idea of Class. *British Journal of Sociology*, 63 (3), 472–490.

Taylor, Y., 2007. *Working-Class Lesbian Life: Classed Outsiders.* Basingstoke: Palgrave.

Taylor, Y., 2009. *Lesbian and Gay Parenting: Securing Social and Educational Capital.* Basingstoke: Palgrave.

Taylor, Y., 2012. *Fitting into Place? Class and Gender Geographies and Temporalities.* London: Routledge.

Taylor, Y. 2015. *Making Space for Queer Identifying Youth.* Basingstoke: Palgrave.

Taylor. Y., Falconer, E., and Snowdon, R., 2014. Queer Youth, Facebook, and Faith: Facebook Methodologies and Online Identities. *New Media and Society*, 16 (7): 1138–1153.

Taylor, Y. and Scurry, T., 2011. International and Widening Participation Students' Experience of Higher Education, UK. *European Societies*, 13 (4), 583–606.

Taylor, Y. and Snowdon, R., eds., 2014a. *Queering Religion, Religious Queers.* London: Routledge.

Taylor, Y. and Snowdon, R., 2014b. Making Space for Young Lesbians in Church? *Journal of Lesbian Studies*, 18 (4), 393–414.

Weeks, J., 2007. *The World We Have Won: The Remaking of Erotic and Intimate Life.* London: Routledge.

Weeks, J., Heaphy, B., and Donovan, C., 2001. *Same-Sex Intimacies.* London: Routledge.

Wilcox, M. M., 2009. *Queer Women and Religious Individualism.* Bloomington, IN: Indiana University Press.

Yip, A. K. T., 1997. Dare to Differ: Lesbian and Gay Catholics' Assessment of Official Catholic Positions on Sexuality. *Sociology of Religion*, 58 (2), 165–180.

Yip, A. K. T. and Page, S., 2013. *Religious and Sexual Identities: A Multi-faith Exploration of Young Adults.* Farnham: Ashgate.

Section 6

Sex and gender/sexual relationships

Chapter 16

Enabling fluid forms of sexual citizenship?

Navigating the presence and absence of queer sex in *Skins*

Kyra Clarke

In the first episode of Season Six of the UK television show *Skins* (2007–2013),[1] Franky (Dakota Blue Richards), wearing a short red dress, dances with her friends by a pool at a private house in Morocco. She is watched by her boyfriend, Matty (Sebastian de Souza), and by the party's host, Luke (Joe Cole). When Matty interrupts her, wanting to talk, she seems disgruntled and annoyed. Finding a quiet space, he apologises, referring to an argument they had as they arrived to party with friends in Morocco, and Franky responds, 'It's OK Matty, it's fine'. When he tries to kiss her, her body language suggests anger and disinterest. She is silent, and he moves away. He comments, 'we were having a fucking classic summer holiday'. Franky affirms this, and he continues, 'so what's going on?' Still staring straight ahead, Franky asks, 'Do we have to do this?' He looks at her, 'What? It's us. We're great together'. Finally, Franky turns to him. 'Is this what it's like? Being with someone?' Matty is defensive: 'You loved it, Tunisia, the beach, making love to me'. Franky replies, 'It gets boring Matty. All the fucking, and the talking, and just all the stuff, OK?' While Matty argues, 'That's not fair', Franky responds, 'What's fair got to do with it?' She stands and walks away. In contrast to Franky's exchange with Matty, when she arrives on the roof moments later there is a sense of danger and exhilaration in her conversation with Luke, who she has only just met. While she comments that she 'should go find [her] boyfriend', she flirts and doesn't step away when he steps closer. While Matty and Franky are depicted in close-up, distance is created between them: they sit side by side. In contrast, Franky is responsive to Luke: they face each other, shots filmed incrementally closer suggesting intimacy and accompanied by music which rises in pitch until they start to dance.

In many ways, I initially felt cheated watching Franky in Season Six of *Skins*. With her androgynous/genderqueer appearance, Season Five Franky represented ambiguity and difference, highlighted when she stated that she was not into boys or girls, or bisexual, but rather 'into people' and was depicted as desired by bad boy Matty and queen bee Mini. In an interview with co-creator Jamie Brittain on *AfterEllen*, the lesbian/bi women popular culture news website, Heather Hogan (2011a) commented, 'I'll bet you'll be surprised to hear that half of *AE*'s readers want Mini and Franky to end up together, and half of them want

Franky and Matty to end up together'. Brittain's response highlighted ambiguity, commenting with regards to Franky and Matty, 'I'm quite proud of the fact that you really don't know what either of them are going to do next', and suggesting that 'Mini is confused. Liv called it a "girl crush" and maybe that's all it is. Or maybe it's something more'. In a subsequent article, Hogan (2011b) notes that her statement about Franky and Matty was viewed as problematic by readers, and yet she emphasises the queer potential of this pairing: as a genderqueer bisexual/pansexual character, a relationship between Franky and Matty has the potential to show 'that gender non-conformity and non-heterosexuality aren't two parts of a package deal' (Tom1906 in Hogan 2011b). Hogan concludes making a statement about queer representation: 'A genderqueer character being courted by the femmeiest femme and the brooding bad boy. Where else on TV is that even a *possibility*? (Answer: Nowhere.)' However, when in Season Six Franky takes to wearing dresses and having sex with multiple guys[2] this ambiguity appears to be lost, her queerness reduced to 'just a phase' (Monaghan 2016). While the lack of narrative and character consistency might itself be perceived as 'queer' (Joyrich 2014), at first glance these acts imply regression in representations of queer sexuality on *Skins*.

Historically, queer characters on television have been represented rarely, and then most often 'as monsters or victims, objects of revulsion and pity or perhaps as a one-off "lesson" in tolerance' (Beirne 2012, p. 3; Monaghan 2016). Similarly, bisexual characters are described 'as traitors, as a menace, as a myth, as sexually indiscriminate and irresponsible, as hopelessly confused, as bottomless pits of desire' or 'not discussed at all' (Moorman 2012, p. 121; Monro 2015). Queer characters are present throughout the six seasons of *Skins*, a show known for being controversial (Masanet and Buckingham 2015). Such characters were not simply presented as 'positive' or 'as role models or transmitters of politicised messages' (Davis 2004, p. 134); instead, depicting 'teenage independence, rebellion and nihilism' issues were 'portrayed not as problems to be solved (as they typically are in US series) but as everyday facts of teenage life' (Berridge 2013, p. 786). Although queer characters are occasionally physically and verbally abused in *Skins*, they are not presented as victims (Marshall 2010), and there is little focus on 'coming out' where 'disclosing' sexuality is 'linked to a subservient subject position' (Dhaenens 2013, pp. 306–307). The six seasons are broken into three 'generations', a term used by the show's creators and fans alike to differentiate between the three separate casts of characters who were replaced every two seasons. In replacing the cast in this way, Monaghan notes that '*Skins* provides a snapshot of adolescent life from a variety of different perspectives' and 'resists neat closure of its narrative threads, eschewing the sense of linear progression that is typical of the teen genre' (2016, p. 65). *Skins* represents Millennials, with characters presumably born in the 1990s, and yet, while representing characters who are ostensibly part of the same demographic (millennial) generation, the experiences of the characters within the three 'generations' of the show are not equivalent and positive linear changes are not made as the seasons progress. Although the representation of queer characters may have increased on television, Beirne argues that 'this has not constituted a steady narrative of progress; rather, it has been marked by advances and retreats, breakthroughs and hiccups, sometimes even all within the same program' (2012, p. 3, Meyer 2010, Monaghan 2016). In this chapter, I argue that demonstrating what is normal and accepted in *Skins* and what is not through discussion of 'cheating' in relationships can give us some idea of where sexual citizenship currently stands with regards to lesbian, gay, bisexual, transgender and queer (LGBTQ) acceptance and representations.

The term sexual citizenship relates to the intersection between one's sexual life or sexuality as well as belonging and participation in the society in which one lives. All citizenship has conditions attached: 'one is expected to do certain things – *obligations* – in return for certain *rights*' (Plummer 2005, p. 90). Although the concept of having rights and responsibilities as a citizen suggests equality (every citizen has the same rights and responsibilities), this is not experienced by everyone in the same way: citizenship is gendered, racialised, sexualised and based on heterosexual and male privilege, with 'a long history of ... being entwined with justifications for Western superiority and colonialism' (Johnson 2017, p. 170). Citizenship is often perceived as requiring heteronormativity and monogamy and this impacts lesbian and gay citizenship with rights generally provided to the domesticated couple (Richardson and Monro 2012). In contrast to this perception of normativity, by considering moments of cheating, such conventions might be disrupted. As Ahmed (2010) writes, 'acts of deviation mean getting in trouble but also troubling conventional ideas of what it means to have a good life' (pp. 115–116). As a 'presence' of queer sex, they take the text in different directions, challenging mononormativity, the 'structures that privilege (alone or in combination) the couple form, "fidelity" and sexual/romantic love' (Kean 2015, p. 700), and potentially open a space to contemplate the limitations of traditional relationships. Indeed, Gregg argues that 'anxieties about adultery are always anxieties about security' including 'worries about losing what little can be counted on' (2013, p. 309). In this space, moments of cheating enable contemplation of change. Labelling behaviours cheating reinforces conceptualisations of 'appropriate' behaviour and yet it is also a moment of transgression in which behaviours are placed in question. As Weeks (1998) notes, feminism as well as gay and lesbian advocacy has involved moments of transgression and citizenship, with 'transgression appear[ing] necessary to face the status quo with its inadequacies, to hold a mirror up to its prejudices and fears', suggesting that it is the publicness of such transgressions that offers the possibility to enact change and 'protect... the possibilities of a private life' (p. 37). Against this background, in this chapter I explore the various ways *Skins* confuses the public and private dimensions of relationships. As Richardson and Monro argue, the public/private is 'a socially produced binary', both 'deeply connected to and regulated by public discourses and social institutions' (2012, p. 67), and such public dimensions impact and inform characters experiences. Far from comparing representations of queer sexuality and sex by providing a statistical analysis of each time a character has sex and defining the 'queerness' of these acts (an impossible task), in this chapter I draw from a series of transgressive moments in *Skins* in which issues of 'cheating' are raised to consider ways of rethinking sexual citizenship in youth.

Moment (Generation One): Tony 'cheats' on his girlfriend Michelle by giving Maxxie 'head'

On a school trip to Russia, Tony (Nicholas Hoult) propositions Maxxie (Mitch Hewer) as an act of 'friendship' when Maxxie's best friend Anwar (Dev Patel) suddenly decides he has a problem with Maxxie being gay (1.6).[3] In the first episode of *Skins*, Maxxie was introduced somewhat stereotypically as a tap dancing, artistic, attractive boy who takes his mates out to show them *his* world at the Big Gay Night Out: a banal night at the pub. In the room they share on camp, Anwar admires and complements the quality and detail of the picture Maxxie drew of them together, arm in arm, reinforcing Maxxie's artistic nature. However, Anwar is soon disoriented as he turns the page of Maxxie's sketchbook to find a drawing of a penis and hastens to compare it to his own. Later, Anwar asks Maxxie not to bring a man back to the room noting he does not want to see him 'do a guy' and justifying this position based on his religion: 'I'm just a Muslim, gay's just wrong'.[4] When Maxxie explains the situation to Tony soon after, his response is to offer to give him 'head' to 'cheer [him] up'. Surprised, Maxxie questions Tony, noting as a friend he is supposed to be helping him with his problem. Tony's proposition is not presented as based on desire for Maxxie, he declares that it is intended to distract Maxxie from his best friend Anwar's homophobia, and yet, rather than backing off, when Maxxie critiques this, Tony kisses him, explaining 'we're in Russia, I want to try something new'. Maxxie comments that he is not a hobby, and asks about Tony's girlfriend Michelle (April Pearson). Indeed, a half-naked Tony is inviting Maxxie to bed when Michelle enters and Maxxie takes the opportunity to leave. In contrast to Anwar's discomfort (and perhaps jealousy at Maxxie's presumed sexual activity contrasting with his own virginity), Tony assumes Maxxie will want to have sex with him, implying his own acceptance of Maxxie's sexuality in the process. In this way, although viewers have not seen Maxxie have sex, both Anwar and Tony present Maxxie and thus 'gay' 'as an intensely sexualized category' (Richardson and Monro 2012, p. 80). While Maxxie initially refuses Tony's advances, after a melancholy conversation with Anwar in which their friendship is not reconciled, Maxxie returns to their room. Michelle lies asleep on the bed and Maxxie comments, 'Tony, you've got to stop fucking around'. Tony puts his finger to his lips, 'I dare you'. He removes both their shirts, kissing Maxxie's lips before moving to his chest and down his body. The shot cuts to a close-up of Michelle's face, clearly awake, watching, shocked. Viewers hear the sound of a zipper, then Tony is shown standing up. Maxxie gently touches his chin and confidently comments, 'Tony, we've finally found something you're not actually good at', intimating fellatio. Tony exclaims 'What?' and in a long shot Maxxie does up his pants and leaves the room.

In defining intimate citizenship, Plummer includes 'the *control (or not) over* one's body, feelings, relationships; *access (or not) to* representations, relationships, public spaces' (1995, p. 151 in Plummer 2005, emphasis in original). Intimacy, he writes, can include 'an array of arenas in which we "do" the personal life' (Plummer 2005, p. 77). Berridge (2013) has argued that *Skins* is conservative in its representation of gender and sexuality, and here representations of queer sex are restrained: although sexuality and even sex have a presence, it is marked by absence when placed beside heterosexuality. The sex act between Maxxie and Tony emerges from Anwar's desire to not watch two boys have sex (he would have been happy seeing Maxxie have sex with a girl) and as viewers we see no more than the kiss between Maxxie and Tony, in contrast to two heterosexual couples shown having sex in beds in this episode. Discussing representations of sexuality on television, Davis argues that 'queer sexual activity... is minimal, in contrast to excessive, occasionally graphic, heterosexual coupling' (2004, p. 130). While viewing Michelle's reaction to the sex act between Maxxie and Tony is important for the narrative, in light of the disgust Anwar conveyed for viewing sex between men it is significant that neither Maxxie's nor Tony's experience of sex here is shown (it is only implied through sound and Maxxie's comments), suggesting that viewers might also not want to see sex between men. Such representation is similarly limited in Season Two. While Maxxie is shown to be chased and then passionately kissed by the bully Dale (Matthew Hayfield) (2.1), this depiction is limited to starting to remove a shirt and a comment about Dale having 'the magic touch' the next morning. While Maxxie is shown to be sexually confident and in control besides 'the still-closeted and self-loathing Dale' (Berridge 2013, p. 797), Berridge suggests this depiction fails to acknowledge 'serious social issues ... perpetuating the dominant myth of male sexuality as natural and unstoppable' (p. 799). In a television show that does not hesitate to show drug and alcohol use and naked heterosexual couplings, such limited representations are significant.

As a gay man, there are also social restrictions on Maxxie's sexual behaviour. In the next episode (1.7), Michelle publicly breaks up with Tony, and realising she saw them together Maxxie asks Michelle not to tell, explaining it will impact other people's perception of him. This perception is reinforced by Michelle's retort that they might think he is 'a dirty little slut who fucks around with other people's boyfriends'. The description 'slut' attaches to Maxxie's confession. After Tony presents his paper on 'The Role of Sex in Power Relationships' in his psychology class, commenting 'sex plus power equals fun', prompting a distraught Michelle to leave, Maxxie stands, explaining 'it's all my fault'. He describes the situation to gasps and laughs from the class, and Tony shakes his head and rolls his eyes. Maxxie concludes, 'I'm really, really sorry for being a slut, OK?' While Maxxie accepts the descriptor 'slut', historically, the term 'props up a sexual double standard, marks female sexuality as deviant, and works to control girls' behaviour', enforcing 'sexual norms' (Attwood 2007, p. 235). But Maxxie's apology and statement he is a 'slut' is placed in direct contrast to Tony's actual behaviour: Tony is reported to cheat on Michelle with many girls and deliberately kissed one of these girls in front of Michelle to make trouble (1.5). In contrast, this is the first representation of Maxxie having sex. Why is Maxxie the slut? Indeed, Tony is generally left unscathed by the act of sex with Maxxie, although he is ostracised by the group for betraying/hurting Michelle, this does not make Tony 'gay'. Tony tells his best mate Sid (Mike Bailey) in explanation 'fuck all ever happens in this shitty little town, you've got to improvise. ... So I messed around with Maxxie a bit, so what? He was bored, I was bored, Michelle was bored, and now we're not'. His statement raises questions of whether he was interested in experimenting, or merely using Maxxie to make trouble. Although viewers are aware that Tony has been cheating on Michelle with other girls, it takes Michelle seeing the interaction between Tony and Maxxie to acknowledge this behaviour. Earlier in the episode Michelle's best friend tried to talk to her about the girls Tony had been having sex with, and Michelle explained her reasons for being with him: 'He's exciting, and he must love me because he could have anyone he wants', continuing 'he always wants me the most'. However, her confidence is placed in question when it is suggested he might like boys as well. Michelle's reaction is left deliberately ambiguous: does she break up with Tony because having sex with a guy crosses a line, because she finally acknowledges his cheating behaviours, or because she no longer wants to be a pawn in his game?

The limited representations of sex between men in the first generation of *Skins* (Seasons One and Two) are exemplified towards the end of Season Two. In a study period, Maxxie introduces his boyfriend, James (Sean Vevey), to the group (2.8). While including an acknowledgement of sex – Sid asks, 'what's he like then', and James responds 'he's good, really good' – this introduction is overshadowed by Cassie (Hannah Murray) arriving at school and passionately kissing Sid (her boyfriend), as Maxxie and James sit quietly, hand in hand. Generally the heterosexual kiss is so 'banal' that it seems invisible, 'perpetuating heteronormativity' (Morris and Sloop 2006, p. 3), however here, placed beside the clear absence of the homosexual kiss, heteronormativity is arguably made visible (Clarke 2017). Viewers are not shown Maxxie and James having sex, and I would argue that the ending of this first generation of *Skins* suggests that to be a sexual citizen is to be in a stable, monogamous, desexualised relationship: Season Two ends with Maxxie and James moving to London and Anwar spontaneously joining them. In the light of the Season One storyline, this ending seems significant: Anwar's friendship with Maxxie is more important than his discomfort at sharing a living space with a homosexual couple. And yet, given the lack of representation of sex between Maxxie and his boyfriend it might also imply desexualisation now that Maxxie is in a coupled relationship. As Bell and Binnie suggest, the duties that accompany citizenship often mean the responsible 'good citizen' conforms to 'the requirements of homonormativity and heteronormative privilege'. At the same time this may enable change: making LGBTQ people mainstream, Bell and Binnie suggest, may make available 'new trajectories' (2006, p. 871).

Moment (Generation Two): fallout after Naomi 'fucked the dead girl'[5]

After a season of coming to terms with their sexuality, Season Three, Episode Nine of *Skins* concludes with Emily (Kathryn Prescott) publicly declaring her love for Naomi (Lily Loveless) at the school ball and Naomi echoing the sentiment. However, early in Season Four this happy relationship is placed in jeopardy when it is revealed that over the summer holidays Naomi had sex with a girl (Sophia) who subsequently takes her own life (4.2). Emily discovers the affair reading Sophia's diary, and viewers hear Sophia recount their affair, accompanied by hand-drawn images and an animated kiss between two girls. Telling Naomi that she 'ruined it', Emily emphasises the fragility of their relationship, commenting 'you don't want anyone to care'. When Naomi cries, 'I was scared', Emily retorts 'you're always scared', highlighting Naomi's reluctance throughout Season Three to acknowledge her attraction to Emily. The repercussions of Naomi's affair are felt throughout Season Four: both Naomi and Emily talk about the difficulties of relationships.[6] Indeed, discussing this scene, Monaghan (2016, p. 71) argues that *Skins* offers something often not seen in more typical 'idealised depictions of teenage experience' with queer girl characters rarely allowed to 'feel... "shit"' in relationships. In depicting a relationship between Emily and Naomi over two seasons, the serialised nature of television allows *Skins* to explore the difficulties and complexities of their relationship in an extended form (Monaghan 2016). Portraying Emily and Naomi's relationship in this way arguably accords sexual citizenship with access to unconventional depictions of a relationship between girls. But this also places the normative coupled form in question. When Emily returns home following this revelation, she sits with her father (John Bishop). He hugs her as Emily cries 'I don't know why she did that' and 'I hate her' and tells her his regrets having cheated on her mother when he was 19, explaining 'people do stupid things when they're trying to pretend they're not trapped'. While Emily suggests she is not tough like her mother, a comment that implies she might not be able to remain with Naomi, he reassures her, 'that's OK too'. In a context where Emily's relationship is not accepted by her mother,[7] this conversation with her father and his attempt to equate their relationships in a moment of bonding appears to 'normalise' Emily and Naomi's relationship, at the same time as cheating and feeling trapped in relationships is produced as ordinary.

Although Naomi and Emily remain together throughout the season, their relationship is plagued by uncertainty. Emily kisses and dates other girls, shown to be dreadfully unhappy and often crying, while Naomi spends much of the season stoned. When Emily thinks she might have drunkenly cheated in the final episode of Season Four, waking up beside a topless girl, Mandy (Karina Minhas), in the bed she shares with Naomi, she appears mortified (4.8). It is Naomi's conversation with Mandy, and the suggestion that Emily might end up with someone else that spurs Naomi to action.[8] As Kipnis writes, 'adultery is ... at heart a drama about change. It's a way of trying to invent a world, and a way of knowing something about what we want' (2000, p. 34). Following Mandy's comment, 'If you don't want her, I do', Naomi arrives at a party and entering, immediately tells Emily in front of the group, 'I've loved you since the first time I saw you'. The music fades as she explains she had sex with Sophia based on the 'hold' she felt Emily had over her, concluding, 'You were trying to punish me back and it's horrible, it's so horrible because … I love you so much, it's killing me'. Tight close-ups of the girls' faces are shown as they both cry, staring at each other. The music, which faded out as Naomi spoke, starts again and Emily steps forward to kiss Naomi. The kiss is filmed closely. While the absence of music during Naomi's speech is used to focus on her emotion and words as she explains her behaviour, suggesting authenticity, as it begins again it signals celebration. The scene reinforces mononormativity with a happy ending for the couple, at the same time as it implies the restrictions of such relationships, with Naomi relating her feelings of being trapped by Emily and her acceptance of them.

The representation of this closely filmed kiss between two attractive young women is particularly significant: sex between attractive women is often critiqued as entertainment for a heterosexual male audience, at the same time as lesbian characters are often 'desexualised' with 'their relationships and intimate lives' ignored (Breire 2012, p. 3). Elsewhere, I have argued that 'the media's eroticisation of girl same sex kissing leads to questions as to how desire between attractive young women may be portrayed without it being fetishised' (Clarke 2017, p. 135). In *Skins*, this is primarily negotiated by critiquing male characters who express a desire to see the girls together. When Emily stops Katie from teasing Naomi by explaining she chose to kiss Naomi while on drugs because she 'felt like fucking kissing someone' (3.3), Cook (Jack O'Connell), the anti-hero of Generation Two, laughs, 'be even better if you showed us', and is shut down by Effy (Kaya Scodelario). Similar critique of male characters viewing sex between girls as entertainment occurs in the next episode (3.4) when Katie's boyfriend Danny (Henry Garrett) comments 'orgy' upon hearing the girls are going to a pyjama party. Katie's behaviour is placed in question here: while Katie is unhappy about her sister's attraction to Naomi, she seems happy to play into a performative sexuality for her boyfriend, behaviour which is again critiqued by Effy, who rolls her eyes and walks away. Later, when sneaking to see what happens at Pandora's party, Cook tells JJ that 'pyjama party means only one thing, girls getting friendly' and JJ responds, 'even I know that only happens in overblown and possibly illegal teen dramas', with the implication being such as *Skins*. However, when JJ walks in on Emily and Naomi kissing later in the episode he doesn't know what to do. These kisses between the girls are not intentionally public; JJ is not meant to be there, and they don't see him. Reflecting on the structure of *Skins*, Monaghan (2016) argues such moments of 'multi-perspectivalism allows the audience to get a better sense of the issue' (p. 74), depicting various characters 'reacting to and reflecting on the Emily/Naomi relationship' (p. 72). Indeed, it is not just JJ who sees such moments, but also Effy and Katie. In this way, *Skins* negotiates a space for a sexual relationship between the girls to be represented, and two episodes later, when the girls are shown having sex for the first time (3.6), in contrast to the representation of Maxxie in Generation One, the focus is on Naomi's face rather than someone watching. In this way, *Skins* may be perceived to carve a space for representation of sex between girls by pedagogically framing concepts of appropriate viewing behaviour, while ironically nevertheless producing entertainment. To do so, however, may be perceived as sexual citizenship, enabling access to representations of same-sex-attracted young women outside of a hypersexual or desexualised space.

Moment (Generation Three): everybody loves Franky?

I opened this chapter with Franky fighting with Matty, then dancing with Luke. While Matty focusses on past experiences – 'You loved it, Tunisia, the beach, making love to me' – Franky tells a different story: these same elements get boring when repeated over time. Franky's conversation with Matty asks the question: is coupledom the only way to be, or can we imagine other ways? The day after the party her friends question her behaviour with Luke, and Franky explains that 'nothing happened'. Grace (Jessica Sula) comments that Franky should 'sort it out' with Matty, and when Franky asks 'Why?' she is told 'He's your boyfriend, and well, last night you were acting like a bit of a slut'. While the young women restate the boundaries of heteronormativity and monogamy, disciplining Franky's behaviour by suggesting it was 'slutty', Franky rejects this condemnation, questioning 'is that what life's all about then? Not upsetting our boyfriends?' As Franky leaves, Mini (Freya Mavor) comments quietly to the girls 'I liked it better when she might or might not have been a lesbian'. Now in a relationship with Matty, Franky is perceived by her friends as heterosexual, her sexual orientation problematically determined by her sexual partner (Moorman 2012). In Season Five, with her androgynous appearance, Franky did not conform to the expectations of her friends, and while the girls attempted to define Franky's sexuality, their questions sat in contrast with their own sexual ambiguity: 'these girls flirt with Franky or at the possibility of something with Franky' (Clarke 2017, p. 193). Although dressed in a more feminine manner, in Season Six Franky continues to disrupt romantic and gendered scripts of behaviour and thus creates difficulty for her friends, difficulty that is exemplified at the party at the beginning of Season Six. As someone who is 'into people' and refuses labelling of her sexuality, Franky offers an opportunity to think of her relationships outside of mononormativity: rather than focussing on the gender of her partners, we might contemplate the concurrence of her attractions. As Monro notes, people often fail to understand the differences in 'sexual scripting' that attraction to people of more than one gender and polyamory can create (2015, p. 42): in a world where television relationship drama is often produced through 'cheating', what would attractions to multiple people, at one time, look like, and how might this challenge our understandings of relationships? In contrast to Matty's statement that 'they are great together', suggesting an unchangeable relationship (6.1), in Season Five, Mini warned Franky that Matty 'just wants to fuck [her] and then fuck [her] up', to which Franky replied 'good' (5.8). Although Matty takes this relationship seriously, as Halberstam writes, 'being taken seriously means missing out on the chance to be frivolous, promiscuous, and irrelevant' (2011, p. 6) and while Matty tells his brother Nick (Sean Teale) 'I think maybe she can't do it, ... be with someone', it might be questioned whether Franky ever really wanted a relationship of this nature. Later in the episode (6.1), Franky leaves with Luke. Although Matty initially watches them go, he is encouraged to chase after them by Liv (Laya Lewis) who is worried about Franky's safety. Matty's and Luke's driving becomes increasingly erratic and Matty loses control, the car rolls, and Grace is killed. Within the narrative, this does not simply condemn Franky's flirtation with Luke, it also creates ambiguity: who was responsible here? For some viewers it might be questioned why Franky, who has spent the entire previous season lusting over Matty, suddenly takes up with Luke; why no one speaks of Luke's role in the accident; and why Matty places the lives of his passengers in danger. I have previously considered the ways in which this third generation (Seasons Five and Six) contemplates grief, belonging and connections to others, and while community is in no way idealised, it is placed in contrast to individualism, which is repeatedly questioned and identified as impossible (Clarke 2017). Perhaps then, Franky demonstrates a need for alternative conceptualisations of sexual citizenship which allow for multiple flirtations, attractions and connections to those around her.

One such conceptualisation might be found in the work of Monro (2015) and her understanding of bisexual citizenship. In many ways, Franky's conceptualisation of her sexuality is queer within an understanding of queer theory which resists 'the allegedly stable relations between chromosomal sex, gender and sexual desire' and 'locates and exploits the incoherencies in those three terms which stabilise heterosexuality' (Jagose 1996, p. 3). As Monro notes, the term 'queer' is used 'by non-heterosexual people internationally to denote multiple, non-categorised, or non-normative sexual and gender identities' (p. 47). Franky is indeterminate: she explicitly notes that she is not bisexual, and yet her statement that she is 'into people' (5.7) aligns with the broad definition of bisexuality proposed by Monro: 'attraction to people of more than one gender' (2015, p. 23). Considering sexual citizenship for LGBTQ people, Monro notes the need for a broader understanding that accounts for bisexual people and includes recognition of identity, and 'support for full equality for people in same-sex relationships' as well as 'acceptance that desire can be fluid, ... an understanding that sexuality can be changeable and that people with more fluid or complex identities also require citizenship rights' (Richardson and Monro 2012, p. 70), which goes beyond the homonormative/heteronormative concepts of sexual citizenship noted earlier. While to label Franky and sexual citizenship in this way potentially restricts the behaviours included, Franky's statement is not simply a statement of desire for people of multiple genders but may be a critique of mononormativity: she might not want to choose between attractions. I use this definition strategically, to account for a form of sexual citizenship that has room for fluidity and ambiguity.

Throughout Season Six, Franky's behaviour can be hard to account for. She refuses the possibility of a relationship with Matty, repeatedly breaks up with him, has passionate and then violent sex with Luke, leaves what quickly becomes an abusive relationship, and starts a relationship with Nick, while maintaining a flirtation with the pregnant Mini. Although Liv calls Franky a 'slut', Liv had sex with the same number of people in Season Five but in more casual encounters. This leads to the question: what is slutty about Franky's behaviour? Is it the sex, or the intense nature of her relationships which flirt with 'love' and its meaning? Lying close together, arms around one another on a single bed in a hostel for pregnant women and single mothers, Franky and Mini talk intimately about their relationships with men (6.9). Asking if Franky has dumped Nick, Franky doesn't directly answer, but comments 'I don't want to keep hurting him'. When Mini asks if Franky is still in love with Matty, Franky explains that Matty makes her feel like she has no control. Mini questions 'isn't that what love feels like' and Franky responds 'I don't know why you're so obsessed with that word. I don't know what it means'. In *Skins*, characters are shown to be 'in love' with more than one person at one time: Matty loves Liv and Franky (5.8), while Franky loves Matty and Nick (6.10). At the same time, these relationships are 'constrained and framed by discourses of love and normative conceptualisations of relationships' (Clarke 2017, p. 202). The final conversation between Liv and Franky (6.10) may be perceived as reinforcing mononormativity. Liv aggressively comments that Franky should go and talk to Nick and Matty, telling her 'just because your life's fucked up it doesn't give you the right to fuck up everyone else's'. Franky refuses responsibility, replying 'I didn't ask anyone to fall in love with me' and Liv responds 'no, but you let them, didn't you Franky'. After Liv leaves, Mini supports Franky and yet she comments that Franky 'need[s] to sort [her] shit out'. An interaction with (the dead) Grace solidifies this. When Franky runs from Nick and Matty at a party, Grace appears seated on a couch, patting the seat beside her. Crying, Franky sits, and Grace runs her hand along Franky's face. Franky asks her what to do, and Grace tells her to stop running: 'tell the truth and all will be hunky dory'. Grace smiles and gently kisses Franky on the lips, before disappearing. These comments from the girls suggest a need for Franky to live a more ordered, less messy life. As the boys burst into the room, Franky starts to run, then stops, explaining to Nick and Matty, 'I love you, both'. Their response is ambiguous: Nick asks, 'Can we not sort something out here?' and Matty comments 'don't end it with us, please'. Throughout this season of *Skins*, Franky has questioned why she was put up for adoption and whether something is wrong with her, whether she can love and be loved. To many in the show, her behaviour seems pathological; however, what if it is just a different way to engage with others that she does not yet have the words for? Indeed, Nick and Matty's use of 'we' and 'us' suggests that rather than Franky needing to choose between the brothers, some arrangement might have been negotiated between the three: she could love them both. As Kean (2015) argues, mononormativity 'makes it difficult to be single, or in a relationship with more than one person, or a person whose sexual-romantic relationship is less important than friendships, business partnerships or "carer" relationships' (p. 702). Mononormativity is so ingrained that even in a television show that embraces transgression and controversy, the possibility of polyamory is only tangentially considered with the suggestion of this relationship between Franky and both Nick and Matty. This highlights the limitations of current forms of sexual citizenship which are unable to represent possibilities beyond normativity. While this is only one reading of this scene, it demonstrates the restrictions placed on our relationships, and the normative understandings which reproduce mononormativity and do not allow for more complex, and perhaps ambiguous relationship forms.

Discussing designations and labels Albury notes that although they 'are supposed to indicate sexed and gendered identity, they actually tell us very little about what people do with their bodies, or what their desires, pleasures, or fantasies might be' (2015, p. 654). Franky's assertions and interactions with girls are in the context of relationships with men, attractions which persist alongside one another. Although I was initially frustrated that Franky is only shown to have sex with men, she exists among a range of queer characters: Alex (Sam Jackson), a young man who has explicit, casual sex with men; Matty, who makes a flippant comment about having sex with men for money while homeless; not to mention the Generation Three kisses between Franky and Mini, Liv and Grace; and, within the broader history of *Skins*, broken-hearted Cassie who has mindless sex with girls, and three generations of male characters who negotiate significant and explicit love-based friendships. The range of fluid relationships between characters provides an opportunity for thinking through 'bisexuality' over the life of a season and, more generally, the fluidity of attractions, desires and relationships across the three generations of the show. Discussing temporality and bisexual representation, Moorman notes a need for representations to include explicit identifications, reiterations or representation of 'intimate relations with both men and women', suggesting one method for conveying bisexuality is for characters to 'not be engaged in a monogamous relationship at the film's end' (2012, p. 122). Indeed, Generation Three is the only one to end without a happy (coupled) ending for its queer characters, perhaps enabling this fluidity[9]: in refusing the attention of Nick and Matty the ending leaves the 'queer' Franky open to alternative relational possibilities. Considering the constant fluctuations in our sexual and intimate lives, Attwood (2006) suggests sexual citizenship is concerned with the ways we might talk about, relate to and negotiate change, with the potential to impact and influence multiple spaces, particularly areas we 'accept as "natural"' – between public citizenship and private life, love and sex, self and other, freedom and responsibility' (p. 91). In contemplating moments of transgression and the presence and absence of queer sex in *Skins*, we can envisage relationships which trouble conventional notions of sexual citizenship and how we 'do' personal life, demonstrating the space to go beyond 'cheating' and mononormativity to consider a broader range of relational possibilities and explore, acknowledge and enable greater fluidity.

Notes

1 Created by Brian Elsley and his then 19-year-old son Jamie Brittain in 2007, the UK teen television drama *Skins* (2007–2013) follows three 'generations' of millennial teens in their final year of college/high school (www.imdb.com/title/tt0840196/). The show was particularly controversial for its representation of teenagers drinking, taking drugs and having sex.
2 Considering issues of gender, it is significant that when Franky first kisses Matty, she is wearing a dress, a representation outside of her earlier androgyny (5.8).
3 All in-text references to *Skins* refer to season and episode.
4 This is resolved at the end of Season One, with Maxxie accepted after revealing his sexuality to Anwar's religious father (1.9).
5 This quote comes from Season Four, Episode Four as Naomi explains their relationship turmoil to the group and Emily's parents.
6 For an excellent discussion of this relationship and its depiction, see Monaghan (2016), Hunn (2012).
7 With suggestions both of homophobia, and a fear that her daughter will be hurt by Naomi.
8 As a prompt for Naomi into action, this has precedence. In Season Three, it was only after Emily's twin sister Katie (Megan Prescott) revealed that Emily had sex with JJ (Ollie Barbieri) that Naomi relented and attended the ball where the girls declare their love for each other. While Emily explains to JJ that she is a lesbian and has sex with him as a friend and a favour, the implication is that Naomi is only willing to acknowledge her love for Emily when she fears she might lose her.
9 For discussion of this ending, see Clarke (2017).

References

Ahmed, S., 2010. *The Promise of Happiness*. Durham, NC: Duke University Press.

Albury, K., 2015. Identity Plus? Bi-curiosity, Sexual Adventurism and the Boundaries of "Straight" Sexual Practices and Identities. *Sexualities*, 18 (5–6), 649–664.

Attwood, F., 2006. Sexed Up: Theorizing the Sexualization of Culture. *Sexualities*, 9 (1), 77–94.

Attwood, F., 2007. Sluts and Riot Grrrls: Female Identity and Sexual Agency. *Journal of Gender Studies*, 16 (3), 233–247.

Beirne, R., 2012. Introduction: Queer Women in Television Today. In: R. Beirne, ed. *Televising Queer Women: A Reader* (2nd ed.). London: Palgrave Macmillan, 1–10.

Bell, D. and Binnie, J., 2006. Geographies of Sexual Citizenship. *Political Geography*, 25, 869–873.

Berridge, S., 2013. "Doing It for the Kids"? The Discursive Construction of the Teenager and Teenage Sexuality in *Skins*. *Journal of British Cinema and Television*, 10 (4), 785–801.

Clarke, K., 2017. *Affective Sexual Pedagogies in Film and Television*. New York, NY: Routledge.

Davis, G., 2004. "Saying It Out Loud": Revealing Television's Queer Teens. In: G. Davis and K. Dickinson, eds. *Teen TV: Genre, Consumption and Identity*. Basingstoke: Palgrave MacMillan, 127–140.

Dhaenens, F., 2013. Teenage Queerness: Negotiating Heteronormativity in the Representation of Gay Teenagers in *Glee*. *Journal of Youth Studies*, 16 (3), 304–317.

Gregg, M., 2013. Spouse-Busting: Intimacy, Adultery, and Surveillance Technology. *Surveillance and Society*, 11 (3), 301–310.

Halberstam, J., 2011. *The Queer Art of Failure*. Durham, NC: Duke University Press.

Hogan, H., 2011a. Exclusive: "Skins" Boss Jamie Brittain Talks Series 5, His Legacy and Leaving the Series He Co-created. *AfterEllen*, April 1. Available from: www.afterellen.com/people/86315-exclusive-skins-boss-jamie-brittain-talks-series-5-his-legacy-and-leaving-the-series-he-co-created [Accessed 11 September 2017].

Hogan, H., 2011b. Is Mini McGuinness Gay as a Window? *AfterEllen*, April 18. Available from: www.afterellen.com/tv/87165-is-mini-mcguinness-gay-as-a-window [Accessed 11 September 2017].

Hunn, D. F., 2012. "The Dark Side of Naomily": *Skins*, Fan Texts and Contested Genres. *Continuum*, 26 (1), 89–100.

Jagose, Annamarie. 1996. *Queer Theory*. Carlton South, VIC: Melbourne University Press.

Johnson, C., 2017. Sexual Citizenship in a Comparative Perspective: Dilemmas and Insights. *Sexualities*, 20 (1–2), 159–175.

Joyrich, L., 2014. Queer Television Studies: Currents, Flows, and (Main)streams. *Cinema Journal*, 53 (2), 133–139.

Kean, J., 2015. A Stunning Plurality: Unravelling Hetero- and Mononormativities through HBO's *Big Love. Sexualities*, 18 (5/6), 698–713.

Kipnis, L., 2000. Adultery. In: L. Berlant, ed. *Intimacy*. Chicago IL: University of Chicago Press, 9–47.

Marshall, D., 2010. Popular Culture, the "Victim" Trope and Queer Youth Analytics. *International Journal of Qualitative Studies in Education*, 23 (1), 65–85.

Masanet, M. and Buckingham, D., 2015. Advice on Life? Online Fan Forums as a Space for Peer-to-Peer Sex and Relationships Education. *Sex Education*, 15 (5), 486–499.

Meyer, M., 2010. Representing Bisexuality on Television: The Case for Intersectional Hybrids. *Journal of Bisexuality*, 10 (4), 366–387.

Monaghan, W., 2016. *Queer Girls, Temporality and Screen Media: Not "Just a Phase."* London: Palgrave Macmillan.

Monro, S., 2015. *Bisexuality*. London: Palgrave Macmillan.

Moorman, J., 2012. Gray Matters: Bisexual (In)visibility in *The L Word*. In: R. Beirne, ed. *Televising Queer Women: A Reader*. 2nd ed. Basingstoke: Palgrave Macmillan, 119–134.

Morris, C. E. and Sloop, J. M., 2006. "What Lips these Lips have Kissed": Refiguring the Politics of Queer Public Kissing. *Communication and Critical/Cultural Studies*, 3 (1), 1–26.

Plummer, K., 2005. Intimate Citizenship in an Unjust World. In: M. Romeo and E. Margolis, eds. *The Blackwell Companion to Social Inequalities*. Abingdon: Blackwell, 75–99.

Richardson, D. and Monro, S., 2012. *Sexuality, Equality and Diversity*. Basingstoke: Palgrave Macmillan.

Skins, 2007–2013. Created by B. Elsley and J. Brittain. UK: Company Pictures, Storm Dog Films.

Weeks, J., 1998. The Sexual Citizen. *Theory, Culture and Society*, 15 (3–4), 35–52.

Chapter 17

'Some teachers are homophobic, you know, because they just don't know any better'

Students reimagining power relations in schools

Katie Fitzpatrick and Hayley McGlashan

KATIE: *I'm sitting in a high school classroom nibbling on snacks and listening to the talk of a group of students. They are meeting here together at lunchtime to make plans for an intervention with teachers. Meera explains: 'some teachers are homophobic, you know, because they just don't know any better. We can help them understand.'*

HAYLEY: *I'm talking to two queer students about their experiences with teachers at their high school.*

HAYLEY: Have either of you experienced biphobia, homophobia or transphobia from a teacher?

RAVEN: Yeah.

SOCRATIS: Especially our biology teacher.

RAVEN: Yeah.

SCORATIS: He's so heteronormative.

RAVEN: We are talking about reproduction and that...

SOCRATIS: 'Every girl is going to go and have children with a guy', he just says stuff like 'all women want children'. And that's another problem I have be-cause not all women want children and then he's like 'you will date a man when you are older'.

HAYLEY: Have either of you ever challenged him?

SOCRATIS: No, I don't really mind, I just feel sorry for him for being so uneducated.

These two 'moments' derive from our critical ethnographic research in two different schools. Both schools are large, diverse, multi-ethnic state schools in Auckland, New Zealand. The group meetings were with students in Gay-Straight Alliance (GSA) groups (sometimes called queer-straight alliances, QSAs), which we henceforth refer to throughout the chapter as 'queer groups'. These groups provide a space for students who identify as lesbian, gay, bisexual, trans, queer and intersex (LGBTQI) and others who are questioning to meet together to gain support. Both groups are also explicitly activist in terms of the actions students undertook within their schools. In this chapter, we explore how students in these groups at two different schools are reimagining power relations in schools between teachers and students. We argue that this is significant in the sense of shifting discourses of teacher-student relationships and the positionality of students – and young people more generally – in schools. Such a reimagining impacts how education might be viewed in terms of the roles of teachers and students, and the perceived capabilities of young people. We argue here that the participants we talked with are disrupting two current (but divergent) discourses about youth in education. The first is a perception that young people have underdeveloped brains and are, therefore, untrustworthy and incapable of looking after their best interests. The second is the argument that young people – especially those who identify as queer or LGBTQI – are marginalised in schools. We do not contest the notion of marginality as such but rather suggest that some young people are going beyond subjectivities of marginalisation and resistance to take up 'expert' subjectivities.

We begin the chapter with an overview of these two discourses and how they affect the positioning of young people in schools currently. We then describe the critical ethnographic methodology we each employed and explain the specific methods relevant to this chapter. Finally, we outline two key themes underpinning students' approaches to issues of power in their schools: students reimaging themselves as experts; and students contesting power within the groups. We end with some thoughts about what this might mean for school practice and LGBTQI students.

Constructing adolescence and youth: brain development and marginality

In an article in the journal *Developmental Science*, David Moshman (2011) rebuts common assumptions about the capability of teenagers to make thoughtful, independent and agentic decisions. He argues that teenagers are young adults with the same capacities as adults (but perhaps with less experience). While many sociologists and post-structuralist scholars have operated on such an assumption for a long time, other youth researchers continue to maintain that brain development is a defining feature of 'adolescence'. The argument that the adolescent brain is incapable of rational decision-making has also made its way into popular discourse. For example, in their recent *New York Times* bestselling book, Jensen and Nutt (2015) make the following statement:

> The problem for teens is that their underdeveloped frontal cortex means they have trouble seeing ahead or understanding the consequences of their independent acts, and are therefore ill equipped to weigh the relative harms of risky behaviour.

(p. 104)

Moshman (2011) points out that, while distinctions between children and adults have been clear for a long time (centuries), adolescence as a life stage is both quite recent and largely a fallacy. He notes that

This is not to say there is no development beyond age 12. Quite the contrary, developmental progress in reasoning, rationality, morality, and identity over the teen years and beyond is common….But, development beyond age 12 is highly individualized. Adolescents develop to varying degrees in diverse domains and cultural contexts. Individual differences beyond age 12 are substantial, but age accounts for very little of the variance.

(p. 172)

This argument is important to consider because many schools, and high schools in particular, are organised on the assumption that young people cannot make decisions for themselves, or, if they do, these need to be circumscribed, controlled and monitored. With respect to learning about health-related concepts such as sexuality, drugs, alcohol and mental health, an overwhelmingly large proportion of school resources and research assumes that young people need to be guided towards the right (i.e. morally correct) attitudes and behaviour (Fitzpatrick and Tinning 2014, Gard and Pluim 2014). These tend to boil down to a series of rules that young people should adhere to: not do drugs; drink moderately, if at all; and (ideally) not engage in sex. If they do engage in sex then contraception should be used to prevent pregnancy and disease.

In her study of how teenagers employ strategies to deal with ageism in schools, however, Gordon (2007) notes that

Despite dominant discourses that naturalize the stages of the life cycle and render what is referred to as "the teenage years" or "adolescence" as an immutable and inevitable part of the human development process, a closer look reveals that both the teenager and the adolescent are also socially constructed categories with traceable histories.

(p. 633)

Moshman (2011) maintains that dominant discourses of adolescence, while largely mythical, are also durable because '[r]egardless of the evidence for adolescent competence, allegations of adolescent irrationality never end' (p. 171). This might explain the tendency for teachers and schools to go about 'protecting' young people from themselves, from their own irrational decision-making and, inevitably, focus school programmes on risk and its avoidance (Evans and Davies 2004, Allen 2007a, 2007b). Such a discourse – of teenage irrationality – sits alongside another set of assumptions, from a different ontological basis, about youth in schools: the notion that many young people, and especially those who do not conform to social norms, are excluded and marginalised in schools.

Exclusion and marginality

Decades of research and scholarship from critical studies in education and gender sexuality studies shows that young people are subject to, perpetrators of and resistant to various (complex) power relations in schools. Chapter length does not allow us to explore the breadth of this field of research. In relation to the students who are at the heart of this chapter, we touch on one aspect of this field dealing with the exclusion and marginality of LGBTQI youth in schools.

The power relations implicit in school environments (Halsey et al. 1997) make researching sexuality at school a contentious process due to the ways in which sexuality, young people and schooling are socially constituted and understood. Quinlivan (2013) states that 'Exploring the role that queer research can play in interrogating heteronormativity within schooling contexts has been seen as necessary and also problematic' (p. S59). She argues that 'Given the structural, ideological and affectively normative cultures of schools, researching queer sexualities and difference will produce conundrums' (p. S57). One such conundrum is the positioning of LGBTQI youth in binary terms: as either victims or agents (Blackburn 2007).

There is, of course, a large body of research focussed on the negative experiences of LGBTQI youth in schools (see Savin-Williams 1994, D'Augelli 1998, D'Augelli et al. 2002, Savin-Williams 2005, Chesir-Teran and Hughes, 2009). Such research has the explicit intention of exposing relations of power that marginalise and oppress LBGTQI students; as a result, it tends to focus on negative outcomes. This has an unintended outcome of positioning these youth as victims. Mayo (2014) questions this approach and insists that 'LGBTQ students and communities need to be understood beyond the lens of victimization. LGBTQ communities are vibrant and resilient, and have long histories of resisting homophobia and transphobia' (p. 1). Researchers drawing on the work of Foucault tend to position queer youth as 'holding productive capabilities of power which produce thoughts and actions and a sense of agency' (Allen 2005, 12). Foucault favours a conceptualisation of power as capillary: 'the point where power reaches into every grain of individuals, touches their bodies and inserts itself into their actions and attitudes, their discourses, learning processes and everyday lives' (Foucault 1980, p. 39). Within this framework, all individuals hold power and have the ability to exercise that power.

Foucauldian scholar Frohard-Dourlent (2016) argues that teachers need to 'interrupt' the regulation of trans and gender non-conforming students in schools. She notes that 'Such interruptions are important because educators' capacity to disrupt systems of gender and sexual conformity undermines the foundations of bullying and other forms of gender policing' (Frohard-Dourlent 2016, p. 63). This is a common call in the literature, for the holders of institutional power in schools (teachers and administrators) to act against the marginalisation of LGBTQI (and other) students. Less is written about how students themselves disrupt power relations, especially as a group. When this is explored, it tends to be focussed on how students employ various forms of 'resistance' and how, even when students take up alternative subjectivities, the norms are reinstated or made more powerful (Youdell 2005).

This discourse of resistance is consistent with the broader field of critical studies in education (for example, Kincheloe 2007, 2008, Steinberg 2007). One

approach to the negative positioning of LGBTQI youth in schools is the formation of (and research around) GSA or QSA (Quinlivan 2013, 2015) groups. While
these vary considerably in both make-up and intention (Mayo 2009; Talburt
and Rasmussen 2010; Youdell 2011; Kosciw et al. 2012; Quinlivan 2013) they
are commonly extracurricular, student-centred groups where LGBTQI students,
along with their heterosexual and questioning allies, gather for conversation,
learning activities and mutual support (Mayo 2013). Quinlivan (2013, 2015) and
others (for example see Mayo 2009, 2013; Talburt and Rasmussen 2010) have
highlighted how critical approaches to learning in QSA groups can allow for the
exploration of fluid subjectivities and non-normative understandings of gender
and sexuality. Such approaches are commonly led by staff or adult facilitators
(Mayo 2013; McGlashan and Fitzpatrick 2017).

Some scholars draw on Foucauldian analyses to conceptualise power in schools
as 'a shifting nexus of relations that act web-like through institutions, practices,
and material subjects' (Allen 2005, p. 12). These relations 'reflect and constitute
the broader sociopolitical discourses in operation, including those that uphold
the constructed superiority of heterosexuality' (Ferfolja 2008, p. 108). Those who
conform to heteronormative understandings of sex, gender and sexuality have
productive forms of power.

In the sections that follow, we explore how a group of young people in two
different schools reimagine power relations beyond resistance or marginality, and certainly beyond the discourses (discussed earlier) of the limitations of
'adolescence'.

Two critical ethnographic studies

For several years, we as authors have engaged in ethnographic research with
young people in schools (for example, see Fitzpatrick 2011, 2013, Fitzpatrick
and May 2015, McGlashan and Fitzpatrick 2017). This chapter is informed by
findings from two separate critical ethnographies in large, culturally diverse, co-
educational, state high schools (years 9–13; students aged 13–18) in Auckland,
New Zealand. We each conducted ethnographic fieldwork in our respective
school during the 2016 year. It is interesting to note here that these two studies
are separate ethnographies; we had not initially planned to intersect in the analysis but after sharing the conversations we each had with the student groups, we
saw important connections and similarities across the two sites.

Patiki College

Katie conducted fieldwork in a school we will refer to as Patiki College (the names
of schools and individuals in this chapter are all pseudonyms for ethical reasons).
Patiki is a very diverse (both ethnically and socioeconomically) state school in
Auckland, with a student roll of over 1500. Katie's fieldwork at Patiki is part of
a larger ethnographic study of four different schools, exploring the intersection

between school-based health education classes and students' culturally located health perspectives, actions and ideas. As part of this study, a year was spent in senior high school health education classes, interviewing teachers and students, and attending health-related student group meetings (such as the queer group and feminist group).

Kahukura High School

Hayley conducted her study at a school we call Kahukura High School, which is a large (2000+) multicultural, co-educational, state school in Auckland. Her study aimed to explore how lesbian, gay, bisexual, trans and queer (LGBTQ) students actively negotiate their queer identities within the schooling environment, and how the school supported them in so doing. Hayley was focussed most intently on the queer group at this school and spent most of her time at related meetings, events and talking with students and teachers associated with this group. She also explored the teaching of sex education across all year levels.

So, while the two schools constitute both in-depth studies in and of themselves (and Katie's project was part of a larger study of four schools), in this chapter, we only draw on the data from the queer student groups in each school.

In both of the studies described, we employed critical ethnography. Thomas (1993) describes critical ethnography as 'conventional ethnography with a political purpose' (p. 4). This approach places the focus on issues of equity, juxtaposing an in-depth epistemological account alongside an analysis of societal issues. In these studies, a critical ethnographic approach allowed locally contextualised data using techniques traditionally developed by ethnographers, such as interviews, observations and immersion in the field of study. It requires social theory to be applied to the research materials (Fitzpatrick and May 2015).

Madison (2012) argues that 'critical ethnography begins with an ethical responsibility to address processes of unfairness or injustice within a particular lived domain' (p. 5). Madison (2012) describes an ethical responsibility as a 'compelling sense of duty and commitment based on moral principles of human freedom and well-being, and hence a compassion for the suffering of living beings' (p. 5). Critical ethnographers aim to disrupt the status quo and unsettle both neutrality and taken for granted assumptions by bringing to light underlying and obscure operations of power. The methodology therefore requires researchers to move from 'what is' to 'what could be' (Thomas 1993, Carspecken 1996, Noblit et al. 2004).

In our wider, school-based ethnographic studies, we also employ narrative inquiry (Clandinin and Connelly 2000), utilising observations, focus groups and semi-structured interviews to weave together narratives of students' experiences and descriptions of moments at school that illustrate schooling cultures. Narrative research is a form of inquiry requiring the researcher to examine the lives of the individuals through the stories they tell about their lives (Clandinin and Connelly 2000). Narrative inquiry also 'becomes a way of understanding experience…In this view, experience is the stories people live. People live stories, and in telling of these stories, reaffirm them, modify them and create new ones' (Clandinin and Connelly 2000, p. xxvi). While we do not include extended narrative descriptions in this chapter, we do include small or partial extracts from longer stories.

Methods

The empirical materials we draw on in this chapter are a result of each being immersed in our separate schools for 3–5 days per week throughout the 2016 school year. During this fieldwork, we engaged in conversations with teachers, students and senior leaders (principals and deputy principals, curriculum leaders, etc.), and experienced school life by observing classroom lessons, assemblies, award evenings, school performances, cultural groups and a range of student-led groups. An initial period of each study was spent developing an understanding of the context and culture of the school. This time was vital for each of us to establish positive relationships with the respective teachers and students in our schools since relationship building is a key feature of critical ethnography (Thomas 1993, Madison 2005). Once an understanding of reciprocity had been established with participants, both authors began to facilitate focus group discussions and interviews with students and staff.

Both queer groups at the two ethnographic sites began as teacher-directed initiatives which were seen to be 'safe spaces' for those who identified as non-heterosexual or non-cisgendered. In 2016, the year we completed the fieldwork, however, the students were directly contesting teacher power, both in terms of the wider school, and in relation to decision-making within the groups. We outline two themes from the research that exemplify how these students were reimagining power relations in their schools and contesting (or ignoring) discourses of 'adolescence' and marginality.

'I just feel sorry for him' – students reimagining themselves as the experts

Katie

The bell rings and I walk over to the health education classroom. It always seems to be raining when I'm at school, or maybe the rain is just more noticeable when I'm here. Four students are already in the room, getting out their own lunches, as well as a few items to share: chips and biscuits are on offer on the table. Meera starts off the conversation by welcoming everyone and there are a few minutes of general chat and eating. Ideas are casually tossed around for the next activity the group will undertake. Martin suggests that the queer group do a promotion for the teachers. He talks for a while about how teachers need help to understand terms 'like, you know, words like pan sexual, trans'. Meera, the group leader, explains that

Like, many students might come up to a teacher that they like and trust, I know that's what I did. And a student might be like 'I don't know what's happening but I think I might be intersex' and the teacher is like 'oh, what's that?' Then it's going to be awkward, but if they know [what intersex means] then they can, like, help the student and be like 'this is something that maybe the counsellor could do...'

Martin then asks, 'so, are we looking at doing maybe a Powerpoint presentation [to the staff] and looking at definitions?' Elise jumps in: 'Maybe our own definitions. Not like what we think it is but like, because some of the dictionary definitions are like, you know. Sometimes they can go into the whole science-y side you know. So, it's like less technical? yeah, so it's easier to understand'.

In this discussion, students at Patiki College were planning to intervene in homophobia at their school. Their conversation highlights that they do directly experience issues of exclusion and marginality in their schools consistent with decades of research in this area, as discussed earlier. However, rather than adopting subjectivities of resistance, they instead see themselves as 'experts' and the teachers as ignorant. Elise even assumes that they should 'translate' the dictionary definitions in order to engage the teachers in learning about various gender and sexual identities. This requires a particular assumption about teachers, age, relations of power and authority in their schools. Instead of seeing themselves as the victims, as marginalised, these students see themselves as more knowledgeable than their teachers, and they feel a responsibility to educate them about issues of sex, gender and sexuality, and the collapse of these categories in everyday school contexts (Youdell 2005).

A similar form of subjectivity was also evident in discussions with students at Kahukura High School, where Hayley was doing fieldwork. As the examples we began this chapter with highlight, students actually 'feel sorry' for teachers who are homophobic.

Hayley

In an interview with Hayley, Prisha and Troy discussed the following:

PRISHA: I feel teachers are not controlled as much as the students are, obviously. They have the freedom to wear what they want, have what tattoos and piercings they want and, I feel, that allows them to feel more, like, who they are and who they can be. And I feel that is why a lot of students, as they come through high school, feel so restricted into this social norm thing because the norms are placed on us and we can't really express our identity. We are all just expected to be the same. That's why, as we leave high school - that is where people, they start to find themselves really.

HAYLEY: Break free?

TROY: Yeah, it could also attribute to kind of, not quite ignorance, but assuming there is not really a big problem with students finding it hard to express themselves because they can all wear what they want. But they only kind of see what goes [on] around them. They don't really interact with students that much on that level and then don't understand us or even understand youth. Like they [the teachers] actually need to be educated on diversity, especially sexuality and gender and then truly understand the importance of being able to express our identities.

Prisha begins by describing some aspects of asymmetrical power in her school and questioning specific examples about choice. Troy goes further by stating that he thinks teachers actually need more education about sexual and gender diversity, and he notes that teachers do not understand young people. These examples are significant because the discourse of power evident in these discussions goes beyond notions of resistance or marginality, and certainly beyond the limitations of notions of 'adolescence'. In some ways, these young people are not even attending to the idea that they should resist or speak back to these power differentials. They are (almost, wilfully) ignorant of the positioning of young people as unreasonable and irrational, and of queer youth as marginalised victims. Instead (and perhaps only for a moment), they assume themselves to be the teachers: the more knowledgeable, more educated and benevolent. This is not a subjectivity of resistance, but one of leadership that invokes particular power-knowledge relationships. Instead of seeing the school as a site of teacher power, they identify the lack of knowledge held by some teachers and, crucially, they take up the responsibility to address this lack (especially in the case of students at Patiki College).

Some research on GSAs and QSAs focuses on the marginalisation of LGBTQI students in schools (see, Savin-Williams 1994, D'Augelli 1998, D'Augelli et al 2002, Savin-Williams 2005, Chesir-Teran and Hughes, 2009). While this work highlights important issues of power and oppression, this risks positioning students as victims (Talburt and Rasmussen 2010, Allen 2015, Mayo 2017). Students are, of course, both subjects of, and subject to, forms of power that frame them in particular ways. Such subjectification is based on traditional regimes of truth that enmeshed in educational institutions. Mayo (2013) argues that complex hierarchical structures continue to be created around age, sex, gender, race and class in school. In this sense, teacher power is centred around their role to 'expand students' knowledge, facilitate students' activism, and encourage students' reflection on significant interactions with peers and family' (Mayo 2013, p. 266). The students in these schools were, instead, creating a new regime of truth formed by their own subjugated knowledge. Foucault (1980) states that knowledge and power are one, and that 'we are subjugated to the production of truth through power and we cannot exercise power except through the production of truth' (p. 93). These queer students worked to exercise this power by drawing on their knowledge about LGBTQI issues, language, definitions and concerns, and then sharing this knowledge with their peers and teachers. In this sense, they sought productive forms of power by opening up and disseminating subjugated understandings of sex, gender and sexuality.

Students contesting power within the queer group: the issue of pronouns

While students saw teachers in the wider school as in need of education about gender and sexuality, they also contested power relations between teachers and students in the queer groups. In each of these groups, teachers played quite different roles. At Patiki College, a health education teacher provided support to the queer group, to offer advice on ideas and provide students with a classroom and resources or permission when needed. The teacher did not always attend meetings and was very much in the background of the group meetings she did attend. The group was wholly run and instigated by the senior (year 12 and 13; 17–18 years old) students. At Kahukura High School, however, the group was very much facilitated by the school counsellor, Magdalena. There were various power struggles in the group between the students' ideas and intentions for group meetings, and Magdalena's. Here we focus on the naming of pronouns as a site for students to (again) position themselves as more knowledgeable.

Several students in the group at Kahukura wanted to begin each meeting with 'a round' of names and pronouns. This involved each student naming themselves and their preferred gender pronoun in turn (he, she, them…). Magdalena – the counsellor and group facilitator – had initially resisted this and, because she actively facilitated the group, she stopped this from happening in the earlier parts of 2016. She explained that she found the naming of pronouns confronting for students and felt that rejecting this practice was 'protecting' the transgender, non-binary and non-gender conforming students (from having to choose a particular pronoun and thus a gender identity). This is consistent with the notion of 'risky truth telling' in Foucauldian thinking (Mayo 2017) whereby parrhesia (truth telling) is used to name one's own truth (even if it is risky to do so). Magdalena, however, also stated that naming pronouns conflicted with her own intention to break down, rather than reinscribe, gender binaries. In an interview with Hayley, Magdalena stated, 'I don't sit comfortably with any level of binary thinking in terms of supporting students I really aim to discourage labelling binary thinking and just want to broaden language around gender and sexual identity as much as I can'.

The naming of gender pronouns is significant and can be viewed as a way to name and expose the silencing of gendered binaries. Naming the pronouns can be a way to unhinge the sex-gender-sexuality constellation (Youdell 2005), by exposing and challenging assumed connections between biological sex, gender identity and sexuality. For some students, it was also a way to publicly claim an alternative identity to that previously ascribed to them. Naming pronouns in public spaces can be a form of parrhesia (in the sense of truth telling); in situations of unequal power, where speaking one's own truth requires courage. Mayo (2017, p. 101) explains that 'Parrhesia is also an act of ethical self-formation: it requires one to make one's experience and context an object for thought and that one take responsibility for one's thinking and move into action, even if the action of speech puts one at risk'. At several points in the year, students in the Kahukura group sought to take control of the meetings and insisted that group members each introduce themselves with their preferred pronoun. This happened, in particular, when the queer groups from the two schools met together.

Students from Patiki College travelled to Kahukura one school day so that the two queer groups could meet together. The meeting focussed on Inka – one of the senior students in the Kahukura group – and her 'coming out' speech, but to start the session Tiata suggested they do a round of names and pronouns, and share one thing they like about the queer group. The students introduced themselves:

PRISHA: Hi I am Prisha and I use female pronouns and this [group] is where we can all come to and kind of just like unleash! And we always have hot cups of milo and yeah, just a really nice warm welcoming place.

TROY: I'm Troy and I use male pronouns and one of my favourite things about the Rainbow group is it is a place where everyone is genuinely friendly and you can get together and talk about stuff that you might not be comfortable with anyone else.

INKA: I'm Inka and I use she/her pronouns and it is going to sound really weird, but possibly my favourite thing about the [queer] group is being here. It is good to see, like, young members of the school community, you know, like finding out about this stuff and being ok with who you are because that is not really something that I had, so yeah good on you guys.

MANI: Hi I'm Mani and I use male pronouns and one thing I mean I like everything about the [queer] group, but something I really enjoy is I feel really safe here and that no one is judging people…

IRA: Hi I'm Ira and I use female pronouns and this group makes me happy…

SARI: I'm Sari and I use any pronouns and my favourite thing about the [queer] group is that it is better than sitting in the library.

MEERA: Hi I'm Meera and I use female pronouns and my favourite part about [the queer group] is that it is a great learning platform and you can really educate yourself on the LGBTQ community and then spread it further.…

TIATA: I'm Tiata, 'she' and 'they', and what I like about this group is it is an open place to be yourself and you can have great opportunities to do things…

The students continued to introduce themselves and name their preferred pronouns.

Pronouns are significant because they relate to what constitutes an 'intelligible subject' (Butler 2005). One of Butler's primary political tasks was to 'insist upon the extension of this legitimacy to bodies that have been regarded as false, unreal, and unintelligible' (p. 24). Drawing on both Butler and Foucault, Youdell (2005) states that 'identity categories, including those of gender and sexuality, *constitute* subjects. These categorical names are central to the performative constitution of the subject who is unintelligible, if not unimaginable, without these' (Youdell 2005, p. 252). The students resisted the teacher's exclusion of pronouns but also played with the naming (or not) of pronouns to claim or reject intelligibility. During the year, some students would change their choice of pronoun (sometimes weekly) and would claim 'he', 'she', 'they', 'non-binary', 'any pronoun'. Shifting between pronouns disrupted the notion of stable gender identities and allowed students to name and claim non-normative, fluid and transgressive gender and sexual identities (Elliot 2009).

At times, the process of naming gender pronouns was not a comfortable or easy task but it served to expose taken-for-granted gender binaries and the unconscious heteronormative articulation of sex-gender-sexuality (Butler 1999, Youdell 2005). Significantly, students at Kahukura High School insisted on the naming of pronouns, regardless of the counsellor's attempts to avoid this practice. Foucault's notion that power is '...exercised rather than possessed' is key in this regard. He notes that 'it is not the 'privilege', acquired or preserved... but the overall effect of its strategic positions - an effect that is manifested and sometimes extended by the position of those who are dominated' (Foucault 1995, pp. 26–27). We are not then suggesting that students were overcoming all forms of marginality, and the general silencing of queer identities in schools. On the contrary, other aspects of these same studies – Hayley's study in particular – demonstrate how schools remain difficult spaces for queer students (see McGlashan and Fitzpatrick, 2018 for a discussion of these issues). But, needless to say, the fact that queer groups also gather for support and 'safe space' speaks volumes about the schooling experiences of their members more generally.

Mayo (2017) argues though that 'Subjectivity doesn't proceed linearly and it may be better to imagine in different registers and relationships as intersecting articulations. The process is not a certain one and instead a complex constellation of feelings and relational connections to one another and missed connections as well' (p. 47). For us this highlights both the importance of attending to the kinds of moments we have drawn attention to in this chapter, moments when LGBTQI students reimagine themselves as the experts in schools, but it is also a reminder to keep such moments in perspective, because subjectivities are constantly under development, and wider school contexts – including cultures of exclusion – are powerful. Nevertheless, these students are making significant connections between themselves as queer students, as experts who are more educated than their teachers and as subjects who are able to insist on practices that are meaningful to them.

Conclusion

The young people in our two studies were engaged in imagining schools and themselves in a wholly different fashion to the dominant view of young people as irresponsible, underdeveloped brains in need of protection. These teenagers have instead reflected on some of the key issues in their schools and come to the conclusion that homophobic practices are based on ignorance, in particular, the ignorance of teachers. They assumed then that, if teachers were better informed, then things might be different. This is interesting in light of a wealth of research exploring not only adolescence but also power relations in schools.

In the context of this book, research on gender, sex and sexuality power relations suggests that young people tend to be frustrated with a lack of meaningful sex education in schools (Allen 2005, 2007a, 2007b) and that sexuality, and youth views are largely silenced. In the case of LGBTQI students, a great deal of research explores how such young people are marginalised and excluded in school contexts (Ferfolja 2008, Kosciw et al. 2012, Mayo 2014). How the queer youth in our two ethnographic studies conceptualised themselves in relation to power then is, perhaps, quite radical, and not in a way commensurate with traditional critical pedagogical work. While critical pedagogical approaches to schooling (a body of work we are both deeply sympathetic to) assume that resistance is both an element of cultural subjugation, and a means to overcome oppressive practice and silencing, it seems to us that these young people have moved beyond a politics of resistance, towards a position of 'expertise' within their schools.

This is significant for several reasons. First, it suggests that teenagers may know more about some things than teachers do; second, that knowledge is powerful and that discrimination is based in ignorance; third, that young people in schools can impact the environments they find unhelpful and unsupportive by educating their teachers and insisting about the practices they find meaningful. What is especially interesting about the young people we talked to is that, despite what we know about schools continuing to be unsafe spaces for queer youth, they do not see themselves as victims. They see themselves as holding knowledge that is powerful, and they feel able (at times at least) to go about educating teachers in the wider school and taking control of practices in their queer groups. This is not to claim that 'knowing' will mean the end of discrimination in schools, but it is to suggest that these young people see hope in educative practices, and that they see themselves as more knowledgeable than their teachers.

References

Allen, L., 2005. 'Say Everything': Exploring Young People's Suggestions for Improving Sexuality Education. *Sex Education*, 5 (4), 389–404.

Allen, L., 2007a. Denying the Sexual Subject: Schools' Regulation of Student Sexuality. *British Educational Research Journal*, 33 (2), 221–234.

Allen, L., 2007b. Doing 'It' Differently: Relinquishing the Disease and Pregnancy Prevention Focus in Sexuality Education. *British Journal of Sociology of Education*, 28 (5), 575–588.

Allen, L., 2015. Picturing Queer at School. *Journal of LGBTQ Youth*, 12 (4), 367–384.

Blackburn, M. V., 2007. The Experiencing, Negotiation, Breaking, and Remaking of Gender Rules and Regulations by Queer Youth. *Journal of Gay & Lesbian Issues in Education*, 4 (2), 33–54.

Butler, J., 1999. *Gender Trouble: Feminism and the Subversion of Identity*. London: Routledge.

Butler, J., 2005. Bodies that Matter. In: M. Fraser and M. Greco, eds. *The Body: A Reader*. London: Routledge, 62–65.

Carspecken, P., 1996. *Critical Ethnography in Educational Research: A Theoretical and Practical Guide*. New York, NY: Routledge.

Chesir-Teran, D. N. and Hughes, D. L., 2009. Heterosexism in High School and Victimization among Lesbian, Gay, Bisexual, and Questioning Students. *Journal of Youth and Adolescence*, 38, 963–975.

Clandinin, D. J. and Connelly, F. M., 2000. *Narrative Inquiry: Experience and Story in Qualitative Research*. San Francisco, CA: Jossey-Bass.

D'Augelli, A. R. 1998. Developmental Implications of Victimization of Lesbian, Gay, and Bisexual Youths. In: G. Herek, ed. *Stigma and Sexual Orientation: Understanding Prejudice against Lesbians, Gay Men, and Bisexuals*. Thousand Oaks, CA: SAGE, 187–210.

D'Augelli, A. R., Pilkington, N. W., and Hershberger, S. L., 2002. Incidence and Mental Health Impact of Sexual Orientation Victimization of Lesbian, Gay, and Bisexual Youths in High School. *School Psychology Quarterly*, 17, 148–167.

Elliot, P., 2009. Engaging Trans Debates on Gender Variance: A Feminist Analysis. *Sexualities*, 12 (1), 5–32.

Evans, J. and Davies, B., 2004. Sociology and Health in a Risk Society. In: J. Evans, B. Davies, and J. Wright, eds. *Body Knowledge and Control: Studies in the Sociology of Physical Education and Health*. London: Routledge, 35–51.

Ferfolja, T., 2008. Discourses that Silence: Teachers and Anti-lesbian Harassment. *Discourse: Studies in the Cultural Politics of Education*, 29 (1), 107–119.

Fitzpatrick, K., 2011. Stop Playing Up! Physical Education, Racialisation and Resistance. *Ethnography*, 12 (2), 174–197.

Fitzpatrick, K., 2013. *Critical Pedagogy, Physical Education and Urban Schooling*. New York, NY: Peter Lang.

Fitzpatrick, K. and May, S., 2015. Doing Critical Educational Ethnography with Bourdieu. In: M. Murphy and C. Costa, eds. *Theory as Method in Research: On Bourdieu, Education and Society*. London: Routledge, 101–114.

Fitzpatrick, K. and Tinning, R., eds., 2014. *Health Education: Critical Perspectives*. London: Routledge.

Foucault, M. 1980. *Power/Knowledge: Selected Interviews and Other Writings, 1972–1977*. New York, NY: Pantheon Books.

Foucault, M. 1995. *Discipline and Punish. The Birth of the Prison*. New York, NY: Random House.

Frohard-Dourlent, H., 2016. I Don't Care What's Under Your Clothes': The Discursive Positioning of Educators Working with Trans and Gender-nonconforming Students. *Sex Education*, 16 (1), 63–67.

Gard, M. and Pluim, C., 2014. *Schools and Public Health: Past, Present, Future*. Lanham, MD: Lexington Books.

Gordon, H. A., 2007. Allies Within and Without: How Adolescent Activists Conceptualize Ageism and Navigate Adult Power in Youth Social Movements. *Journal of Contemporary Ethnography*, 36 (6), 631–668.

Halsey, A., et al., eds., 1997. *Education, Culture, Economy and Society*. New York, NY: Oxford University Press.

Jensen, F. E. and Nutt, A. E., 2015. *The Teenage Brain: A Neuroscientists Survival Guide to Raising Adolescents and Young Adults*. New York, NY: Harper Collins.

Kincheloe, J., 2007. City Kids - Not the Kind of Students You'd Want to Teach. In: J. Kincheloe and K. Hayes, eds. *Teaching City Kids: Understanding and Appreciating Them*. New York, NY: Peter Lang, 3–38.

Kincheloe, J., 2008. *Critical Pedagogy Primer*. New York, NY: Peter Lang.

Kosciw, J. G., et al., 2012. *The 2011 National School Climate Survey: The Experiences of Lesbian, Gay, Bisexual and Transgender Youth in Our Nation's Schools*. New York, NY: Gay, Lesbian, and Straight Education Network (GLSEN).

Madison, D. S., 2005. *Critical Ethnography: Method, Ethics, and Performance*. Thousand Oaks, CA: Sage.

Madison, D. S., 2012. *Critical Ethnography: Method, Ethics, and Performance* (2nd ed.). Thousand Oaks, CA: Sage.

Mayo, C., 2009. The Tolerance that Dare Not Speak Its Name. In: A. Darder, M. P. Baltodano, and R. D. Torres, eds. *The Critical Pedagogy Reader* (2nd ed.). New York, NY: Routledge, 262–273.

Mayo, C., 2014. *LGBTQ Youth and Education: Policies and Practices*. New York, NY: Teachers College Press.

Mayo, C., 2017. *Gay-Straight Alliances and Associations among Youth in Schools*. New York, NY: Palgrave Macmillan.

Mayo Jr., J. B., 2013. Critical Pedagogy Enacted in the Gay-Straight Alliance: New Possibilities for a Third Space in Teacher Development. *Educational Researcher*, 42 (5), 266–275.

McGlashan, H. and Fitzpatrick, K., 2017. LGBTQ Youth, Activism, and School: Challenging Sexuality and Gender Norms. *Health Education Journal*, 117 (5), 485–497.

McGlashan, H. and Fitzpatrick, K., 2018. 'I Use Any Pronouns and I'm Questioning Everything Else': Transgender Youth and the Issue of Gender Pronouns. *Sex Education*, 18 (3), 239–252.

Moshman, D., 2011. Adolescents Are Young Adults, Not Immature Brains. *Applied Developmental Science*, 15 (4), 171–174.

Noblit, G. W., Flores, S. Y., and Murillo, E., Jr, eds., 2004. *Postcritical Ethnography: Reinscribing Critique*. Cresskill, NJ: Hampton Press.

Quinlivan, K., 2013. The Methodological Im/possibilities of Researching Sexuality Education in Schools: Working Queer Conundrums. *Sex Education*, 13 (1), 56–69.

Quinlivan, K., 2015. Acknowledging and Working Doublebinds: The Im/possible Work of a High School Queer/Straight Alliance. In: A. Gunn and A. Smith, eds. *Sexual Cultures in Aotearoa/New Zealand Education*. Dunedin: Otago University Press.

Savin-Williams, R., 1994. Verbal and Physical Abuse as Stressors in the Lives of Lesbian, Gay Male and Bisexual Youths: Associations with School Problems, Running Away, Substance Abuse, Prostitution and Suicide. *Journal of Consulting and Clinical Psychology*, 62 (2), 261–269.

Savin-Williams, R., 2005. *The New Gay Teenager*. Cambridge, MA: Harvard University Press.

Steinberg, S., 2007. Preface: Where are We Now? In: P. McLaren and J. Kincheloe, eds. *Critical Pedagogy: Where Are We Now?* New York, NY: Peter Lang, ix–x.

Talburt, S. and Rasmussen, M. L., 2010. 'After Queer' Tendencies in Queer Research. *Journal of Qualitative Studies in Education*, 23 (1), 1–14.

Thomas, J., 1993. *Doing Critical Ethnography*. Newbury Park, CA: SAGE.

Youdell, D., 2005. Sex-Gender-Sexuality: How Sex, Gender and Sexuality Constellations are Constituted in Secondary Schools. *Gender and Education*, 17 (3), 249–270.

Youdell, D., 2011. *School Trouble: Identity, Power and Politics in Education*. London: Routledge.

Chapter 18

The proliferation of gender and sexual identities, categories and labels among young people

Emergent taxonomies

Rob Cover

Introduction

Recently, we have witnessed the popular diversification of sexual identity labels emerging through young people's interactive engagement online in a search for a more descriptive and more inclusive language to represent sexual identity, desire, behaviour, attractions and relationships. A number of online sites associated with young adults such as *Tumblr*'s social justice network and dating sites that include *OkCupid* and queer *Facebook* groups inhabited often by younger persons have been active in developing new labels for sexual identities that more specifically describe sexual interest and taste, gender articulations and attractions (Bell 2013). An Australian-based *Facebook* group for young queer people, for example, requests that on joining, members list their preferred 'gender pronouns, gender identity and sexual preferences' to ensure, as one user described it, 'accurate and ethical conversations'. Unlike the assumptions of masculine/feminine and straight/lesbian, gay, bisexual and transgender (LGBT) that might be recognised in looking at a user's name, image or other details, these self-descriptions present a very broad set of new terminologies, such as 'non-binary, panromantic and boysexual' or 'male, genderqueer, asexual'.

While some rejection of older hetero/homo dichotomies occurs in online queer political and social groupings, this proliferation of new, complex schemata of sexuality and gender labels is primarily notable in online, interactive communication sites used by younger persons internationally under the age of 25. These present a new, interesting, unexpected and valuable challenge to heteronormative and homonormative regimentary categorisations of masculine/feminine and heterosexual/homosexual, both of which rely on binary exclusions, notions of fixed identity across time and a prohibition on 'grey areas', changeability and complexity. What has emerged in the array of dozens of new gender and sexuality descriptors and categories is a new 'taxonomy' or 'lexicon' of gender and sexual identity that provides new opportunities for young people to articulate their gendered and sexual selves in terms of new ways of belonging and new forms of citizenship.

This digital emergence is not, of course, the first challenge to binary, essentialist models of sexuality and gender. A number of such challenges were articulated in the second half of the twentieth century from within psychoanalytic, Marcusean, post-structuralist perspectives as well as in the activism of various brands of Gay Liberation from the 1970s. A critique of the narrow, binary and essentialist models of gender and sexuality that dominated in academic dialogue in the 1990s was that of queer theory, which used post-structuralist approaches to demystify, deconstruct and de-essentialise the logic of masculine/feminine and hetero/homo binaries, and the ways in which binaries underlie texts, practices, behaviours and language. Although queer theory was principally limited to academic and fringe activist discourses and had little immediate impact on everyday gender and sexual lives or on the approaches taken by LGBT 'rights based' political groups across much of the globe, it is tempting to ask if the new taxonomy of gender and sexuality that overcomes binaries by the proliferation of dozens of new gender/sexual categories is the fruition of that early work. Arguably, there are many similarities between queer theory and the new labels in their objective to overcome narrow identity categories and exclusions. However, the new taxonomy of gender and sexual identities has different origins and its practices are more wedded to the continuation (and proliferation) of identity categories than queer theory's deconstruction. Indeed, the new language emerges from a more accessible, popular and populist logic that, on the one hand, seeks to incorporate diverse behaviours, sexualities and genders but, on the other, relies on the more recognisable and accessible language of liberal-humanist identity categories and citizenship.

Rather than the more 'fluid', deconstructionist and anti-foundationalist approach advocated by 1990s queer theory, the new taxonomy maintains 'categories of identity' at the centre of its logic. The new terminology might, then, be understood as instances of 'micro-minoritisation', whereby the tools of contemporary digital identifications are deployed to produce ever-more-nuanced but ever-more-surveiled, policed, disciplined and regimented sexual identity and gender categories. In other words, this framing of gender and sexual subjectivity allows us to ask if new, broader descriptions of sexuality are just as *regulatory* as the hetero/homo binary distinction was, and might open problematic pathways to new kinds of normativisation and discipline.

New categories and labels of sexual identity

Emerging first in the alternative communities that inhabit parts of the *Tumblr* social networking sites, the past half-decade has seen a substantial proliferation of sexual and gender identities that are responses to a perceived need among sometimes vulnerable younger persons to articulate more accurate, encompassing, and inclusive sexualities and genders (Cover 2012). Many non-heterosexual youth are not able to easily identify with the cultural norms, stereotypes, practices and communities of LGBT cultures, sometimes due to the ways in which these have excluded those who do not fit neatly within racial, gender or neo-liberal consumerist norms (Cover 2013). Other persons do not see themselves 'fitting in' with the twentieth- and early twenty-first-century simplistic dichotomies of gender (masculine/feminine and male/female binaries) and sexuality (hetero/ homo binary with the bi- of bisexuality straddling and thereby reinforcing both sides). With considerable press attention, *Facebook* announced in 2013 that it had altered its gender and pronoun profile options to encompass up to 50 different genders in order to be inclusive to transgender, intersex and gender-diverse persons (Molloy 2014). Soon after, the North American online dating, friendship and social networking site *OkCupid* published in late 2014 an online list of multiple new 'genders' and 'sexual orientations' (Kellaway 2014). The *OkCupid* list of diverse sexual orientations and genders was partly editorial and partly crowdsourced from user comments and contributions, including from younger people. *OkCupid* offers the following lists of new sexual and gender identity categories or labels:

> **Genders**: Agender, Androgynous, Bigender, Cis Man, Cis Woman, Genderfluid, Genderqueer, Gender Nonconforming, Hijra, Intersex, Man, Non-binary, Pangender, Transfeminine, Transgender, Trans Man, Trans-masculine, Transsexual, Trans Woman, Two Spirit, Woman, Demigirl and Neutrois.
>
> (www.okcupid.com/deep-end/identity/more-genders)

> **Sexual Orientations**: Asexual, Bisexual, Demisexual, Gay, Homoflexible, Heteroflexible, Lesbian, Pansexual, Queer, Questioning, Sapiosexual, Straight, Omnisexual.
>
> (www.okcupid.com/deep-end/identity/more-orientations)

Other sites, including pages on *Tumblr* and *YouTube* explanatory videos, as well as sites critical of the emerging language, such as *Age of Shitlords*, have published lists and definitions, in one case as many as 80 categories or labels of sexuality, among which the more traditional terms heterosexuality and homosexuality are only two. Some queer political, social and support-based *Facebook* queer youth groups require participants to identify their genders and sexualities according to lists similar to these at the time of introducing themselves and/or commenting or posting on the site; and in some cases participants of the *Facebook* groups have actively verified (or disavowed) users' posts by examining their prior posts on their own *Facebook* pages.

Just as more traditional non-heterosexual identities such as gay or lesbian have been articulated in the context of resistance to traditional sexuality and gender labelling practices, and as the term queer emerged in the 1990s in opposition to bourgeois stereotyping of lesbian/gay (Buchbinder 1997, p. 150), these new categories are significant in that they have been produced by and within an online youth culture through younger persons debating and engaging in the interactive co-creation of sexual label information, much of which operates in resistance to both older generational definitions. In that context, they are the product of a cultural formation of practices of generationalism which relies usually on an arbitrary set of age and birthdate distinctions (Davis 1997, pp. 1–20), and produces a breakdown of the consensus on (sexual) knowledge between 'adult' and 'youth' (Hebdige 1979, p. 17).

Generations, however, are also a way of making sense of shifts in cultural practices – in this case, practices of understanding, articulating, and inhabiting sexualities and genders – over time. The fact that these practices have sped up such that sexual identity categories that remained culturally sensible for over a century now shift within decades (from, for example, 'queer' to a broader set of sexual identity labels) is more complex and requires further theorisation. At least one element of distinction involves the capabilities of digital communication, networking and the Internet, which play a significant role in connecting disaffected persons to each other in ways that give access to and produce new experiential knowledge (Byron 2015, p. 324). According to the critic Lenore Bell (2013), the fact that these new identity labels emerged first on *Tumblr* may be due to the fact that its unique format is more removed from the everyday real-life social networks than sites such as *Facebook*. *Tumblr's* network of friends is typically less likely to be made up of those known in geographic, physical senses and more through bringing together those who are 'connected by interests, and are not bound by personal interactions in real life… tailored to the individual reader's interests' (p. 33).

Just as the older system of sexual and gender categorisations might have been intensely felt as a set of sensations transcribed into emotion, attraction and desire (Papacharissi 2015, p. 21), these new categories can also be understood as deeply felt attachments and intensities by those who articulate their sexual and gender identities within these contexts. That is, they are not theatrics of taste, style or nuance (e.g., sapiosexual aromantic demiboy) overlaid on a categorical real (e.g., unattached lesbian woman). The fact that these labels and categories have not, in all cases, emerged through civil rights-style claims to recognition does not necessarily suggest that they are not 'emotionally fraught and liable to touch on deep feelings and desires', as Doreen Massey (2004, p. 6) has argued about spatial and geographically based identities and identifications. Indeed, there is a deeply felt attachment to these categories, labels or identities by those who feel they embody them – from a queer theory perspective, this is no different from acknowledging that although the category of 'woman' might be from a post-structuralist perspective a linguistic trope, a norm and a fiction but that powerful cultural demands require a deep-seated belief in it as a category with which to identify and that this identification is very meaningful for a very large number of people (Butler 1990, p. 136).

Indeed, where the nineteenth-century pathologisation of same-sex sexual attraction and behaviour-produced identity, and where twentieth-century formations of communities, rights discourses and multicultural inclusion operated as a response, a twenty-first-century framework of identity labels emerges through multiple claims to sexual citizenship. Arguably, these cultural practices actively encapsulate the proliferation of sexual identity labels in ways that appear to encourage agentic self-definition in terms of personal and collective identities built on multifarious gender and sexual attributes in order to claim recognition, rights and respect (Weeks 1998, p. 36). These new practices of sexual citizenship may *appear* to challenge the dominance of the hetero/homo binary as a parallel manifestation of the same cultural challenges to the categorisation of subjects into heterosexual and homosexual that emerged with queer practices of the 1990s. In queer theory, criticism of sexual identity categories began as a critique of the cultural practices of naming, labelling and categorising, arguing for the value of looking at alternative ways of thinking about sexuality not based on orientations towards a gendered object. For example, Eve Sedgwick suggested in her seminal *Epistemology of the Closet* (1990) that certain

> 'dimensions of sexuality, however, distinguish object-choice quite differently (e.g., human/animal, adult/child, singular/plural, autoerotic/alloerotic) or are not even about object choice (e.g., orgasmic/nonorgasmic, noncommercial/commercial, using bodies only/using manufactured objects, in private/in public, spontaneous/scripted)'
>
> (p. 35)

In other words, the foundationalist logic of sexualities built on the idea of a trajectory from one, stabilised gendered subject to another stabilised gendered object as a normative description of sex, desire and attraction is – in a post-structuralist world of polysemic meaning and unstable signification – no more sensible than any other way in which to categorise sexuality without gender. The new, emerging taxonomy is, in this respect, just as legitimate as any alternative way by which to understand gender and sexuality, and operates as one new 'truth' that may replace older, more familiar 'truths' about gender and sexual selfhood at both cultural and personal levels.

Understanding emergence

Regardless of the extent to which there is no singular, 'true' logic of gender and sexual identity, these new taxonomies have considerable significance for youth health, education, belonging and citizenship, particularly as this new language or lexicon becomes more popular among younger people and newer generations of sexual and gendered subjects. It is, therefore, important to ask how a new set of gender and sexual labels emerges, the conditions that make this emergence possible, and what this might mean for older logics, languages and lexicons of identity.

One useful way forward may be to conceive of the new taxonomy as the emergence of a new 'structure of feeling', in Raymond Williams's culturalist terminology, which operates as a way to describe the public consciousness of a particular historical moment in regard to a particular, much-discussed topic of gender and sexuality. It is pertinent here to pay attention to Williams's (1977) distinctions between the residual, the dominant and the emergent, whereby all are part of the broad structure of feeling of a culture but function in significantly different ways (pp. 122–125). Indeed, it might be argued that homophobic and über-heteronormative accounts of sexuality which claim that the only 'true' sexuality is heterosexual is, in contemporary Western cultures, now a residual cultural practice, formed in the past, active in the cultural process today through a range of debates, public discussions and political struggles but no longer part of the dominant structure. The residual is thereby part of the *process* of debate, but relegated to being a set of views that have limited relevance on the ways of making sense of sexual citizenship and belonging today. For example, openly homophobic attitudes, gay-bashing or ridicule using effeminate stereotypes of gay men or butch stereotypes of lesbian women may appear in the public sphere but are themselves ridiculed in favour of dominant liberal norms.

The dominant structure, in contrast, presents a broadly liberalist account of LGBT identities that actively tolerates lesbian, gay and bisexual identities, stereotypes, cultures, communities and practices. The dominant liberal perspective is actively critiqued by, for example, queer theory and queer radical perspectives for its reliance on categorisation, consumerism, rights-based discourse, separate of public and private, but it remains the most significant way in which people give meaning to sexuality and gender diversity and recognise 'proper' ways of relating to each other.

Both the residual and the dominant differ from the emergent, which Williams described as being marked by new practices that become apparent not as processes wholly isolated and alien from the dominant but that produce new configurations of knowledge, meanings, values, practices and relationships. The dominant may respond to the emergent through incorporation or exclusion (p. 123), or the emergent may come to replace the dominant over time. It is thus possible to understand the new taxonomy of sexual identities as emergent, produced by young people in ways that actively challenge dominant understandings but which do not necessarily work outside the underlying notions of identity coherence and belonging that have operated within the dominant. That is, the new approach retains the prior framework of seeking to manage labels and categories of sexuality, only now through more complex tabulation and taxonomies of possibilities. But this emergent schemata materialises in ways that are to some extent at-odds with the more simplistic identity categories of the dominant cultural formation of liberal-tolerance.

As with many cultural emergences, the new taxonomy suffers from ridicule, which is a mechanism used by dominant perspectives to marginalise the emergent. For example, mocking a so-called 'alphabet soup' as the LGBTQ+ acronym struggles to incorporate a greater number of letters is a common response in discussions of the new labels in contrast to the 'normality' of the dominant language (Bell 2016, Stokes 2016). The emerging language is also often responded to with bewilderment from older online participants less familiar with the language of new sexualities and genders. For example, as one user of a city-based queer *Facebook* group put it in relation to a conversation about correct usage of new sexuality labels: 'I'm learning so much from this group. There's so much I'm ignorant of; lets

[sic] just say thank fuck for Google and Wikipedia'. Some public commentators argue that some of the new terms in the *OkCupid* pantheon of labels are pretentious, illegitimate or fail to form the basis of a meaningful real-world community outside of online sites and networked memes (Allen 2015). Others have pointed to arguments that some of the more amorphous and non-gender-fixed terms are really just new descriptions of bisexuality (Kort 2016), while the most extreme rejections of these terms argue that this expansion leads to sexual orientations trajected towards non-human subjects, inanimate objects or dead persons (e.g., https://answers.yahoo.com/question/index?qid=20071110210521AAMm4Mc).

Notable among those who have actively articulated concerns around emergent sexualities is Lenore Bell (2013), who is suspicious of the authenticity of the claims to complex sexual subjectivities made in queer social justice settings on *Tumblr*:

> A typical social justice queer blog's author will introduce themselves with a descriptive list on their homepage or 'about me' page. Here is an example of what one could typically find: "Sp-arkle-king, asexual-faggot, white-boy dyke, 23 femmboyant, Sagittarius, Masshole… My pronouns are varied. My gender is sometimes… The fact that some of these identities appear to conflict (i.e. 'king', 'dyke', 'femmboyant', 'asexual') is meant to contribute to the image that a deeply original and sincere queer personality is at work.
>
> (p. 34)

Bell's suspicion can be read as being centred on whether or not these identity labels presented in their complexity and newness are authentic and felt attachments and, perhaps, whether they are a kind of pretentious theatrics in which younger people attempt to be 'more unique' (or more interesting) than others.

Questioning the authenticity of an emergent language is, alongside ridicule and bafflement a common response to dismiss that which is emerging. Bell, however, is concerned here with the way in which the new lexicon of sexuality and gender emerges in online settings such as *Tumblr*, arguing that this is a wholly distinct setting from both an embodied 'real life' and from the kinds of social networking that tend to be more representative of 'real life' narratives such as *Facebook* and *Twitter* (pp. 33–34). Problematic here is that Bell deploys a real/virtual binary in order to critique the authenticity of the new taxonomy, *as if* sexualities that are more commonly articulated vocally, bodily and in face-to-face contexts are somehow 'more real' or 'more authentic' than others. Distinguishing between the real and the virtual is to draw on what is now a defunct dichotomy that has less relevance in determining identity play than it might have done in the text-based Web 1.0 internet and chat rooms of the 1990s (Cover 2016).

While Bell and other critics do not take emergent sexual identities as 'serious' expressions of self, what matters is that they *are* deeply felt attachments to new categories or labels of sexual subjectivity. For example, a contributor to *OkCupid's* identity spectrum definition for 'demisexual' (an orientation for 'a person who does not experience sexual attraction unless they form a strong emotional connection with someone', with demi- referring to 'halfway between' sexual and asexual) points to his/her identity through evoking its 'truth' as a kernel of selfhood governing practices of desire and attraction: 'I have to have a connection with you in order to be aroused. This is generally true for me…I rarely just see someone and want to fuck them'. Attachments to these identity labels are no less authentic than the attachments felt by older and contemporary generations to the then dominant categories of sexual selfhood that were, themselves, just as much historical fabrications as the new categories. To view a new, emergent logic or language as less authentic than that which is represented within the dominant is to unethically disavow the meaningfulness of the logic or language to a younger generation who find it represents their gender or sexual lives in ways better than the old regime.

The cultural production of new sexualities

While digital media has enabled the production of new labels for sexuality and gender, it is not necessarily helpful to understand this media as the 'source' or 'cause' of new gender and sexuality labels; rather, it has provided the conditions for the co-creative and networked capacities for groups of young people to develop collaboratively new frameworks for discussing, articulating, performing and feeling sexual subjectivity. It is important to ask what might be the cultural conditions that prompt the contemporary emergence of new sexual subjectivities, since these arise neither by accident nor by deliberate design but, as with all cultural shifts, through positionings and tensions between historical continuities and ruptures. In this context, I want to discuss two factors which may be considered to be among cultural structures, norms, and disciplinary and biopolitical circumstances that enable the new production of altered sexual subjectivities: (a) the neo-liberal framework through which categories of citizenship are 'productively consumed' rather than articulated and (b) the culture of authenticity and the emergence of greater distinctiveness of categories in light of the breakdown of more simplistic norms. Together, these two 'responses' to the cultural conditions of the dominant that have driven the emergence of the new taxonomy of gender and sexuality labels might be understood in terms of populism. That is, this particular formation of 'micro-minority' gender and sexual citizenship is grounded in a populist language that seeks to solidify identity and rejects the 'expert' or 'academic' queer theoretical arguments for contingency, fluidity, temporality and anti-essentialism that are arguably too complex for everyday language and make little sense within broader, more established frameworks of everyday life such as consumerism and authenticity – both of which are less easily undone.

Neoliberalism

Consumption and consumerism increasingly play a role in the general shift in the construction of identity and the performance of identity categories, in contrast to a more strict, broadly felt perception of 'inner authenticity' or belonging centred on kinship ties and geographic community. Consumption is understood as the means by which subjectivity is grounded, felt and articulated in late contemporary capitalist cultures (Jameson 1985). Liberal notions of citizenship shape dominant understandings of subjectivity, often through the fixation on questions of freedom and belonging – these have conditioned one aspect of the dominant approach to social relationality and identity that continues into the emergent setting in the form of sexual citizenship. Weeks (1998) argues that sexual citizenship is reflective of a postmodern world in which the self can continually be remade. A neo-liberal framing of sexual and gender subjectivity then is one in which minorities are encouraged 'to define themselves both in terms of personal and collective identities by their sexual [and gender, diverse] attributes, and to claim recognition, rights and respect as a consequence' (p. 36). For Weeks, the notion of sexual citizenship opens up new possibilities for the self and identity by a re-characterisation of transgression as a 'constant invention and reinvention of new senses of the self' that persistently challenge dominant institutions and traditions. Such a transgression, of course, is the mimicking of transgression: it is the purchase and consumption of the affect of transgression without transgressing anything.

Through surveillance, marketing and representation, contemporary culture plays a central role in processes of normativisation and measurement (Foucault 2007, p. 63). The compulsion to do so produces a particular kind of *productive self* in the terms of neoliberalism's culture of economic measurement. In governance terms, the practices of individual subjective production, circulation and consumption serve to encourage, foster and promote neoliberalism's particular regime of truth such that it subsumes *ways of thinking in all other fields aside from the economic*. This framework includes ways of thinking about the self, subjectivity and identity, which involve 'generalizing it throughout the social body and including the whole of the social system not usually conducted through or sanctioned by monetary exchanges' (Foucault 2008, p. 243). Every social and identity activity falls under the framework of an economic rationality, including the governance of the self (p. 286). Within this framework the *homo oeconomicus* or 'economic man' is produced. This is not, for Foucault, the classical economic man who is understood to be a partner in exchange. Rather, this is a neo-liberal remodelling of the subject as that which manages itself within the bounds of the biopolitical and the economic as an *investment and* an *entrepreneur of the self* in which the production of selfhood occurs only through participation in an ever-expanding market (p. 226).

Important here, then, is the fact that for *homo oeconomicus* to produce oneself not only as a subject but as a sexual subject requires a marketplace of sexual and gender categories. In this context, a series of micro-minority sexual identities becomes available as a felt response to the contemporary neo-liberal call for 'choice': a subject seeks to produce oneself through finding and choosing the most productive way of describing/articulating sexual selfhood, where older models based on hetero/homo categorical exclusivity are unproductive in that they require intensive conversational explanatory frameworks. Labels such as 'sapiosexual' or 'agender demisexual' are not only part of the range of choice but also are productive in that they allow a potentially more efficient stereotype of sexual identity to be enunciated in a few words rather than a longer explanation of complex sexual specificity – an economisation of sexual 'explanatory' discourse. In this sense, sexual citizenship is a way of understanding the right to exist according to an articulation, affiliation or identification with a category but within the dominant neo-liberal mode. Here, a proliferation of labels of gender and sexuality are not only productive but are encouraged as a response that allows greater investment in the self as a gendered and sexual self, and in a way which helps to ensure that *all* subjects can purchase a suitable identity.

Cults of authenticity

Although neoliberal, late-capitalism and postmodern accounts of identity are often described as the antithesis of an older, residual authenticity that is now lost in favour of the *laissez-faire* production of the self through consumption (e.g., Jameson 1985), a cult of authenticity continues to govern the 'language of the language' of sexual and gender identity labels. That is, articulating identification within the new market of labels, subjects are actively produced as subjects who must articulate that identity *as if* authentic, in order to fulfil the continuing cultural demand for coherence, intelligibility and recognisability. Indeed, this dominant liberal-humanist 'truth' of selfhood remains necessary in contemporary Western culture for social participation and belonging. Authenticity is an aspect of the performance of identity – whether under the old, dominant taxonomy or the new emergent one. Judith Butler's (1997) framework for performativity argues that identities are produced through repeated and stylised acts that are recognised as an inner identity core. Performance occurs in such a way to disavow their own citation from a language that precedes the subject (pp. 9–10). This provides subjects with a sense of their own authenticity. Butler (1990) pointed out that it is possible to expose the foundational categories of sex, gender and desire as consequences of power formations, resulting in the critical knowledge that 'those identity categories… are in fact the *effects* of institutions, practices, discourses with multiple and diffuse points of origin' (p. ix). In other words, the language that constructs the categories of sex, gender, bodies and sexuality is by no means stable but changes, reacts to the 'making available' of alternative languages – such as emergent sexuality labels – and undergoes sometimes disruptive shifts in the logic on which that discourse is founded. In this case, the logic of the hetero/homo binary is replaced by a new lexicon, range or set of axes of sexuality labels and gender categories.

What remains, however, is the identity process: the fact that subjects continue to cite a category in order to produce a sexual subjectivity as part of the demand for sexual identity coherence, even though what is coherent now is not necessarily that which was recognisably coherent in the past. In this context, then, the imperative for authenticity in the light of the failure of the hetero/homo distinction to operate seamlessly for all subjects results in a cultural demand for more complex categories through which subjects can perform an identity that, illusively, appears or feels *more authentic*. For example, one teenage user of a *Tumblr* page dedicated to addressing difficulties of 'coming out' as demisexual noted the pain felt when adults disavowed the authenticity of the user's demisexuality, 'calling me "our little prude" every time I showed the real me. The other friends don't understand me being demi because I used to talk like that. and both situations are incredibly shitty'. New sexualities, then, can be understood as identifications with labels through which one can account for the anomalies of attractions that run counter to the stereotyped logic of the labels heterosexual or homosexual, even though language of identity and practices of articulation and coming out are retained. A wider range of categories answers the call for greater authenticity of gender and sexual identity.

Conclusion

If, as I have argued, the new regime of sexual categories and labels is just as regimentary, regulatory and normativising as older sexual regimes of the twentieth century, then what are the available alternatives for a more genuine diversity? It is important not to prescribe these alternatives from within contemporary frameworks of sexuality; in that respect, they may remain at least partly unknowable. As with the older regimentations of hetero/homosexuality, the new taxonomy is marked by the fact that gender as the object of desire remains *definitionally* built into each of the sexual labels or categories and thereby produces a taxonomy that is built on exclusions rather than the breadth of sexual potentialities. As Ken Plummer has remarked, there is a need to look for new stories that 'take us beyond the limiting categories of the past' (Plummer 1995, p. 160). New stories that open the field of possibilities for inclusive sexualities might rely on a post-categorisational framing of sexuality through a concept of 'fluidity', which is to hark back to one strand of Gay Liberation's proto-queer imperative for a liberation built on a 'new diversity, an acceptance of the vast possibilities of human experience' (Altman 1971, p. 115) and to make productive use of the later 1990s learnings of post-structuralist queer theory which de-authenticated all notions of categories as being 'real' (albeit still meaningful) and 'helpful' because they tended to regiment towards norms that create new kinds of exclusions. In this context, we might argue that a youth gender/sexuality lexicon based on micro-minority categorisations is an unproductive shift away from the potentialities of Gay Liberation and queer theory, because it dangerously results in greater surveillance, greater exclusion and potentially greater stabilisation of heteronormative identity regimes rather than creating possibilities for the acceptance and appreciation of contingency and diversity.

Indeed, it is important to bear in mind that there are multiple temporalities and structures of feeling at stake: an imperative for social change that overcomes both hetero/homo and micro-minority sexual categorisations on the one hand

and, on the other, a parallel framework in which exclusions from sexual normativity continue to mean unliveability and death for some young subjects (Cover 2012). A framework for a queer post-citizenship politics must disavow not only the efficacy of the hetero/homo and masculine/feminine binaries, but also the new, emergent categorisations that continue the regimentation of sexualities. However, to do so ethically, it must do so in a way which does not undo the forms of resilience, pleasure, identity, belonging, protection and citizenship produced and made available by both the dominant liberal-humanist LGBT logic and the emergent new taxonomy of multiplicities of gender and sexual identity labels.

References

Allen, S., 2015. Pretentious Is Not a Sexual Orientation. *The Daily Beast*, 18 April. Available from: www.thedailybeast.com/articles/2015/04/18/pretentious-is-not-a-sexual-orientation.html [Accessed 3 May 2016].

Altman, D., 1971. *Homosexual Oppression and Liberation*. New York: New York University Press.

Bell, L., 2013. Trigger Warnings: Sex, Lies and Social Justice Utopia on Tumblr. *Networking Knowledge: Journal of the MeCCSA Postgraduate Network*, 6 (1), 31–47. http://ojs.meccsa.org.uk/index.php/netknow/article/view/296/136 [Accessed 18 January 2016].

Bell, M., 2016. Why be LGBT when you can be LGBTIQCAPGNGFNBA? The story of an escalating acronym. *The Spectator*, 5 November. Available from: www.spectator.co.uk/2016/11/why-be-lgbt-when-you-can-be-lgbtiqcapgngfnba/ [Accessed 17 December 2017].

Buchbinder, D., 1997. *Performance Anxieties: Re-Producing Masculinity*. St. Leonards, NSW: Allen & Unwin.

Butler, J., 1990. *Gender Trouble: Feminism and the Subversion of Identity*. London and New York, NY: Routledge.

Butler, J., 1997. *The Psychic Life of Power: Theories in Subjection*. Stanford, CA: Stanford University Press.

Byron, P., 2015. Troubling Expertise: Social Media and Young People's Sexual Health. *Communication Research and Practice*, 1 (4), 322–344.

Cover, R., 2012. *Queer Youth Suicide, Culture and Identity: Unliveable Lives?* London and New York, NY: Routledge.

Cover, R., 2013. Conditions of Living: Queer Youth Suicide, Homonormative Tolerance and Relative Misery. *Journal of LGBT Youth*, 10 (4), 328–350.

Cover, R., 2016. *Digital Identities: Creating and Communicating the Online Self*. London: Elsevier.

Davis, M., 1997. *Gangland: Cultural Elites and the New Generationalism*. St. Leonards: Allen & Unwin.

Foucault, M., 2007. *Security, Territory, Population: Lectures at the Collège de France, 1977–78*, trans. G. Burchell, ed. M. Senellart. Basingstoke: Palgrave Macmillan.

Foucault, M., 2008. *The Birth of Biopolitics: Lectures at the Collège de France, 1978–79*, trans. G. Burchell, ed. Michel Senellart. Basingstoke: Palgrave Macmillan.

Hebdige, D., 1979. *Subculture: The Meaning of Style*. London: Methuen.

Jameson, F., 1985. Postmodernism and Consumer Society. In: H. Foster, ed. *Postmodern Culture*. London: Pluto Press, 111–125.

Kellaway, M., 2014. OKCupid Unveils New Options for Gender, Sexuality. *The Advocate*, 18 November. www.advocate.com/business/technology/2014/11/18/okcupid-unveils-new-options-gender-sexuality [Accessed 11 December 2014].

Kort, J., 2016. Are 'Heteroflexible' and 'Homoflexible' Shades of 'Bisexual'? *Huff Post Queer Voices*, 2 February. www.huffingtonpost.com/joe-kort-phd/are-heteroflexible-and-homoflexible-shades-of-bisexual_b_4549126.html [Accessed 8 May 2016].

Massey, D., 2004. Geographies of Responsibility. *Geografiska Annaler: Series B, Human Geography*, 86 (1), 5–18.

Molloy, P. M., 2014. Facebook Expands Gender Options for Trans and Gender-Nonconforming Users. *The Advocate*, 13 February. www.advocate.com/politics/transgender/2014/02/13/facebook-announces-expanded-gender-options-transgender-and-gender [Accessed 17 December 2014].

Papacharissi, Z., 2015. *Affective Publics: Sentiment, Technology, and Politics*. Oxford: Oxford University Press.

Plummer, K., 1995. *Telling Sexual Stories: Power, Change and Social Worlds*. London and New York, NY: Routledge.

Sedgwick, E. K., 1990. *Epistemology of the Closet*. Harmondsworth: Penguin.

Stokes, D., 2016. We Need to Move Beyond LGBT Alphabet Soup And Slurs. *HuffPost*, 8 February. www.huffingtonpost.com/dashanne-stokes/we-need-to-move-beyond-lg_b_10465840.html [Accessed 12 December 2017].

Weeks, J., 1998. The Sexual Citizen. *Theory, Culture & Society*, 15 (3–4), 35–52.

Williams, R., 1977. *Marxism and Literature*. Oxford: Oxford University Press.

Afterword

Youth and scenes of sexual citizenship

Susan Talburt

What is sexual citizenship and why, or how, does it matter to youth? We are all sexual citizens but some more obviously so than others. Attached to the nation state, citizens are subjects of rights, subject to responsibilities and subjected to regulation. In a sort of contract, the state grants rights to citizens who then have responsibilities to the collective, the nation and the future. These responsibilities, whether to work, to vote, to marry or to reproduce, render us subject to regulation. For those whose lives and actions align with the norms those regulations would enforce, the rights and responsibilities of citizenship seem and feel natural, invisible and taken-for-granted. For those whose lives and actions do not conform to appropriate forms of productivity, reproductivity and sociality, citizenship can be more fraught. Citizenship can become a site of denial, exclusion and repression. Or citizenship can be something to strive for, an ideal to attain. Being both affective and material, citizenship and non-citizenship can work as a promise or a threat.

Citizenship has always tacitly been a sexual category, but the emergence of 'new identities', usually gay and lesbian, has made it visibly so. The idea of the sexual citizen names identities, social actors and collectives that have materialised in response to exclusion and repression, revealing the state's heteronormativity as they struggle for rights. As construed in much social theory, the sexual citizen becomes such through conduct (acts), identities or relationships, which may later become the basis for rights claims (Richardson 2000). As Foucault (1990) and others have taught us, many sexual acts (and object choices) morphed into identities over the course of the late nineteenth and twentieth centuries. More recently, lesbian and gay identities' rights claims have emphasised relationships, specifically marriage. Young people's citizenship practices are implicated in these shifts.

Two decades ago, Jeffrey Weeks (1998, p. 36) described something of a dialectic in sexual politics: 'a moment of transgression, and a moment of citizenship'. Social movements articulated narratives of exclusion that brought sexual difference explicitly into public discourse and 'place[d] new demands on the wider community for the development of more responsive policies' (p. 47). A 'constant invention and reinvention' (p. 36) of individual consciousness and collective action disrupted the public sphere to make 'a claim to inclusion, the acceptance of diversity, and a recognition of and respect for alternative ways of being, to a broadening of the definition of be-longing' (p. 37). This transgressive moment, Weeks argued, enabled 'the moment of citizenship: the claim to equal protection of the law, to equal rights in employment, parenting, social status, access to welfare provision, and partnership rights, or even marriage, for same-sex couples' (p. 37). Sexuality explicitly asked to join citizenship, to make the previously personal, or private, a public matter. The vernacular and the formal entered into a relationship.

The backdrop of the constitution of the sexual citizen is to be found in multiple informal venues of affiliation, connection and belonging – the park, the bar, the rent party, the consciousness-raising group, the protest, the bedroom, and more recently, the Internet – spaces for practices of everyday life that are often incon-gruent with official citizenship. Communities of sexually minoritised subjects, or what some now call counterpublics (e.g. Warner 2002), engage in cultural and political production, offer material resources and enable actors to sustain lives. In its non-institutional meaning, sexual citizenship connotes informal practices of a subject who seeks and creates spaces to survive and, possibly, to thrive, despite an oppressive, exclusionary state and a dominant society that mark some subjects as disposable. In its institutional meaning, sexual citizenship denotes a subject who has secured some rights and recognition as legitimate. Sexual citizenship, then, is at once formal and informal, oppositional and assimilative. It is never static.

But it is not only formal citizenship that demands particular modes of doing and being. Even the communities that offer resources, a sense of freedom and transformed consciousness entail boundaries; they create duties and responsi-bilities for their members in exchange for belonging. Historically, lesbian, gay, bisexual and transgender (LGBT) communities have asked members to share an identity; adhere to that identity's norms; and participate in and circulate narratives of exclusion that confirm the need for political action, struggles for rights and particular forms of progress. But, like sexual citizenship, communities' norms, forms of belonging and boundaries are not static; rather, they are reor-ganised through actors' relations and movements across shifting sociopolitical landscapes.

The idea of sexual citizenship once named a progressively inclusionary future in which the state and society respond to sexually marginalised subjects' de-mands. With the intensification of neoliberalism, analysis of sexual citizenship opens up questions of 'the extent to which these new moments of citizenship can be understood as a process of assimilation into the mainstream, uphold-ing normative frameworks for social inclusion *or* as having a transformative potential' (Richardson 2017, p. 213). The answer to both options is probably yes. The normalisation of the sexual citizen, *or of some sexual citizens*, has taken place largely in the context of the global entrenchment of neo-liberal modes of governance.

Although neoliberalism has different nuances regionally and nationally, its reach transcends the nation state to produce newly configured 'subjects, forms of citizenship and behavior, and a new organization of the social' (Brown 2005, p. 37).

Neoliberalism infuses a market-based, individualised logic that constructs and interpellates subjects as entrepreneurial actors, responsibilised to care for themselves as they make correct choices in political, social and economic spheres with declining safety nets and supports. As neoliberalism 'erases the discrepancy between economic and moral behavior' (Brown 2005, p. 42), subjects tend to be divided into winners and losers, good and bad, who bear 'full responsibility for the consequences of his or her action no matter how severe the constraints on this action' (p. 42). In this context, citizenship can become a technology for reifying a liberal, sovereign subject who is capable of self-governance; the sexual citizen should perform worthiness through sexual respectability. As Sabsay (2012) argues, sexual citizenship entails

> a complicated process of inclusive othering [that] takes place when this new sexual respectability, that now imaginarily includes some (but not all) former sexual "others" defined by liberal European and US ideals, becomes the benchmark against which every sexual subject must be measured.
>
> (p. 611)

Cathy Cohen (2014) makes explicit the racialisation of sexual citizenship in the USA, where neoliberalism's gutting of the welfare state has depended on 'not only a policy agenda but also a set of ideological commitments and rhetorical strategies meant to create and demonize some "Other"' (p. 4). Animating white fear and animosity, 'bad citizens', such as the welfare queen, the teen mother or the sex worker, are to be regulated more than they are to be granted rights.

In recent years, the seeming culmination of sexual citizenship for lesbian and gay subjects entails a relationship claim (Richardson 2000): the symbolic recognition and material protection of same-sex marriage. Both affective and pragmatic, this relationship-based citizenship evokes what Berlant (2007) calls 'a feeling of aspirational normalcy, the desire to feel normal and to feel normalcy as a ground of dependable life, a life that does not have to keep being reinvented' (p. 281). Franke (2006) describes advocacy for same-sex marriage as challenging the privatisation of sex: 'this is a public argument of a collective nature—we want to be included in "We the People"' (p. 239). This inclusion means that 'the rights-bearing subject of the lesbigay rights movement has now become "the couple"—a We…, a certain kind of citizen-subject who becomes politically legible by and through a particular form of intimate affiliation' (p. 239). Attachment to the nation conflates recognition as a citizen-subject with 'self-governance within the couple and governance of the couple by the state' (Franke 2006, p. 246). But this self-governance, recognition and protection are not available to all. Same-sex marriage, argues Cohen (2014), 'serves to legitimize a process intent on producing a hierarchy of citizenship' (p. 8) that 'falls into a category of a racialized state project that is involved in the differential distribution of rights, that disproportionately disadvantages people who are not married, often people of color' (p. 9).

Having said this, recognition of the coupled adult sexual citizen is intimately connected to the figure of the child, who is said to need the stability and security of an idealised version of marriage:

> Sectors of our community have argued that our unmarriageability inflicts a kind of harm on our children in terms that echo the manner in which familial pathology and illegitimacy were thought to cause injury to African-American children in the Moynihan Report.
>
> (Franke 2006, p. 241)

The progressive moment of formal citizenship has recognised a homonormative couple who is aligned with a national future.

Youth as sexual citizens

Although young people may have formal citizenship status in their nations of birth, youth are transitional subjects, becoming-adults and, hence, becoming-citizens to be granted the rights. Citizen rights and responsibilities, then, are a spatio-temporal domain, something that is to be entered into later in life. Young people are to learn and practice citizenship in their families, schools, places of worship, parks, playgrounds, peer networks and civic engagement projects. As young people develop and are developed, they try on and adapt to new rights and responsibilities, sometimes succeeding and sometimes failing, making good choices and bad ones. This so-called developmental process is neither cumulative nor progressively linear, but marked by discontinuities, regressions and breakthroughs. Given that 'sex' is supposed to demarcate a dividing line between youth and adult, one could ask, What is a youthful sexual citizen? How does the state explicitly recognise youth as sexual citizens? Or, if not citizen, (potential) sexual actors? How do youth practice or exercise their sexual citizenship in their everyday lives? Questions of youth as formal sexual citizens create a blurry space of acts, identities, affects, policies and practices whose outlines can only be inferred by attending to state and institutional practices of regulating the age of consent, protecting their innocence or educating youth sexually, as well as by tracing authorities' fraught and often spectacularised prosecutions related to sexting, cyberbullying, sexual assault and statutory rape.

Young people share the space of neoliberalism with adults, but their individualisation; responsibilisation; and subjection to pressures to self-brand, self-monitor and self-create are differently inflected. They do so under the surveillant gaze of parents, schoolteachers, religious communities and so on, whose job is to keep youth on track as they transition properly to adult citizenship in an orderly, timely manner. Protectionist discourses and practices, whether keeping young people safe from paedophiles, sex talk or the Internet – and, more recently, each other – intersect and collide with calls for youth to be good sexual decision makers and to prepare for productive futures as flexible, self-realising citizen-workers in a global economic context of austerity and precarity.

Given that the state is an ambiguous site of citizenship that regulates more than it grants rights to youth, it is crucial to examine multiple sites of living and subject formation as scenes of citizenship, sexual and otherwise. The chapters in this volume depict numerous venues of citizenship, some of which are enacted in contexts of 'vertical' relations (to the state, work authorities, schools, teachers) and others that represent more 'horizontal' attachments (friends, lovers, schoolmates, Internet groups), although in young people's lives, the vertical and the horizontal are always mutually implicated. Scenes of world-building, community-making and identity exploration are interstitial, the work of bricoleurs who have different relationships to the private/public dichotomy at the heart of sexual citizenship than those of adults.

Public space and the public sphere are fundamentally adult spaces to which youth have less, or differential, access (as in the surveillance of the city park or the shopping mall). Following Mary Gray's (2009) work with rural youth, it might be more appropriate to think of young people's creations of connections, affiliations and belongings – their informal practices of citizenship – as 'boundary publics' located at the edges of, outside of, and sometimes in the public sphere. In contrast to more visible and semi-institutionalised adult counterpublics, boundary publics are less spaces than they are moments of 'iterative, ephemeral experiences of belonging that circulate across the outskirts and through the center(s) of a more recognized and validated public sphere' (Gray 2009, pp. 92–93). Given their lack of capital, authority and resources, youth may momentarily 'hold a space' in their everyday citizenship practices as they borrow, re-mix, poach and transform spaces designed for other purposes, such as church parking lots, commercial spaces, non-profits or 'new media' (see Gray 2009, pp. 92–118). Seemingly purposeless hanging out or purposeful political projects can be scenes of learning, pleasure, disruption or the reification of old and new norms as young people follow and deviate from predictable trajectories of becoming-citizen.

Scenes of youth sexual citizenship

Given that youth can only be tenuously considered sexual citizens, this book intervenes in a largely adult-oriented body of scholarship, asking readers to consider the nature of the resources, discourses and spaces available to young people; the hopes and fears of the institutions that would form young sexual citizens; and shifting sociopolitical landscapes in which desires and practices are formed and enacted. The collection's section titles are suggestive of a range of tangible spaces, 'Kinship', 'Schooling and Education', 'Communication Technologies', which are both tangible spaces and areas of concern, just as are the sections 'Well-being and Health', 'Work' and 'Sex and Relationships'. These spaces and concerns are never wholly formal or informal, public or private, but are porous, as youth, their families, teachers, sex education curriculum writers and others carry their knowledge and practices across domains.

The chapters in this collection demonstrate the ambivalent nature of sexual citizenship, in which formal rights, recognition and protection offer resources for action, and informal spheres are circulating new discourses, but dominant ideas of national futures and neo-liberal governance align to cultivate productive hetero- and now homonormative citizens. Before discussing this ambivalence, let me pause on three chapters that offer helpful questionings of citizenship and rights discourses that are echoed in various ways across the collection. First, Bredström and Bolander analyse the fumblings of liberalism's well-intentioned efforts to refuse narrow nationalisms through anti-racist sex education that emphasises individual freedom of choice by erasing cultural difference. They show how this move to tolerance falls into a universalising human rights discourse whose elision of difference serves 'neo-assimilatory' functions, offering a caution regarding the power of normalisation to create good and bad citizens. Next, Gutierrez-Maldonado critiques sexual citizenship's disembodiment by demonstrating how rights to protection and inclusion fail subjects who are 'too much', whose gendered and racialised performances exceed the singular, un-marked identities that schools and advocacy organisations would protect. He not only reveals the limits of identity-based inclusion but also depicts Larry King's 'uncitizenly' performances as everyday practices of resistance to narrow sexual and gender norms. Both chapters reveal the limits of inclusion and rights and the need for understandings of citizenship that are neither universalising nor static. Alldred and Fox develop just such an alternative to the dominant language of belonging and inclusion/exclusion used to conceptualise sexual citizenship: a new materialist approach that considers assemblages of bodies, things, collectives, norms, laws and ideas as integral to what a body (or thing) can do. Rather than accepting sexual citizenship as a binary status of citizen/non-citizen, they theorise the production of 'citizenship effects', such as inclusion, as elements of open-ended processes of becoming. These arguments – for local, specific and cultural understandings of citizenship and rights; attention to embodiment that transcends acts, identities and relationships; and processual, relational theorising of sexual citizenship that is always emergent, in flux – offer useful tools to conceptualise youth's relations to sexual citizenship.

If sexual citizenship has historically entailed scenes of resistance and transgression, what forms do these take in young peoples' lives under neoliberalism? Noteworthy across the volume is the relative paucity of liberationist politics and the predominance of tactical interventions that put to use discourses of rights, inclusion and protection. While Ferfolja depicts the enduring silencing and invisibility that young lesbian, gay, bisexual, transgender and queer (LGBTQ) teachers negotiate in the context of backlash to the curricular inclusion of sexual and gender diversity in schools, Fitzpatrick and McGlashan present youth who claim expertise and power over their homophobic teachers to challenge hierarchies of adult/youth. Jones historicises trans and intersex youth and activists' uses of protectionist, progressive, expert and universalising discourses as they seek more radical mobilisations for the right to self-identification. In contrast to these institutional tactics, Boon-Kuo, Meiners and Simpson depict young people organising to combat state violence that criminalises and over-incarcerates deviant, disposable youth of colour while also creating community-based forms of safety and belonging. Goudie enacts a poetic call to work against the hauntings of colonial violences through indigenous projects of reclamation that shift protection from the state to community and culture. These struggles are organic to their locations, and it is no accident that the actors engaged in (re)formations of counter-communities and practices are racialised subjects marked for social death (Cacho 2012).

Present in many chapters are ambivalent scenes of action given the relentless normalisation and entrepreneurialism of neoliberalism, which both celebrates the young sexual citizen and shapes the terrain in which they create identities and aspirations. For example, Taylor demonstrates the ways neo-liberal mandates for youth to be future-oriented, enterprising workers collide with LGBTQ and class-based subjectivities and religious and spiritual commitments to produce in some young people aspirations of simply 'getting by', or managing rather than overcoming 'queer precarity'. Heaphy traces how tolerance and rights have contributed to a rewriting of some LGBT subjects' earlier narratives of kinship as movement from a hostile family of origin to a chosen (queer) community, pointing to a rise in individualised orientations to (homo)normative coupledom and family. Narrating a study of neo-liberal sexuality education's individualising anti-bullying projects, Fields, Gilbert, Mamo and Lesko explore how racialised schools market progressivism and inclusion and promote the development of self-regulating individual subjects. Personal responsibility obscures subjects' and communities' interdependence and discourages potentially transformative educational practices and solidarities. At stake in these scenes of work, kinship and schooling is the creation of open futures and affiliations – or their containment.

The extent to which digital media forms enable alternative logics of identity, community and political formations is similarly ambivalent. Abidin and Cover examine YouTube as a paradoxical scene of sexual citizenship, in which gay micro-celebrities become brands by promoting the self and social justice through personal coming out narratives that then create demand for the branded micro-celebrity to take on new responsibilities for self-disclosure as activism. The ambivalent role of the commercial media's potential to challenge the public/private divide is present in Clarke's questioning of whether TV depictions of queer sex among fluid subjects can expand viewers' notions of sexual citizens beyond normative categories and relations. And Cover theorises the proliferation of micro-identities among youth online as rejecting rigid adult (LGBT) identities while enforcing an identitarianism congruent with neo-liberal calls to produce a coherent, authentic and marketable self. Sexual citizenship may enable the proliferation of categories, but their regulation and normativisation remain intact.

Critiques of sexual citizenship as a universalising project of Western liberalism (e.g. Sabsay 2012) often focus more on the ways discourses travel than the ways bodies mobilise these discourses. In less ambivalent chapters, the contributions by Albury and Byron and by Robards, Churchill, Vivienne, Hanckel and Byron demonstrate how young people's collective practices of 'digital sexual citizenship' can temporarily place them beyond the protectionism of risk discourses, enabling new practices that may travel from virtual to 'real' spaces. Yan and Tang portray this movement through the assemblage of religious traditions, morality, colonial legacies and progressive discourses that would govern possibilities for young people, who turn to exercise sexual citizenship in alternative spaces of informal groups and the Internet. Finally, Pullen recasts sexual citizenship as fragmentary and mobile through diasporic subjectivity, whether the queer youth refugee seeking liberalism's promise of citizenship rights or Undocuqueer youth fighting liberalism for social justice.

As this book demonstrates, young people engage formal and informal sexual citizenship amidst a proliferation of venues and discourses about sexuality that often seem to embrace them as subjects of rights but also govern the logics of their possibilities for action. Their movement through spaces and boundaries, to borrow from Alldred and Fox, continues to assemble and reassemble, as do the boundaries and discourses of the young sexual citizen.

References

Berlant, L., 2007. Nearly Utopian, Nearly Normal: Post-Fordist Affect in *La Promesse* and *Rosetta*. *Public Culture*, 19 (2), 273–301.

Brown, W., 2005. *Edgework: Critical Essays on Knowledge and Politics*. Princeton, NJ: Princeton University Press.

Cacho, L. M., 2012. *Social Death: Racialized Rightlessness and the Criminalization of the Unprotected*. New York: New York University Press.

Cohen, C., 2014. *#DoBlackLivesMatter? From Michael Brown to CeCe McDonald: On Black Death and LGBTQ Politics*. Center for Lesbian and Gay Studies, The Graduate School, City University of New York. 12 December. Available from: www.racismreview.com/blog/wp-content/uploads/2014/12/Cohen_CLAGS_Transcript_121214.pdf

Foucault, M., 1990. *The History of Sexuality: An Introduction* (Vol. 1). Trans Robert Hurley. New York, NY: Vintage.

Franke, K. M., 2006. The Politics of Same-Sex Marriage Politics. *Columbia Journal of Gender and Law*, 15 (1), 236–248.

Gray, M., 2009. *Out in the Country: Youth, Media, and Queer Visibility in Rural America*. New York: New York University Press.

Richardson, D., 2000. Constructing Sexual Citizenship: Theorizing Sexual Rights. *Critical Social Policy*, 20 (1), 105–135.

Richardson, D., 2017. Rethinking Sexual Citizenship. *Sociology*, 51 (2), 208–224.

Sabsay, L., 2012. The Emergence of the Other Sexual Citizen: Orientalism and the Modernisation of Sexuality. *Citizenship Studies*, 16 (5–6), 605–623.

Warner, M., 2002. *Publics and Counterpublics*. New York, NY: Zone.

Weeks, J., 1998. The Sexual Citizen. *Theory, Culture & Society*, 15 (3–4), 35–52.

Index

Printed in the United States
by Baker & Taylor Publisher Services